AF762840

Modern Otology and Neurotology

Series Editor
Kimitaka Kaga, National Tokyo Medical Center
National Institute of Sensory Organ
Meguro-ku, Tokyo, Japan

This series plays a role as a clinical reference in the rapidly evolving subspecialty of modern otology and neurotology. Written by prominent academic authorities, this series integrates contents from all fields of medicine and covers every aspect of the field, including surgical issues in pediatric audiology, neurotology and neurology, genetic testing, oncological study in auditory and vestibular organs, geriatric audiology and neurotology, and new clinical application of bone conduction hearing etc. Historical developments and unsolved problems of each field will also be described in detail to help readers' understanding. The editors and contributors hope that this book series will contribute to medical residents and experts of otolaryngology and related clinical medicines in the evaluation of patients with otological and neurotological disorders.

Kimitaka Kaga
Editor

ABRs and Electrically Evoked ABRs in Children

Springer

Editor
Kimitaka Kaga
National Institute of Sensory Organs
National Hospital Organization
Tokyo Medical Center
Audiology Clinic
Kamio Memorial Hospital
Tokyo, Japan

ISSN 2567-2169 ISSN 2567-2525 (electronic)
Modern Otology and Neurotology

ISBN 978-4-431-54188-2 ISBN 978-4-431-54189-9 (eBook)
https://doi.org/10.1007/978-4-431-54189-9

© Springer Japan KK, part of Springer Nature 2022
This work is subject to copyright. All rights are solely and exclusively licensed by the Publisher, whether the whole or part of the material is concerned, specifically the rights of translation, reprinting, reuse of illustrations, recitation, broadcasting, reproduction on microfilms or in any other physical way, and transmission or information storage and retrieval, electronic adaptation, computer software, or by similar or dissimilar methodology now known or hereafter developed.
The use of general descriptive names, registered names, trademarks, service marks, etc. in this publication does not imply, even in the absence of a specific statement, that such names are exempt from the relevant protective laws and regulations and therefore free for general use.
The publisher, the authors and the editors are safe to assume that the advice and information in this book are believed to be true and accurate at the date of publication. Neither the publisher nor the authors or the editors give a warranty, expressed or implied, with respect to the material contained herein or for any errors or omissions that may have been made. The publisher remains neutral with regard to jurisdictional claims in published maps and institutional affiliations.

This Springer imprint is published by the registered company Springer Japan KK, part of Springer Nature.
The registered company address is: Shiroyama Trust Tower, 4-3-1 Toranomon, Minato-ku, Tokyo 105-6005, Japan

Preface

Ever since Dr. D. L. Jewett discovered the auditory brainstem response (ABR) in cats and humans in 1970, ABRs and electrically evoked ABRs (EABRs) have been successfully used as a necessary element of the audiologic and neurotologic diagnostic armamentarium worldwide.

This book is a compendium of our basic and clinical research studies of the ABR and EABR over a 40-year time span and provides up-to-date information of the history, recording techniques, and the neurological substrate underlying these responses. On the diagnostic side, we present the manifestation of changes in these responses in patients with peripheral hearing loss, brainstem and cortical lesions, auditory neuropathy (AN), and inner ear malformations.

In the last 25 years, hearing screening of newborns by ABR has been adopted by many countries worldwide. Because of an increase in a combination of findings, including the ABR, the syndrome of AN, as first reported by Kaga K, et al. and Starr A, et al. in 1996, has gained the attention of many clinicians. Also, cochlear implants for young infants with congenital deafness are performed worldwide. EABRs have become a very valuable tool both in determining the integrity of the implant and in evaluating cochlear nerve function. We herein discuss a few difficult cases of infants with complicated inner ear malformations and/or cochlear nerve deficiencies to illustrate the effectiveness of ABRs and EABRs as a diagnostic imperative.

I trust that with this book readers can gain an insight into auditory brainstem physiology and its various pathologies, as well as hearing disorders, as revealed by the ABR and the EABR. In addition, the EABR is essential in the programming of cochlear implant electrodes.

I thank Ms. Kayoko Sekiguchi, B.S., for her indefatigable contributions for her secretarial work and Dominic W. Hughes, Ph.D. for his scientific acumen and for editing this manuscript in order for us to publish this book within 2 years.

Tokyo, Japan
January, 2022

Kimitaka Kaga

Contents

Abbreviations

ABR	Auditory brainstem response
AABR	Automated auditory brainstem response
ACS	Air conduction stimulation
ACTH	Adrenocorticotropic hormone
AE	Anoxic encephalopathy
AEP	Auditory evoked potential
AFD	Appropriate for date
ALD	Adrenoleukodystrophy
AN	Auditory neuropathy
ANSD	Auditory neuropathy spectrum disorder
AP	Action potential
APGAR	Appearance, pulse, grimace, activity, and respiration named from Dr. Virginia Apgar
AR	Autosomal recessive
ASD	Atrial septal defect
ASSR	Auditory steady-state response
AXD	Alexander's disease
BCV	Bone conducted vibration
BMT	Bone marrow transplantation
BOA	Behavioral observation audiometry
CAG	Cerebral arterial angiography
CC	Chief complaint
CHD	Congenital heart disease
CI	Cochlear implant
CM	Cochlear microphonic
CMTD	Charcot-Marie-Tooth disease
CMV	Cytomegalovirus
CN	Cochlear nucleus
CN	Cochlear nerve
CND	Cochlear nerve deformity
CNV	Contingent negative variation

COR	Conditioned orientation response audiometry
CP	Cerebral palsy
CPA	Cardiopulmonary arrest
CSF	Cerebral spinal fluid
CT	Computerized tomography
CVN	Cochlear vestibular nerve
DCN	Dorsal cochlear nucleus
DIC	Disseminated intravascular coagulation
DPOAE	Distortion product otoacoustic emission
DQ	Developmental quotient
DRPLA	Dentato-rubro-Pallido-luysian Atrophy
EABR	Electrically evoked auditory brainstem response
ECMO	Extracorporeal membranous oxygenation
EEG	Electroencephalography
ECoG	Electrocochleogram
EMG	Electromyogram
EP	Epilepsy
ERG	Electroretinogram
ERT	Enzyme replacement therapy
F-VEP	Flash-Evoked visual evoked potential
GA	Gestational age
GLD	Globoid Cell leukodystrophy
GVS	Galvanic vestibular stimulation
HSAN	Hereditary sensory-autonomic neuropathy
HSCT	Hematopoietic stem cell transplantation
HSMN	Hereditary sensory-motor neuropathy
IA	Infantile autism
IAC	Internal auditory canal
IAR	Interaural asymmetry ratio
IC	Inferior colliculus
ICH	Intracerebral brain hemorrhage
ICU	Intensive care unit
ID	Intellectual disability (= mental retardation)
IPL	Inter peak latencies
LL	Lateral lemniscus
LLR	Long latency response
MAP	Mean arterial pressure
MAS	Massive aspiration syndrome
MELAS	Mitochondrial encephalomyopathy with lactic acidosis
MERRF	Mitochondrial encephalomyopathy with ragged red fibers
MGB	Medial geniculate body
MLC	Middle latency component
MLD	Metachromatic leukodystrophy
MLR	Middle latency response
MMN	Mismatch negativity

MPS	Mucopolysaccharidosis
MRI	Magnetic resonance imaging
NCL	Neuronal ceroid lipofuscinosis
NCV	Nerve conduction velocity
NICU	Neonatal intensive care unit
NPC	Nieman-pick disease, type C
OAE	Otoacoustic emissions
P300	Event-related potential (response) at 300 ms
PDA	Patent ductus arteriosus
PGTC	Primary generalized tonic-clonic seizure
PMD	Pelizaeus-Merzbacher disease
PME	Progressive myoclonic epilepsy
PPHN	Persistent pulmonary hypertension
SCM	Sternocleidomastoid muscle
SEP	Sensory evoked potential
SOC	Superior olivary complex
SON	Superior olivary nucleus
SP	Summating potential
SSEP	Somatosensory evoked potential
SSPE	Subacute sclerosing panencephalitis
SVR	Slow vertex response
TOAE	Transient otoacoustic emission
UHS	Universal hearing screening
VCN	Ventral cochlear nucleus
VEMP	Vestibular evoked myogenic potential
cVEMP	VEMP recorded from the cervical area
oVEMP	VEMP recorded from the extra-ocular muscles
GVEMP	Galvanic VEMP
VEP	Visual evoked potential
VOR	Vestibular ocular reflex
VRA	Visual reinforcement audiometry

Part I
Introduction

Chapter 1
History of ABR and EABR

Kimitaka Kaga

Abstract There are multiple types of auditory evoked potentials (AEPs) and they are classified based on the latency and length of their response time and on the stimuli used to provoke them. The types are: electrocochleography (ECoG), auditory brainstem responses (ABRs), middle latency responses (MLRs), the slow vertex response (SVR), mismatch negativity (MMN), and the P300, an event-related potential. Of these AEP types, the ABR has been widely accepted by audiologists and neurotologists as a valuable aid in the diagnosis and monitoring of neural activity of the eighth cranial nerve. The emphasis of this chaper is to both show the historical development of AEPs, since the discovery of electroencephalography (EEG) in 1924, and to explain the methodology and the specific value of each of these AEP types.

Electrically evoked auditory brainstem responses (EABRs), recorded from cochlear implants, were initially reported in 1979. Thereafter, EABRs have been incorporated into a practical procedure for programming cochlear implants in young children and in patients with inner ear malformation or cochlear nerve deficiency.

Keywords Electrocochleography · ABR · EABR

1.1 Auditory Evoked Potentials (AEPs)

In 1924, a German psychiatrist at Jena University, Hans Berger, described his invention of the electroencephalogram (EEG) recording system and he recorded human EEGs for the first time in history [1] (Fig. 1.1).

In 1930, cochlear microphonic potentials were recorded from the cochlea by Weber and Bray [2]. In Fig. 1.2, the lower trace is the sound stimulus and the upper trace is the resultant cochlear microphonic (CM) which is similar in its pattern to

K. Kaga (✉)
National Institute of Sensory Organs, National Hospital Organization, Tokyo Medical Center, Audiology Clinic, Kamio Memorial Hospital, Tokyo, Japan
e-mail: kimitaka.kaga@kankakuki.jp

© Springer Japan KK, part of Springer Nature 2022

K. Kaga (ed.), *ABRs and Electrically Evoked ABRs in Children*, Modern Otology and Neurotology, https://doi.org/10.1007/978-4-431-54189-9_1

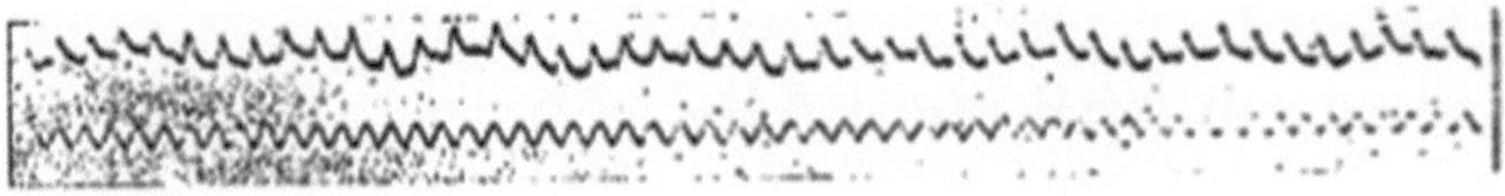

Fig. 1.1 The first recordings of the EEG, by Hans Berger in 1924, were taken from epidural electrodes placed directly on the dura of a patient via a local craniotomy [1]

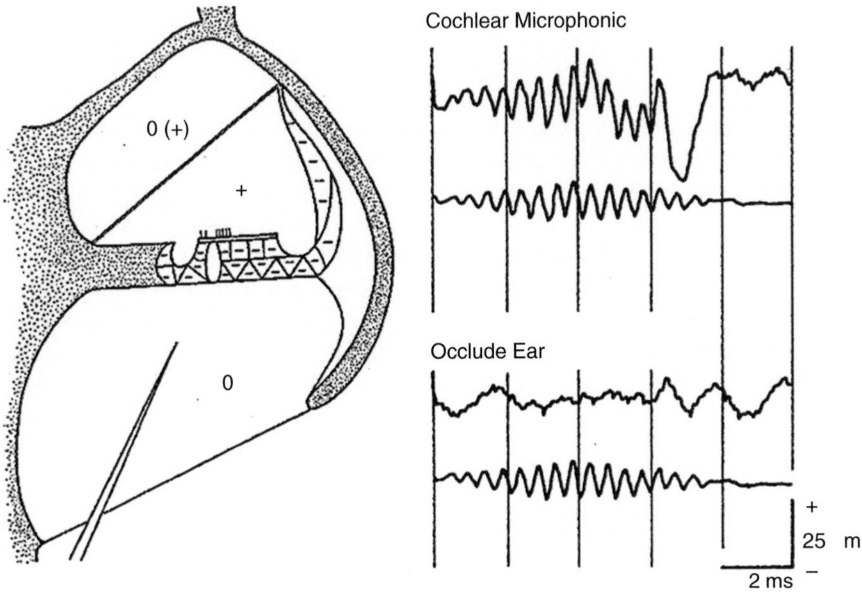

Fig. 1.2 Cochlear microphonic potentials recorded by Weber and Bray in 1930 [2]

that of the sound stimulus. Stimulation of an occluded ear did not elicit a definable CM.

In 1938, Loomis found a K complex on the EEG which is a cortical response to auditory and touch stimuli or inspiratory interruptions during stage II of sleep [3]. In Fig. 1.3, the EEG tracings change simultaneously with the K complex and two phases following the sound stimuli are evident on the EEG recordings.

In 1939, Davis PA, described V potentials on the EEG provoked by acoustic stimuli [4]. In Fig. 1.4, arrows indicate the acoustic stimuli. The V wave indicates that the brain was also responsive to the stimuli.

The K complex and the V potentials elicited on the EEG were ultimately found to be the same response of these brain waves to acoustic stimulation. In 1947, Dawson reported his finding of a long latency response (LLR) which was illustrated by superimposing each EEG tracing following frequent acoustic stimuli [5]. In Fig. 1.5. The amplitude of the LLR is influenced by the depth of sleep level, Stages II and III, with Stage III eliciting more robust responses. After the discovery of the LLR, Geisler, in 1958 [6], found a middle latency response (MLR) around a latency

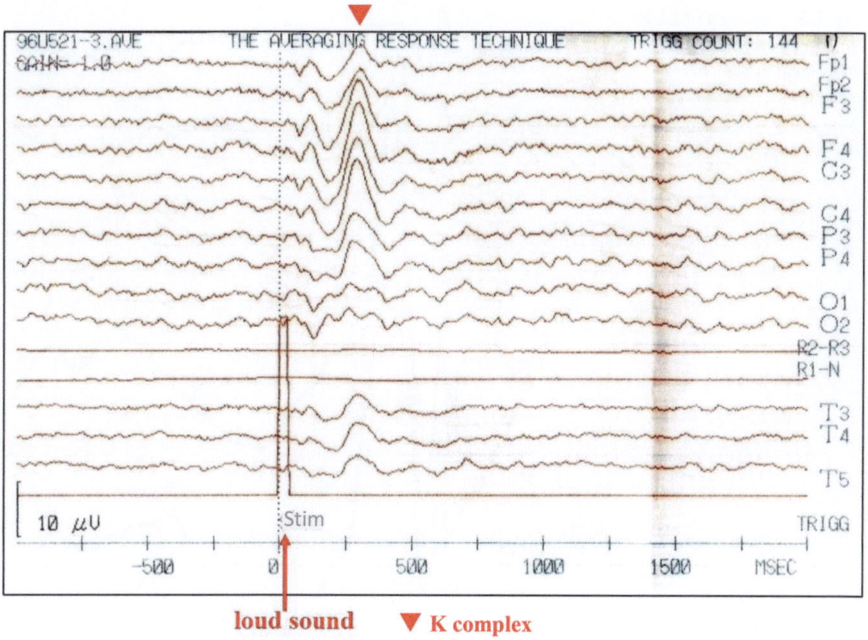

Fig. 1.3 Examples of the K complex in modern EEGs to acoustic stimuli

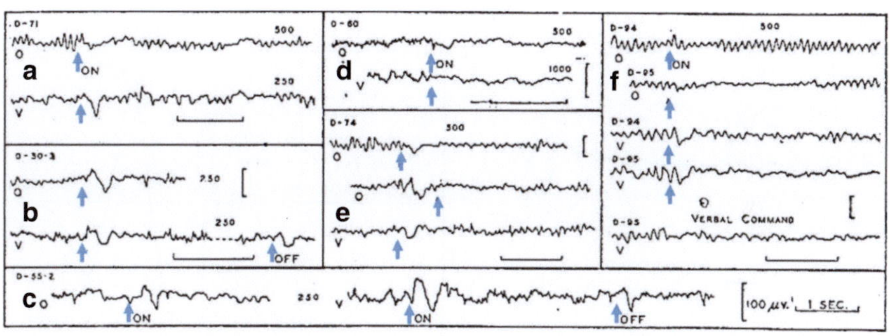

Fig. 1.4 V potentials found on the EEG as reported by Davis, PA [4]. On-effects and modifications of spontaneous rhythms in response to sounds. The frequency employed is indicated in each case. No measurements of loudness were reported. O is the monopolar occipital record; V is the monopolar record from the vertex. The reference electrodes on the ear lobes are connected in parallel. Paired tracings do not represent simultaneous records. Calibrations are for 1 sec. and 100 μV. throughout. (**a**) Resolution of the alpha rhythm and the on-effect in an alpha subject on the alpha rhythm. (**b**) On- and off-effects in a non-alpha subject. Also, note the resolution of beta waves in the vertex record. (**c**) The same as in B but in another subject. (**d**) Resolution of fast (beta) frequencies in another non-alpha subject. (**e**) Typical on-effects. "Anticipatory" reactions are shown in the second tracing. (**f**) Resolution of the alpha rhythm and on-effects from a pair of identical twins, D-94 and D-95, and the effect of a verbal command

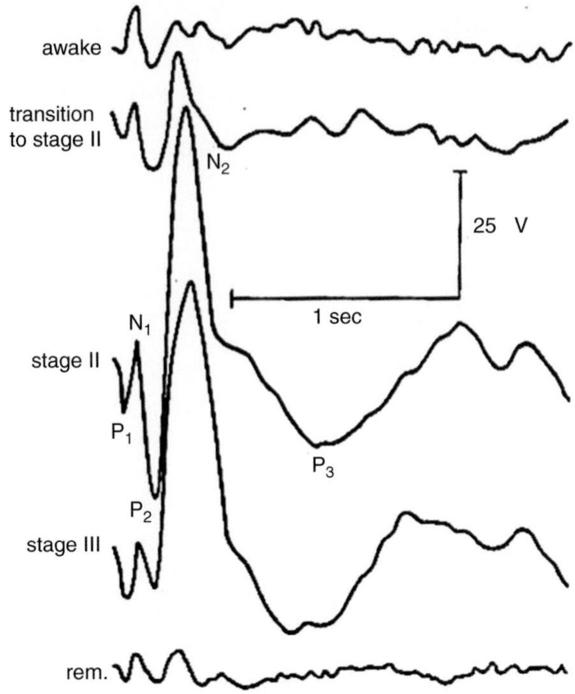

Fig. 1.5 Changes of LLR as a function in depth of sleep levels [5]

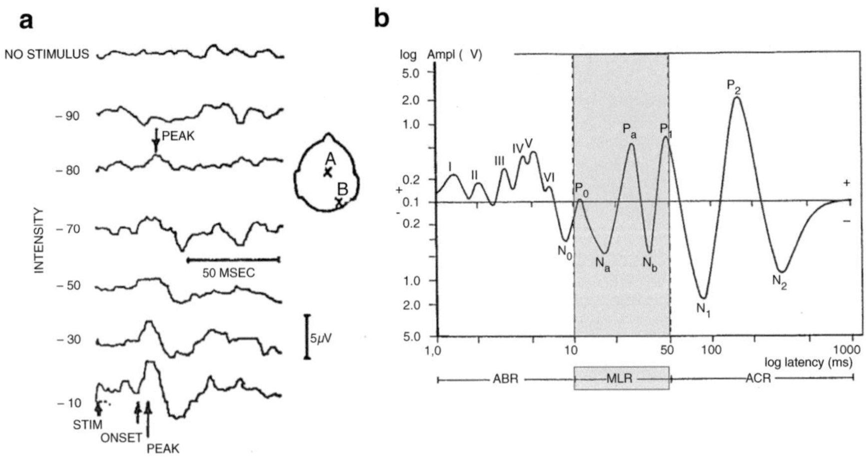

Fig. 1.6 (**a**) MLR responses as reported by Geisler in 1958 [6] (**b**) Under the rubric of AEPs, the shadowed area outlines the MRL

of 10–50 msec following acoustic stimulation (Fig. 1.6). At that time, the auditory brainstem response (ABR) had yet to be discovered. Almost half a century later, the MLR contributed to the finding of an auditory steady-state response (ASSR). In the same year, 1958, Davis H described a summating potential (SP) which was mixed in with and preceded the CM recordings [7] (Fig. 1.7). The polarity of SPs was positive at the basal turn of the cochlea and negative at the third turn of the cochlea.

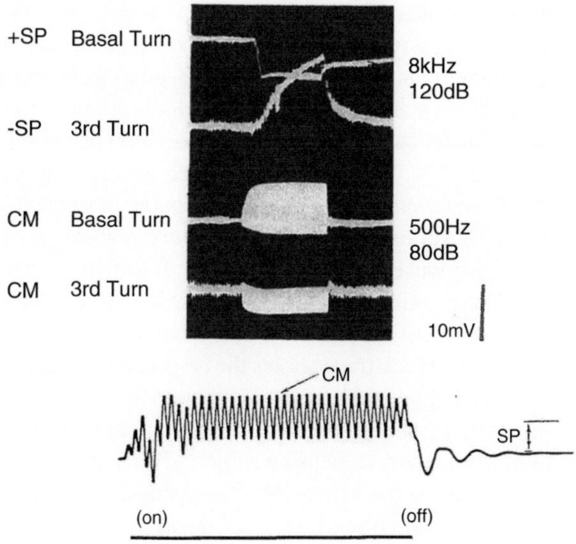

Fig. 1.7 Summating potentials (SP) were found in cochlear microphonic (CM) recordings by Davis H in 1958 [7]

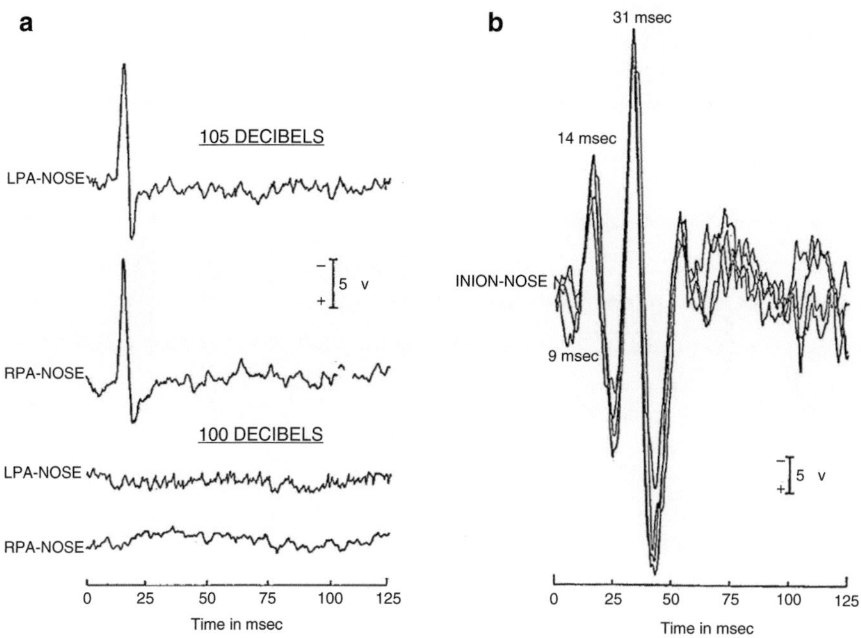

Fig. 1.8 (**a**) The postauricular response was reported by Kiang, N in 1963 [8]. (**b**) Inion response. Both responses are identical to the postauricular muscle response

In 1963, Nelson Kiang discovered a postauricular response to sound stimuli [8] evoked by a loud click (Fig. 1.8). Another name given to this response was the inion response. This response was forgotten immediately but has recently been appreciated as a vestibular-evoked myogenic potential (VEMP).

In 1964, Walter described a contingent negative variation (CNV) response which can be regarded as a type of event-related potential [9] (Fig. 1.9). An irregular but predictable pattern of auditory stimuli is presented to the subject who is tasked to predict the next presence or absence of the next auditory stimulus to which he/she is presented following a visual flash. The subject's expectation of the next auditory stimulus generates the cortical CNV. The CNV was an epoch-making potential that is evoked by activity of higher brain functions involved in perception, judgement, or decision-making.

In 1967, Sutton described a P300 evoked wave, an event-related potential, which is a positive wave occurring 300 msec following a discrete auditory stimulus [10]. Two different stimuli (tones) are presented to a subject. One is a target tone presented rarely, 20% frequency, and a nontarget tone presented frequently, 80%. In Fig. 1.10, the black trace shows the response to frequent stimuli and the dotted trace shows a largely positive response around 300 msec to the rare stimuli [11].

Figure 1.11 shows typical P300 responses comparing rare stimuli with frequent stimuli from a normal hearing subject. The upper trace (a) indicates when each button is pushed button by the right-hand finger, the middle trace (b) shows when each button is pushed button by the left-hand finger. The lower trace (c) is the mentally counted number of rare stimuli. There are recorded P300s to rare stimuli in the three tasks but not to frequent stimuli.

In 1967, an electrocochleographic response (the ECoG) was described simultaneously by Yosie, in Japan [12] and Portman, in France [13]. In Fig. 1.12, the upper trace shows the wave configuration of rarefaction and condensation wave of the

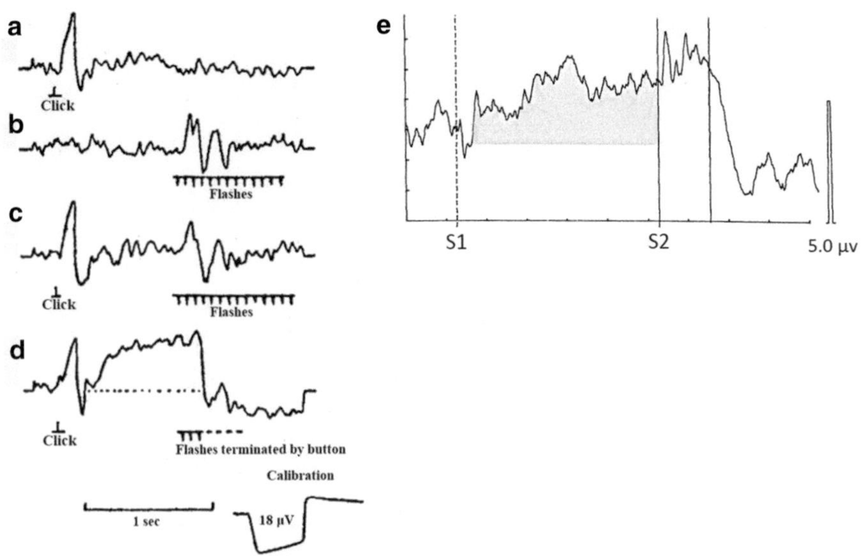

Fig. 1.9 Contingent Negative Variation (CNV), as a type of event-related potential, was reported by Walter, WG in 1964 [9]. (**a**) Auditory evoked potential stimulated by click, (**b**) Visually evoked potential stimulated by flash 1 sec after click, (**c**) Evoked potential (a+b), (**d**) CNV evoked by click and flashes terminated by button (a+b). CNV is called as expectancy wave, (**e**) CNV evoked by click (S1) and flash (S2) terminated by button in a 15-year-old patient with auditory agnosia. CNV is evoked after click (S1)

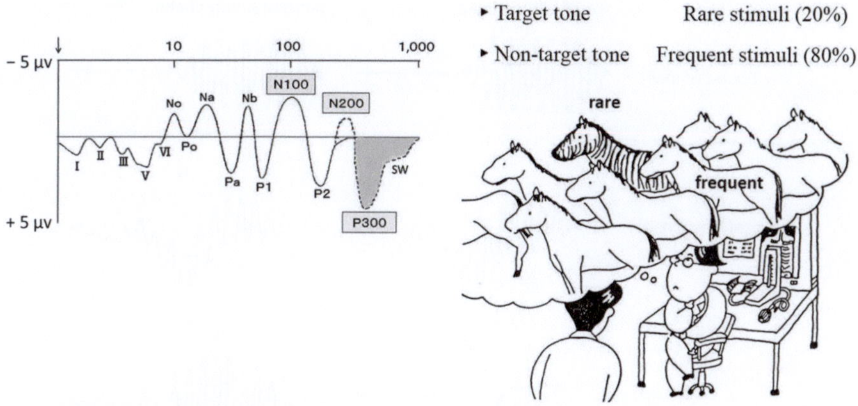

Fig. 1.10 P300, as an event-related potential, was reported by Sutton S in 1967. Two different tones of rare stimuli and frequent stimuli are presented to the listener [10]

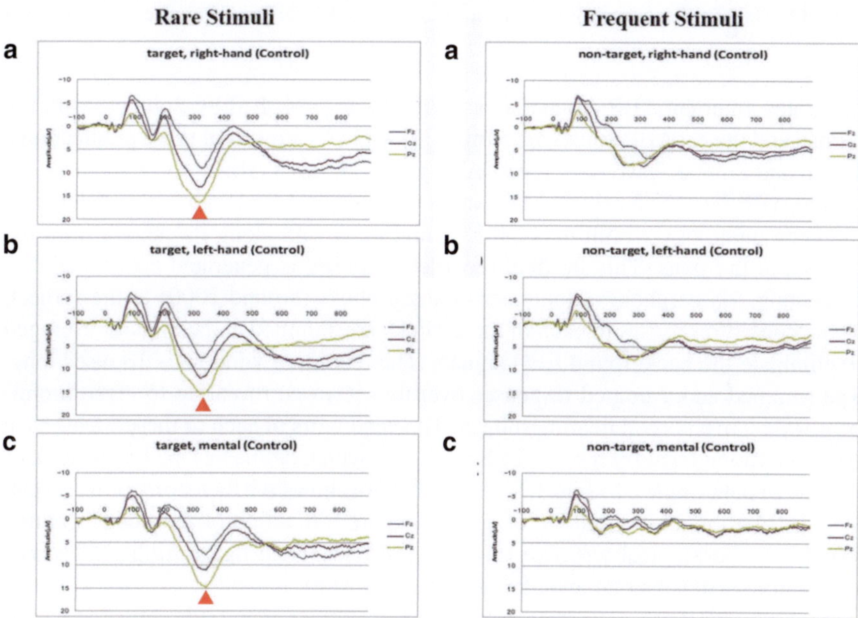

Fig. 1.11 Grand average of P300s recordings from Fz, Cz, and Pz are superimposed following rare stimuli and frequent stimuli in normal subjects [11]. ▲: P300

auditory stimulus. The middle trace shows the evoked responses to these rarefaction and condensation stimuli. The lower trace shows the ECoG by A + B and CM by A - B. The finding of the ECoG soon led to the discovery of the ABR.

1970 was the most important year in the history of the ABR. Jewett, in the USA, and Sohmer, in Israel, concurrently reported, for the first time, their discovery of the ABR [14, 15]. Figure 1.13 shows our examples of human and cat ABRs. Figure 1.14

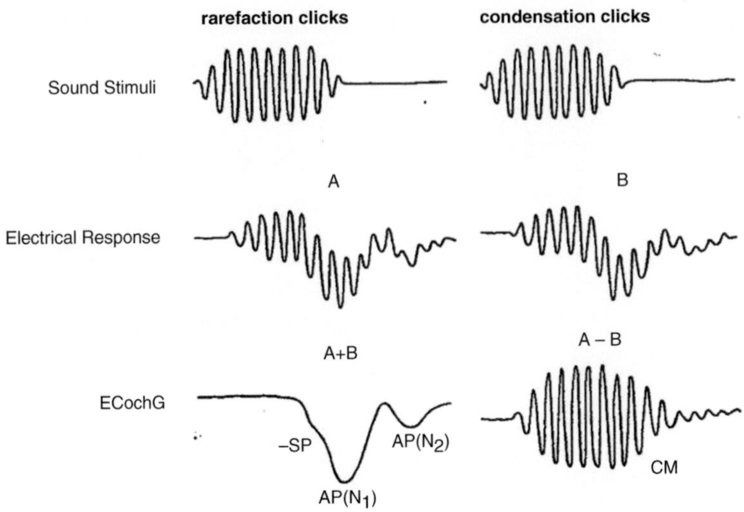

Fig. 1.12 The ECoG as first reported by Yosie, N in Japan and Portman M in France in 1967 [12, 13]

illustrates a human ABR (a) and a cat ABR (b) as published by Sohmer. Both the human and the cat ABR waves are similar in shape. As a result of these publications, Jewett and Sohmer have been regarded as the pioneers of ABR.

The ABR became a new and extremely valuable tool for localizing and diagnosing neuropathology within the eighth cranial nerve and along its' length from the cochlea to the pons. This far-field recorded response is generated acoustically by presenting, via earphones, a number of sharp clicks (around 2000) to the subject. The recorded responses to each of these clicks are summed and computer averaged to eliminate the background EEG signals. The recording window is 10 msec long. The summed and averaged responses over this 10 msec reveal up to seven prominent waves, in a normal hearing subject. The generators of each of these waves have been determined neurophysiologically [14, 16], which delineates the localization of brainstem pathologies. In Fig. 1.15, the left figure shows ABRs recorded from a cat. The distribution and amplitude of each wave are a function of the nuclei through which the neurological response traverses [16]. The right figure further illustrates the neurological substrate underlying each ABR wave.

Since the ABR was discovered by Jewett and Sohmer, many subsequent researchers have applied different names to the ABR, as shown in Fig. 1.16. In 1979, at the US-Japan ABR Seminar in Hawaii, Professor Jun-Ichi Suzuki of Teikyo University in Japan proposed choosing the best nomenclature, among 6, to the participants. They voted and chose ABR and it is now used universally to describe this technique.

In 1978, a new potential was discovered by Kemp [18] (Fig. 1.17) and he called it a transient-evoked otoacoustic emission (TOAE). In the following year, Kemp subsequently described another OAE which he called a distortion product otoacoustic emission (DPOAE) [19] (Fig. 1.18). DPOAEs have since been routinely used in clinical practice and they have contributed to establishing the concept of auditory neuropathy (AN) which was reported by Starr [20] and Kaga [21] simultaneously in 1996.

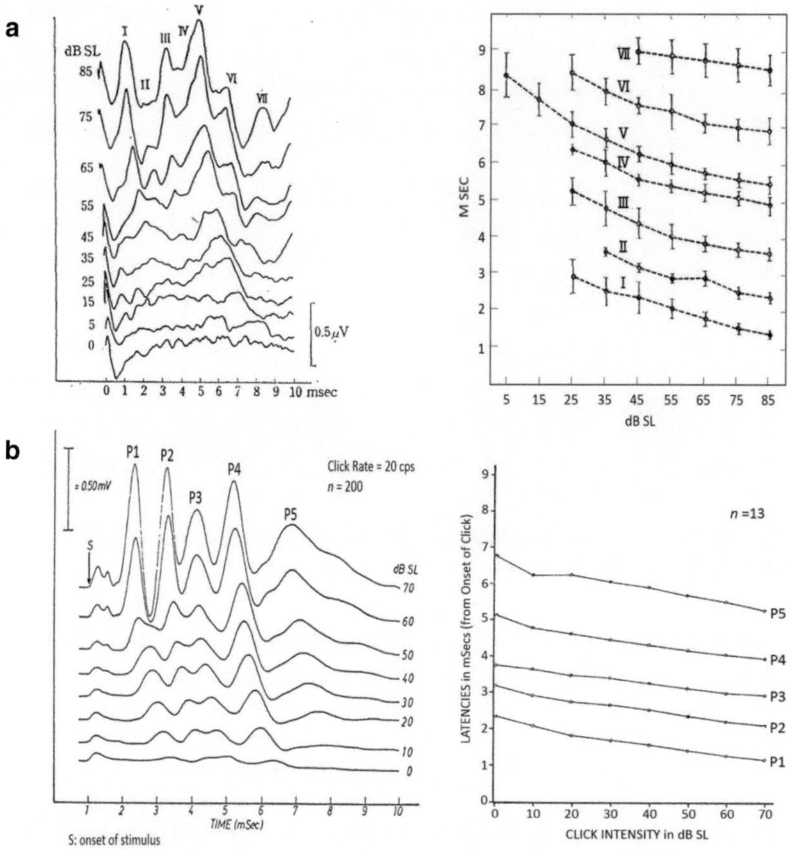

Fig. 1.13 Recordings of the ABR were initially published by Jewett, DL in 1970 [14]. Examples of human and cat ABRs. (a) Human ABRs as a function of stimulus intensity, (b) Cat ABRs as a function of stimulus intensity

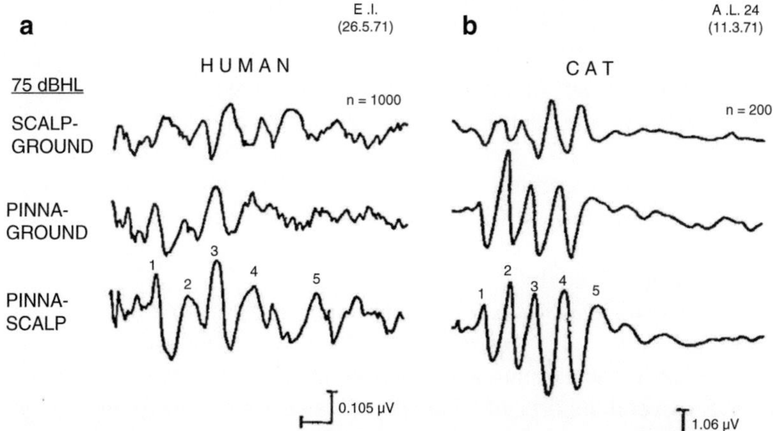

Fig. 1.14 Simultaneously, Sohmer in 1970 published his ABRs [15]: (a) human, (b) cat

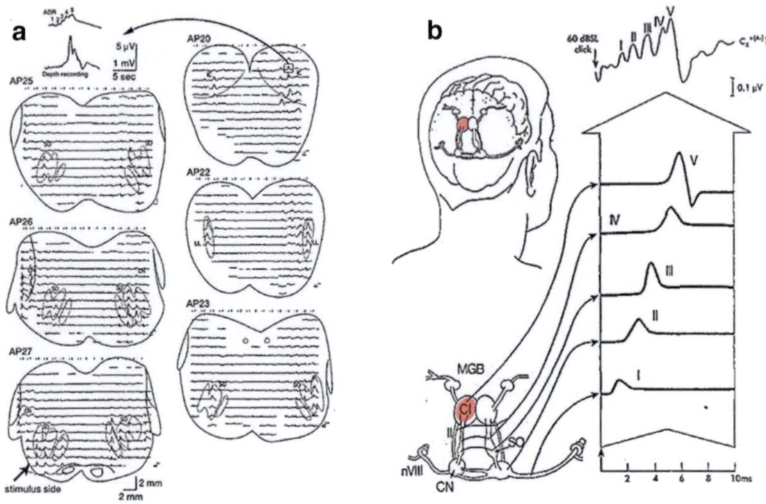

Fig. 1.15 (**a**) The distribution of auditory evoked potentials in the brainstem of a cat [16]. (**b**) is a Schema of the origins of each peak of the human ABR [16, 17]

In 1978, another new potential was discovered by Näätärnen in Finland [22] (Fig. 1.19). He called it a mismatch negativity (MMN) potential and it also is a type of event-related potential, which is automatically elicited by any discriminable change in a repetitive sound or sound pattern. Two different auditory stimuli are presented to a subject. However, button-pushing or mental counting is not used as a task. Deviant and standard stimuli are presented and, automatically, the brain discriminates the amplitude difference between the two. The N200 amplitude is more robust to deviant stimuli than it is to standard stimuli. This difference in response amplitude quantifies the MMN as an index of central auditory system plasticity.

In 1981, Galambos described a 40-Hz ASSR (Auditory Steady-State Response) [23]. The ASSR is somewhat similar to the ABR in that both are electrophysiologic responses to rapid acoustic stimuli, presented via earphones or ear inserts, and these responses are recorded from external electrodes arranged in a particular montage on the scalp. The difference between the two techniques lies in the rate of the presented stimuli. The ASSR sound stimuli are repeatedly presented at a high repetition rate whereas the ABR stimuli are presented at a relatively lower rate. Also, the identification of the evoked ASSR responses (waves) uses a mathematical algorithm to identify these waves, increasing the objectivity in the analysis of these responses. The lower recording, illustrated in Fig. 1.20, shows the stimulus sound wave, called the sinusoidal amplitude modulation, and the upper recording shows the 40-Hz sinusoidal evoked potentials.

In 1992, a vestibular-evoked myogenic potential (VEMP) was discovered by Colebatch and Halmagyi in Australia [24]. This wave configuration is remarkably similar to the postauricular muscle response (Fig. 1.21) [24, 25].

In 1995, several reports of clinically obtained multiple-frequency ASSRs were published in the literature by Picton's Canadian and Australian groups

US-JAPAN ABR Seminar in Hawaii, Jan. 1979

The various names of the ABR prior to the accepted one (ABR).

BSR : Brain Stem Response

BSER: Brain Stem Evoked Response

BAER: Brainstem Auditory Evoked Response

BERA: Brainstem Electric Response Audiometry

BAEP: Brainstem Auditory Evoked Potential

► **ABR : Auditory Brainstem Response**

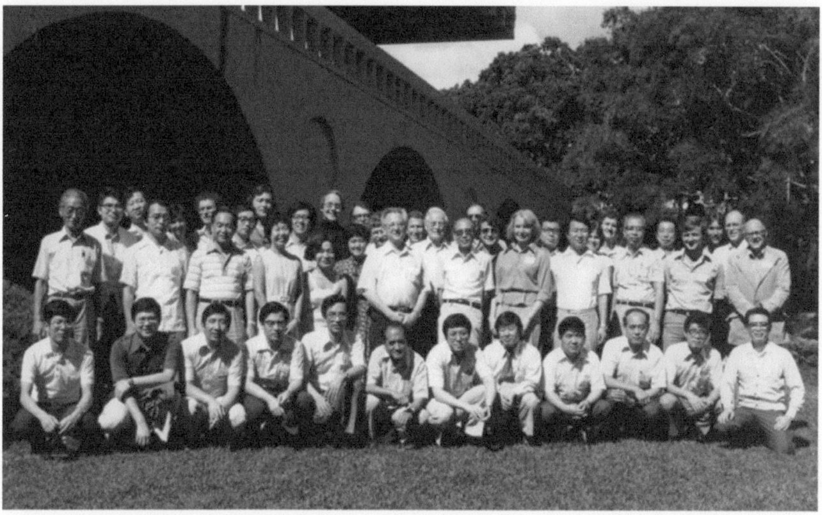

Fig. 1.16 US-Japan ABR Seminar in Hawaii, Jan. 1979

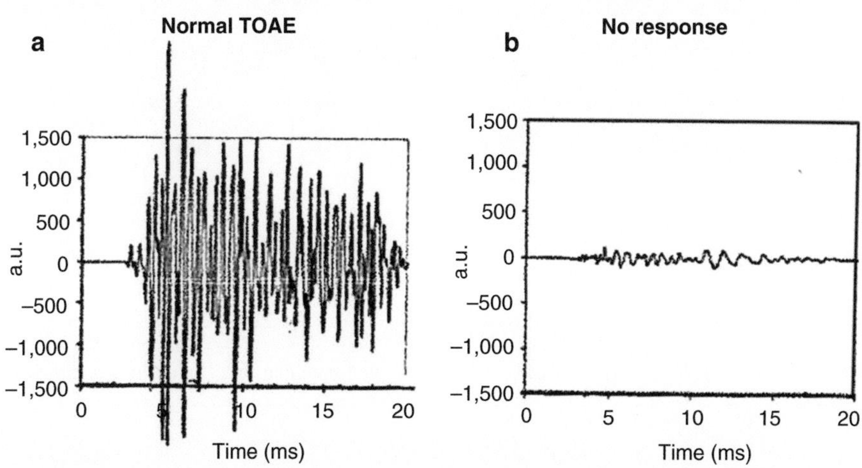

Fig. 1.17 Transient otoacoustic emissions (TOAEs) were discovered by Kemp, DT in 1978 [18] Examples of normal TOAE (**a**) and no response of TOAE (**b**)

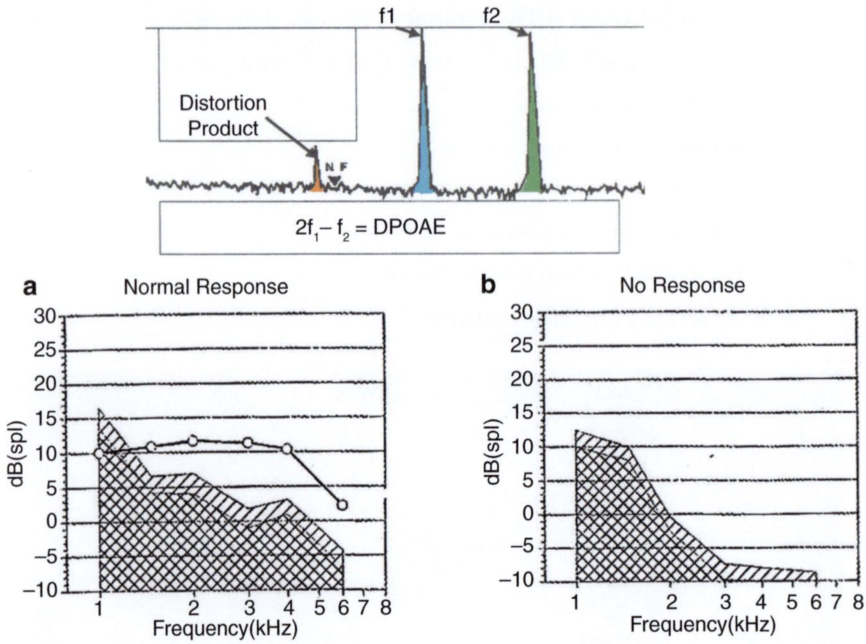

Fig. 1.18 Distortion product OAEs (DPOAEs) were also discovered by Kemp, DT in 1979 [19] and they have been used clinically in the evaluation of cochlear function. Examples of normal DPOAE (**a**) and no response DPOAE (**b**)

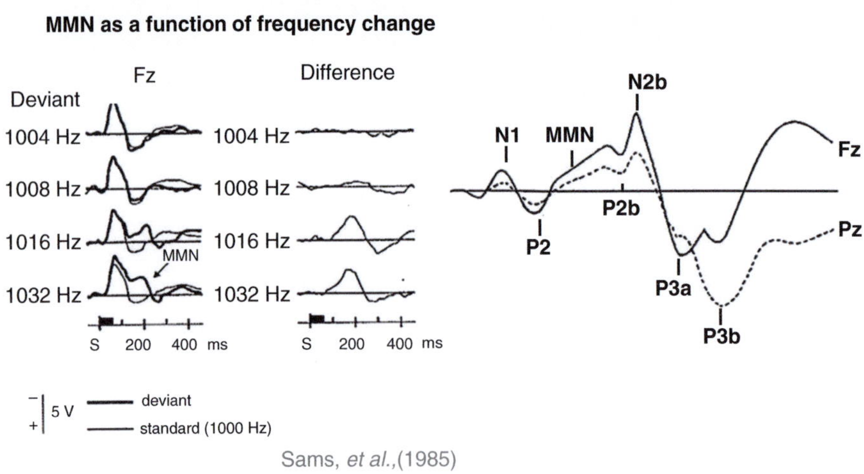

Fig. 1.19 Mismatch negativity (MMN), an event-related potential, was found by Näätärnen in 1978 [22]

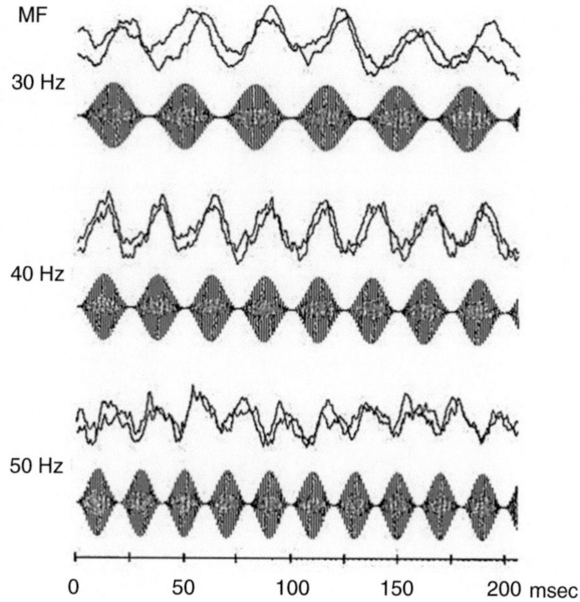

Fig. 1.20 When using stimuli of 30 Hz, 40 Hz, and 50 Hz, the sinusoidal peak amplitude of 40 Hz is larger than the others (Galambos R, 1981) [23]

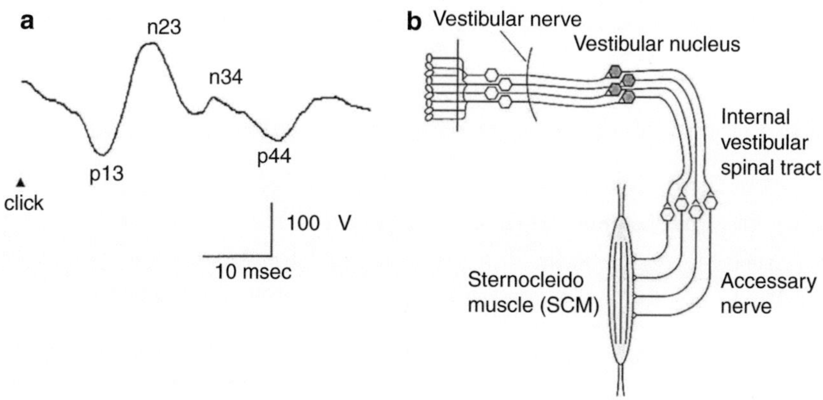

Fig. 1.21 (**a**) Example of a typical VEMP, (**b**) A reaction of the vestibular neural myogenic pathway [24, 25]

simultaneously. Pure tone audiograms were generated by multiple-frequency ASSRs [26]. In Fig. 1.22, the upper ASSR displays a simple audiogram such as a pure tone audiogram. However, the lower ASSR shows an estimated audiogram generated by the algorithm.

Table 1.1 is a chronological presentation illustrating the development of auditory evoked potentials over time. Many years have passed since the discovery and recording of the EEG by Hans Berger in 1924.

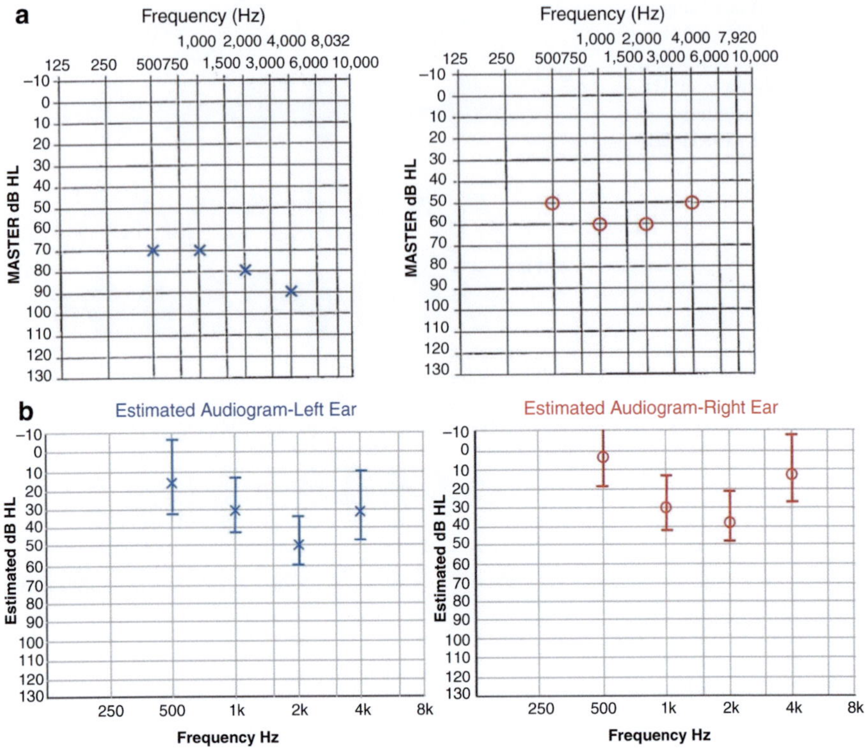

Fig. 1.22 Examples of audiograms (**a**, **b**) generated by multiple-frequency ASSR [26]

Table 1.1 The year of publication of various evoked potentials

Year	Author	Name	Journal
1929	Berger	Electroencephalograph	Archiv für Psychiatrie und Nervenkrankheiten
1930	Weber & Bray, et al	Cochlear microphonic	Proc Natl Acad Sci, USA
1938	Loomis, et al	K complex	J Neurophysiol
1939	Davis PA	V potential	J Neurophysiol
1947	Dawson	Long latency response	J Neurol Neurosurg Psychiat
1958	Geisler, et al	Middle latency response	Science
1958	Davis H, et al	Summating potential	Am J Physiol
1963	Kiang, et al	Postauricular response	Mass Inst Technology
1964	Walter, et al	Contingent negative variation	Nature
1967	Sutton, et al	P300	Science
1967	Yosie et al. Portman et al.	Electrocochleography Electrocochleography	Laryngoscope Rev. Larynogol (Bordeaux)
1970	Jewett, et al. Sohmer & Feinmesser	Auditory brainstem response Auditory brainstem response	Science Isr J Med Sci
1978	Kemp	Otoacoustic emission	J Acoust Soc Am

Table 1.1 (continued)

Year	Author	Name	Journal
1979	Kemp	DPOAE	Arch Oto-rhino-laryngol
1978	Näätänen, et al	Mismatch negativity	In a book edited by Kimmel, et al.
1981	Galambos, et al.	40 Hz ASSR	Proc Natl Acad Sci USA
1992	Colebatch & Halmagyi	VEMP	Neurology
1995	Lins, Picton TW, et al	Multiple ASSR	Electroencepahlogr Clin Neurophysiol

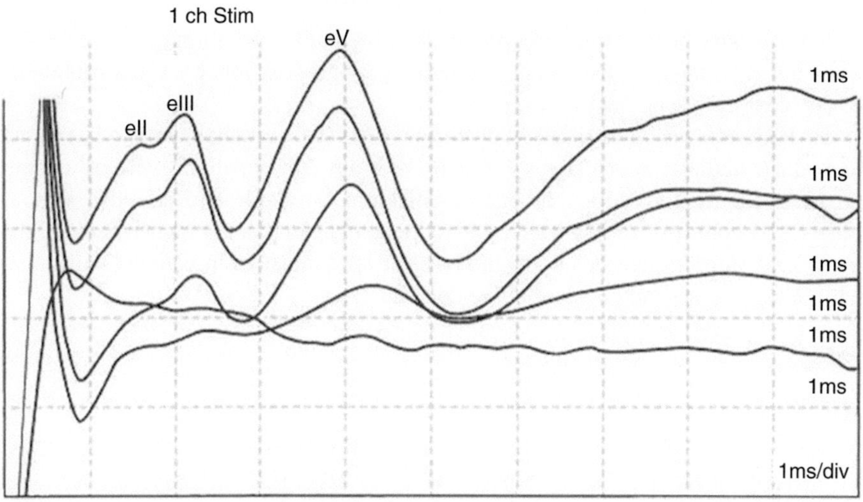

Fig. 1.23 Typical EABRs recorded from an apical electrode of a cochlear implant (MED-EL)

1.2 Electrically Auditory Brainstem Responses (EABRs)

In 1979, the electrically evoked auditory brainstem response (EABR) was first recorded by Starr and Brackman [27] from scalp electrodes in response to biphasic square-wave electrical stimuli of implanted electrodes of the single channel cochlear implant within the cochleas of three patients. Since then, and for over the last 40 years, many clinical studies describing the applications of EABRs of the multi-channel cochlear implant have been reported to evaluate the integrity of cochlear implants during surgery and for later auditory rehabilitation.

In 1985, Gardi presented intracochlear EABRs from three patients who rested quietly on a hospital bed in a darkroom, showing that they could be reliably recorded [28].

The EABR can be used to functionally evaluate the integrity of the auditory brainstem tracts during the initial activation of the cochlear implant and during its long-term use [29].

The evoked positive peaks, eII, eIII, and eV, of the EABR have a slightly different nomenclature than those of the ABR (Fig. 1.23). However, the familiar positive peaks of I, VI, and VII of acoustically evoked ABRs are not discerned in the EABR. Wave I of the ABR is masked by the stimulus artifact. Waves VI and VII of the ABR originate from the brachium of the inferior colliculus and medial geniculated bodies. This discrepancy in nomenclature, i.e., why eVI and eVII have not been recorded in the EABR, is an ongoing research endeavor. Waveforms produced during the EABR are evoked as the result of electrical stimuli to the cochlear nerve and thus differ from acoustic stimuli presented to the ear via headphones or insert earphones. The eV wave latency represents the total transmission time through the brainstem from discreet electrical stimuli of the cochlear nerve. This transmission time is essentially identical to the interpeak latency (IPL) interval (brainstem transmission time) as measured in the click-evoked ABR.

EABRs have been helpful as a practical method in the programming of cochlear implants in young children and in evaluating patients with inner ear malformations or cochlear nerve deficiencies [30].

EABRs, using cochlear implant electrodes mediated stimuli, have also been used to evaluate auditory neuronal responses in the brainstem of patients with or without an inner ear malformation [31–33]. EABRs are a reliable and effective way to objectively confirm cochlear implant function and the implant-responsiveness of the peripheral auditory neurons up to the level of the brainstem in patients with inner ear malformations and cochlear nerve deficiencies.

References

1. Berger H. Über das Elektroenkephalogramm des Menschen. Arch Psychiatr Nervenkr. 1929;87:527–70.
2. Weber EG, Bray CW. Action currents in the auditory nerve in response to acoustical stimulation. Proc Natl Acad Sci U S A. 1930;16:344–50.
3. Loomis AL, Harvey EN, Garret A, Habart III. Distribution of disturbance-patterns in the human electroencephalogram, with special reference to sleep. J Neurophysiol. 1938;1(5):413–30.
4. Davis PA. Effects of acoustic stimuli on the waking human brain. J Neurophysiol. 1939;2:494–9.
5. Dawson GD. Cerebral responses to electrical stimulation of peripheral nerves in man. J Neurol Neurosurg Psychiatry. 1947;10:134.
6. Geisler CD, Frichkopf LS, Rosenblith WA. Extracranial response to acoustic clicks in man. Science. 1958;128:1210–1.
7. Davis H, Deatherage BH, Eldredge DH, Smith CA. Summating potentials of the cochlea. Am J Phys. 1958;195(2):251–61.
8. Kiang N, Grist AH, French MA, Edward AG. Postauricular electric response to acoustic stimuli in human. Mass Inst Technology. 1963;68:218–25.
9. Walter WG, Cooper R, Aldridge VJ, Mccallum WC, Al W. Contingent negative variation: an electric sign to sensorimotor associated and expectancy in the human brain. Nature. 1964;203:380–4.
10. Sutton S, Braren M, Zubin E, John ER. Information delivery and the sensory evoked potential. Science. 1967;155:1436–9.
11. Kaga K, Fukami T, Masubuchi N, Isikawa B. Effects of button pressing and mental counting on N100, N200, and N300 of auditory-event-related potential recording. J Int Adv Otol. 2014;10:14–8.
12. Yosie N, Ohashi T, Suzuki T. Non-surgical recording of auditory action potentials in man. Laryngoscope. 1967;77:76–85.

13. Portmann M, Le Bert G, Aran J. Potentiels cochleaires obtenus chez l'hommeen dehors de toute intervention chiruor'gi-cale. Note: Preliminaire Rev Laryngol (Bord). 1967;88:157–64.
14. Jewett DL, Romano MN, Williston JS. Human auditory evoked potentials: possible brainstem components detected on the scalp. Science. 1970;167:1517–8.
15. Sohmer H, Feinmesser M. Cochlear and cortical audiometry conveniently recorded in the same subject. Isr J Med Sci. 1970;6:219–23.
16. Kaga K, Shinoda Y, Suzuki J-I. Origin of auditory brainstem responses in cats: whole brainstem mapping, and a lesion and HRP study of the inferior colliculus. Acta Otolaryngol. 1997;117(2):197–201.
17. Donkelaar HJ, Kaga K. Chapter 7. The auditory system. In: Hans J Donkelaar ed, Clinical Neuroanatomy, 2nd Edition, Springer Nature, Switzerland; 2020. p. 373–407.
18. Kemp DT. Stimulated acoustic emissions from within the human auditory system. J Acoust Soc Am. 1978;64:1386–91.
19. Kemp DT. Evidence of mechanical nonlinearity and frequency selective wave amplification in the cochlea. Arch Otorhinolaryngol. 1979;224:37–45.
20. Starr A, Picton TW, Sininger Y, Hood LJ, Berlin CI. Auditory neuropathy. Brain. 1996;119:741–53.
21. Kaga K, Nakamura M, Shinogami M, Tsuzuku T, Yamada K, Shindo M. Auditory nerve disease of both ears revealed by auditory brainstem responses, electrocochleography and otoacoustic emissions. Scand Audiol. 1996;26:233–8.
22. Näätänen R, Gaillard AW, Mäntysalo S. Early selective-attention effect on evoked potential reinterpreted. Acta Psychol. 1978;42(4):313–29.
23. Galambos R, Makeig S, Taimachoff PJ. A 40-Hz auditory potential recorded from the human scalp. Proc Natl Acad Sci U S A. 1981;78(4):2643–7.
24. Colebatch JG, Halmagyi GM. Vestibular evoked potentials in human neck muscles before and after unilateral vestibular deafferentation. Neurology. 1992;42:1635–6.
25. Murofushi T, Kaga K, editors: Vestibular evoked myogenic potential. Its basics and clinical applications. Springer, Tokyo; 2009.
26. Lins OG, Picton TW. Auditory steady-state response to multiple simultaneous stimuli. Electroencepahlogr Clin Neurophysiol. 1995;96(5):420–32.
27. Starr A, Brackman DD. Brain stem potentials evoked by electrical stimulation of the cochlea in human subjects. Ann Otol Rhinol Laryngol. 1979;88(4):550–6.
28. Gardi JN. Human brainstem and middle latency responses to electrical stimulation: preliminary observations. In: Schinder RA, Merzenich MM, editors. Cochlear implants. New York: Raven; 1985. p. 351–63.
29. Shallop JK, Beiter AL, Goin DW, Mischke RE. Electrically evoked auditory brain stem responses (EABR) and middle latency responses (EMLR) obtained from patients with the nucleus multichannel cochlear implant. Ear Hear. 1990;11(1):5–15.
30. Brown CJ, Abbas PJ, Fryauf-Bertschy H, Kelsay D, Gants BJ. Intraoperative and postoperative electrically evoked brain stem responses in nucleus cochlear implant users: implications for the fitting process. Ear Hear. 1994;15(2):168–76.
31. Papsin BC. Cochlear implantation in children with anomalous cochleovestibular anatomy. Laryngoscope. 2005;115(S106):1–26.
32. Yamazaki NY, Fujiwara K, Moroto S, Yamamoto R, Yamazaki T, Sasaki I. Electrically evoked auditory brainstem response-based evaluation of the spatial distribution of auditory neuronal tissue in common cavity deformities. Otol Neurotol. 2014;35(8):1394–402.
33. Kaga K, Minami S, Enomoto C. Electrically evoked ABRs during cochlear implantation and postoperative development of speech and hearing abilities in infants with common cavity deformity as a type of inner ear malformation. Acta Otolaryngol. 2020;140(1):14–21.

Part II
ABRs

Chapter 2
Origins of ABR

Kimitaka Kaga and Dominic W. Hughes

Abstract The ABR (Auditory Brainstem Response) is the neurological activity that is generated and transmitted along the auditory neural pathways from the cochlea on its way to the medial geniculate body (MGB) in the brain.

This response, which can be recorded from external electrodes pasted onto the skull and mastoid process of the subject, is therefore called a "far-field recording" which means that the electrodes recording this response are externally placed on the skull, quite distant from the actual neurologic activity within the brainstem.

Stereotypical in that this ABR waveform is remarkably similar in overall form across mammalian species (human, simians, cats, rabbits, etc.). As this response traverses the neurological substrate, it passes through various nuclei which each generate a positive potential (wave), the ABR waveform, related to its source (P1; cochlear nerve, P2; cochlear nucleus, P3; superior olivary complex, P4 and P5; lateral lemniscus nucleus and inferior colliculus, P6; brachium of inferior colliculus, and MGB in the brain). Neurophysiological knowledge of the sources, peak latencies and amplitudes of these seven waves are clinically valuable not only for evaluating peripheral hearing loss but also in localizing lesions within the eighth cranial nerve over its length from the cochlea to the midbrain inferior colliculus.

Keywords ABR · Cochlear nucleus superior · Olivary complex · Inferior colliculus · Medical geniculate body · Auditory cortex

K. Kaga (✉)
National Institute of Sensory Organs, National Hospital Organization, Tokyo Medical Center, Audiology Clinic, Kamio Memorial Hospital, Tokyo, Japan
e-mail: kimitaka.kaga@kankakuki.jp

D. W. Hughes
Neurotology, West Linn, OR, USA

© Springer Japan KK, part of Springer Nature 2022

K. Kaga (ed.), *ABRs and Electrically Evoked ABRs in Children*, Modern Otology and Neurotology, https://doi.org/10.1007/978-4-431-54189-9_2

2.1 Origins of the ABR

2.1.1 Experiment 1: Whole Brainstem Mapping Study in the Cat

The aim of the first experiment was to map out the auditory pathways within the brainstem through analysis and comparison of ABRs to click stimuli by moving the active electrode to various locations in the cats' brainstem and recording responses from each location.

The whole brainstem distribution of the local ABRs over six planes to clicks delivered to the left ear in a cat is presented in Fig. 2.1. This map indicates that large potentials are distributed around and in the auditory brainstem nucleus or tracts on the side contralateral to the stimulus side. The response is displayed more quantitatively in detail in Fig. 2.2, where the diameter of each dot indicates the amplitude of the ABR recorded in each plane and corresponds to each ABR peak latency. The latency for the maximum amplitude of each auditory evoked potential varied from point to point in the auditory brainstem pathway. Therefore, the amplitude of each potential at each spot was defined as the amplitude at the ABR wave peaks obtained anywhere over the scalp in that cat. The results were similar in other cats. They indicate that each ABR wave peak is composed of evoked potentials originating from multiple auditory brainstem nuclei and tracts [1].

2.1.2 Experiment 2: Medial Geniculate Body Mapping Study in the Cat. ABR Wave P6

Medial geniculate body (MGB) field potentials were mapped anteriorly-posteriorly (AP) from 2.0 mm to 8.0 mm over the cat skull by monopolar electrodes inserted every 1 mm. Typical responses are shown Fig. 2.3 from the left MGB to both contralateral and ipsilateral auditory stimuli. This MGB mapping study revealed that large potentials corresponding to the same latency of the ABR wave P6 were recorded from the medio-ventral nucleus of the MGB to the contralateral stimuli.

In Fig. 2.4, the amplitudes of these evoked potentials are illustrated as black dots over the six AP planes of the MGB by measuring amplitude at the latency of P6. The distribution of each potential is localized in magnocellular parts of the MGB and distributed cortically from there. Those responses from the contralaterally stimulated ear were more widely distributed anterior-posteriorly, vertically, and horizontally. The onset and the peak of these MGB field potentials corresponded to the trough of P5 and the peak of P6. This mapping study suggested that contralateral stimuli evoke a response from both MGBs which essentially comprises the ABR wave P6 in the cat.

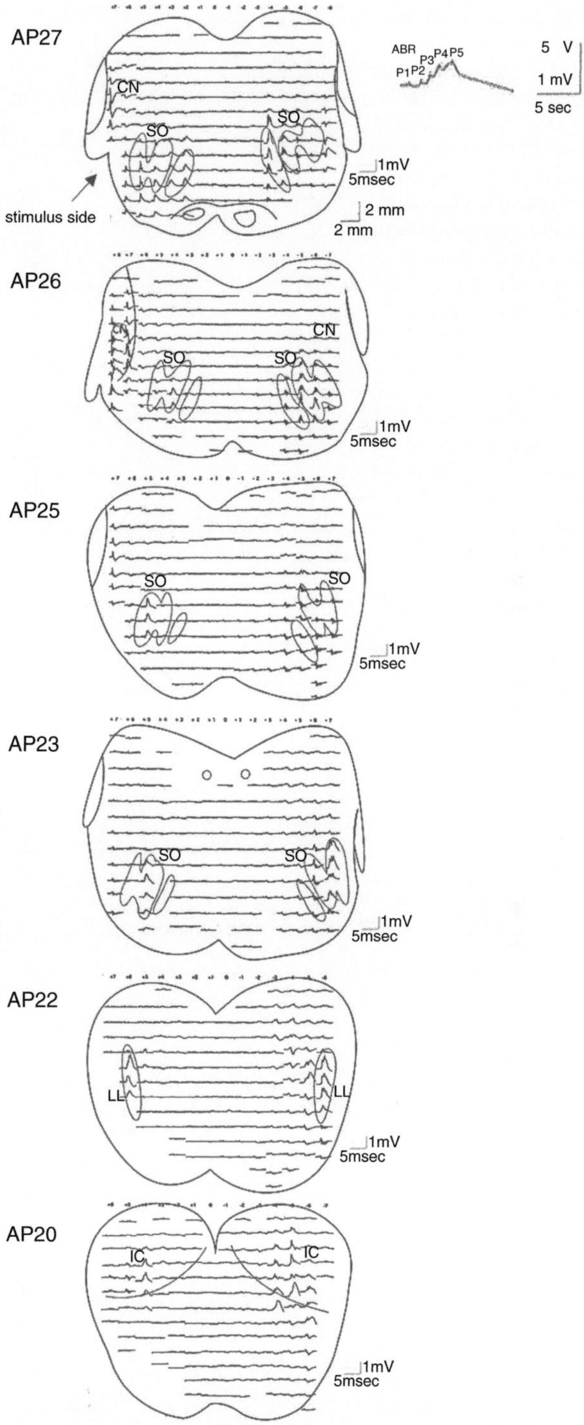

Fig. 2.1 Whole brainstem distribution of the response to auditory stimuli (clicks) from within six levels of the cat brainstem. Stimuli were presented to the left ear of a cat to compare these responses to the simultaneously recorded ABR waveform. Large evoked potentials are evident from various auditory nuclei within the midbrain and brainstem: *SO* superior olivary complex (AP27-AP23); *CN* cochlear nucleus (AP26); *IC* inferior colliculus (AP20); *LL* lateral lemniscus nucleus (AP22). Each AP (anterior-posterior) indicates the coronary plane of the cat brainstem from which recordings were taken

Fig. 2.2 Evoked potential maps of the frontal sections of the brainstem from the level of the cochlear nucleus to the level of the midbrain are constructed using whole brainstem field-potential analysis for comparison with ABR waveform peaks. The diameter of each dot indicates the amplitude of the auditory evoked potentials, which correspond to each wave of the ABR waveform at the corresponding site. Microvolt equivalents are given below. *CN* cochlear nucleus; *VII* facial nerve; *SO* superior olivary complex; *IC* inferior colliculus; *LLV* ventral lateral lemniscus nucleus; *VI* oculomotor nucleus; *LLD* dorsal lateral lemniscus nucleus

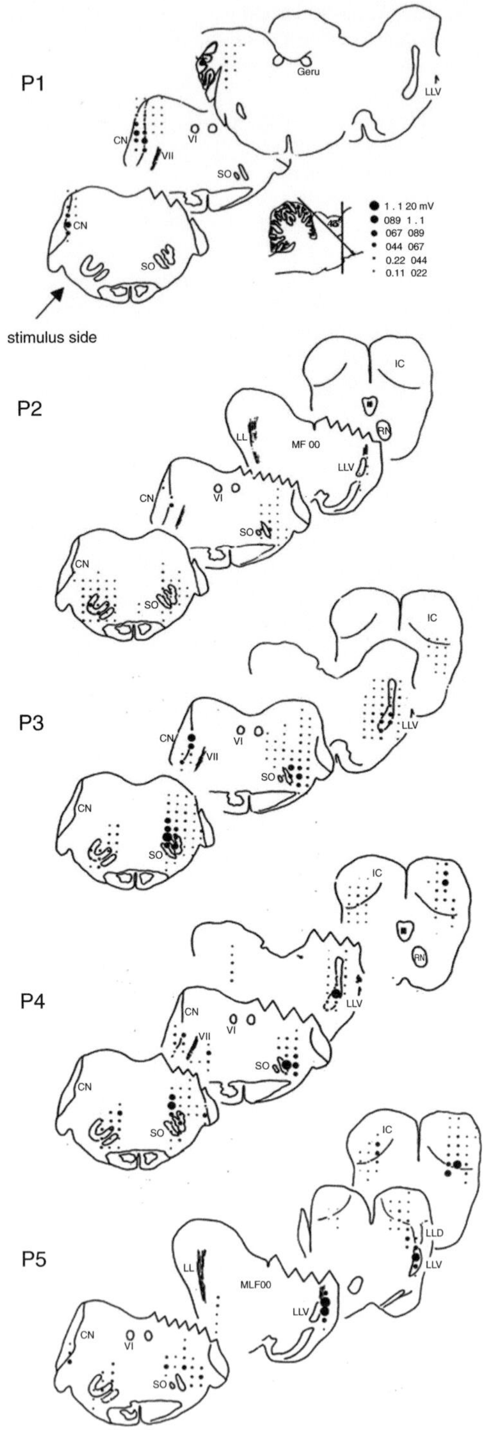

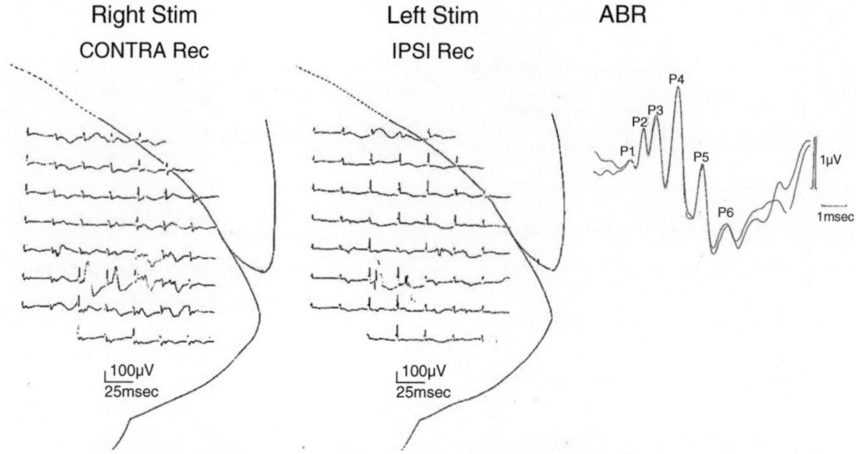

Fig. 2.3 The whole left MGB distribution of the response in six planes to clicks presented to the right ear in a cat and compared with its ABR. Large evoked potentials were recorded from medio-ventral part of the MGB. *CONTRA Rec* contralateral recording, *IPSI Rec* ipsilateral recording

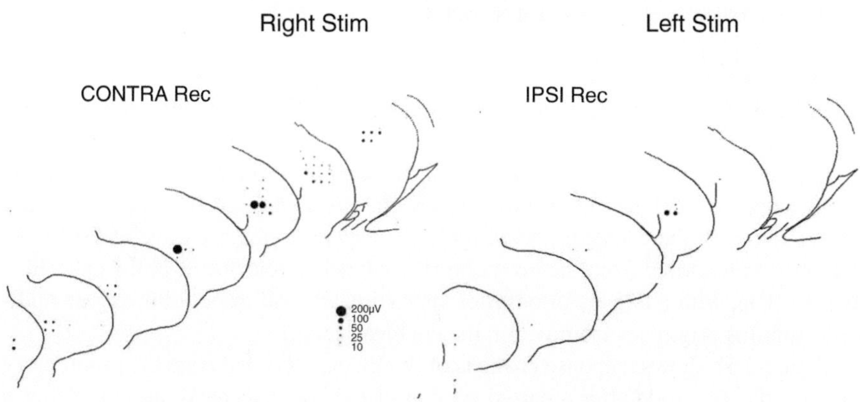

Fig. 2.4 Evoked potential maps of the frontal section of the MGB, from AP 2.0 to 8.0 mm, constructed using whole MGB potentials analysis for comparison with ABR peaks. The diameter of each dot indicates the amplitude of the ABR potential in the MGB, which correspond to wave P6 of the ABR at the corresponding site. Microvolt equivalents are given above

2.2 Experiment 3: Origins of the Six Waves of the ABR Waveform in the Cat as Determined by Depth Recordings and Lesion Studies

2.2.1 Cochlear Nerve (Eighth Cranial Nerve): ABR Wave P1

In Fig. 2.5, ipsilaterally recorded field potentials from cochlear nerve corresponding to N1 of the ECoG (electrocochleographic) response are shown. The ECoG is the

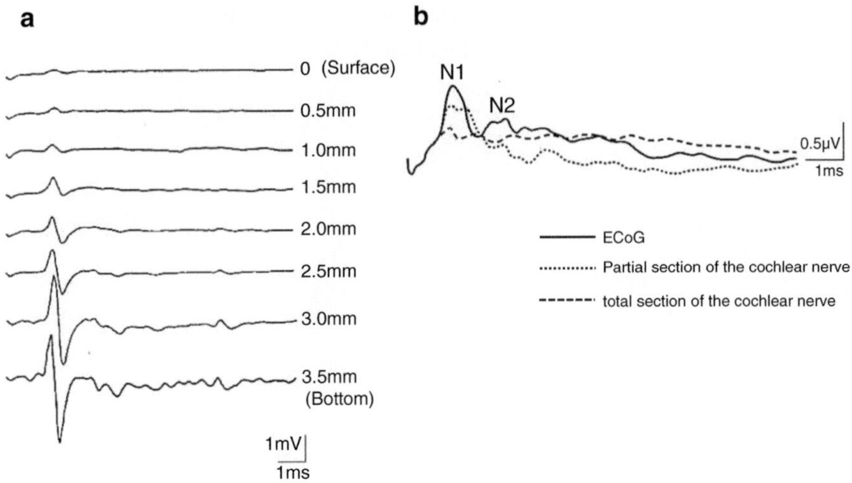

Fig. 2.5 Field potentials from the cochlear nerve (**a**) and ECoGs from the cat promontory (**b**) showing charges in the ECoG after partial and total sections of the cochlear nerve. The thin dotted line (partial section) shows a partial loss of N1 and a complete loss of N2. The thick dotted line (total section) shows a complete loss of N1 and N2

initial recorded response from the cochlea and the eighth nerve to an auditory stimulus (a loud click).

Figure 2.5a shows the recorded potentials from the surface and from within the cochlear nerve to click stimuli presented to the ipsilateral ear. The P1 (or N1 and N2) latencies of the cochlear nerve highly correspond to the N1 wave of the ECoG response as recorded from the promontory, by a needle electrode, in the cat. Thus, Wave I (P1), with a latency of onset of approximately 1.8 msec following an auditory stimulus originates from within the cochlear nerve.

Figure 2.5b shows response changes of the ECoG recorded from the promontory by a needle electrode after a partial section of the cochlear nerve and thereafter a total section of the nerve. After the partial section, amplitude of both N1 and N2 decreased and after total section, N1 and N2 were abolished.

In conclusion, these two studies demonstrated that P1 of the ABR, which is also referred to as N1 of the ECoG, is most likely generated by the cochlear nerve.

2.2.2 *Cochlear Nucleus: ABR Wave P2*

Ipsilateral recorded field potentials from the surface of the cochlear nucleus (0) to its mid-depth (2.4), which correspond to P2 of the ABR, are shown in Fig. 2.6.

In order to establish the validity of P2 of the click evoked ABR waveform arising from the cochlear nucleus, depth recordings were taken from within the cochlear nucleus of a cat. A tungsten electrode was inserted to a depth of 0.3 mm below the

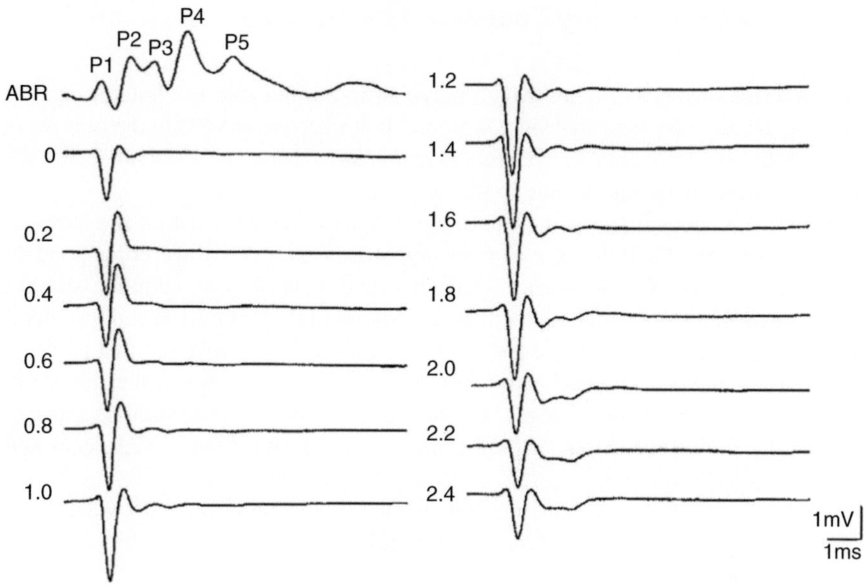

Fig. 2.6 Ipsilateral stimulus responses from the cochlear nucleus (CN) were taken by an electrode from the surface to a depth of 2.4 mm in the cat (bipolar recordings)

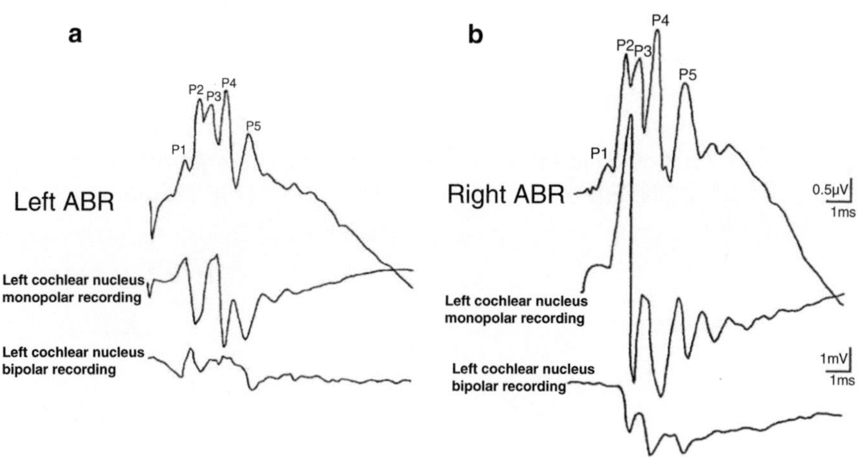

Fig. 2.7 Depth recording from the left cochlear nucleus following acoustic stimulation of the left (**a**) and right (**b**) ears

surface of the left cochlear nucleus. The left ABR and the monopolar and bipolar auditory evoked potentials were recorded from this electrode (Fig. 2.7a) and the right ABR and the monopolar and bipolar auditory evoked potentials were also recorded (Fig. 2.7b). These recordings revealed that P2 of the ABR waveform originates from the bilateral cochlear nuclei.

2.2.3 *Superior Olivary Complex: ABR Wave P3*

The superior olivary complex (SOC) plays an important role in bilateral hearing because the auditory neuronal signals are the first to arrive at SOC in the brainstem and they do so bilaterally with a slight delay in relative latencies which underlies the ability to localize a sound source in space.

Figure 2.8 shows monopolar recordings from an electrode within the superior olivary complex. The latency and intensity of this recorded wave correspond to wave P3 of the ABR following ipsilateral and contralateral auditory stimuli. Contralaterally recorded field potentials correspond to P3 of the ABR and ipsilateral field potentials correspond to P2 and N2 of the ECoG. Thus, we assert that P3 wave of the ABR waveform arises from the contralateral SOCs in the pons of the brainstem.

In Fig. 2.9, ABR wave changes are compared before and after midline transection of the brainstem. After midline transection, the amplitude of P3 decreased remarkably to the stimuli.

In conclusion, these experiments suggest that the origin of the ABR wave P3 is likely the contralateral superior olivary complex.

2.2.4 *Inferior colliculus in the Midbrain: ABR Wave P4 and P5*

In the midbrain, the inferior colliculi receive neuronal signals from the ascending auditory pathways in the brainstem (specifically the superior olivary complex and

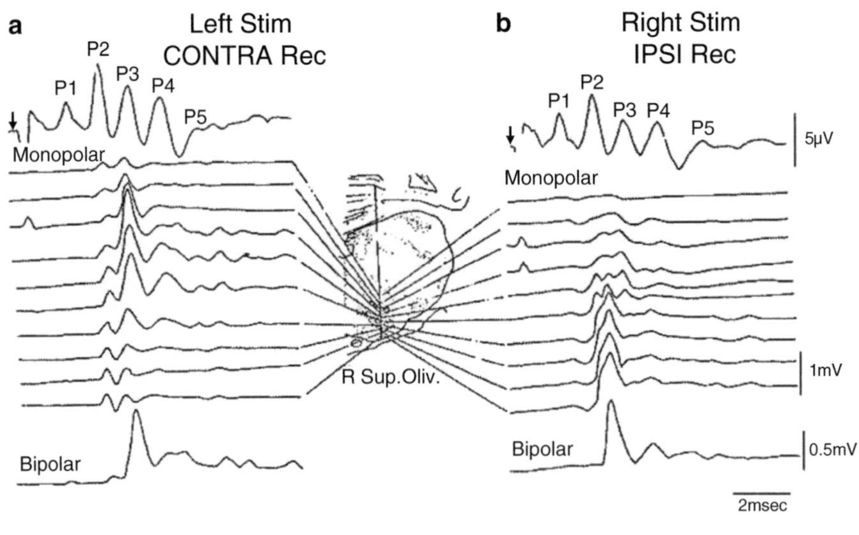

Fig. 2.8 Field potentials recorded from the right superior olivary complex in the cat (monopolar and bipolar recording). (**a**) Left ear stimulation (contralateral recording), (**b**) Right stimulation (ipsilateral recording)

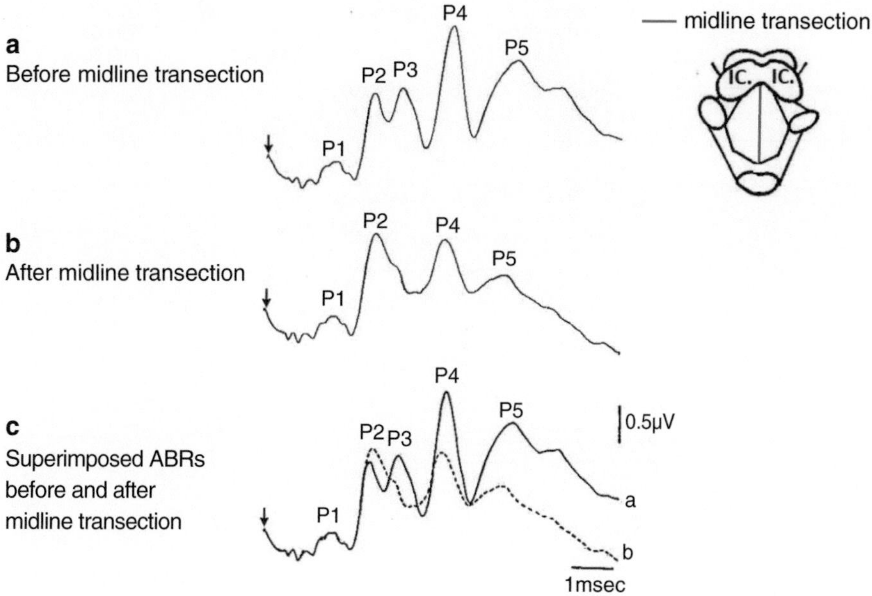

Fig. 2.9 ABRs of a cat to monoaural stimulation before and after midline transection of the brainstem and midbrain. P3 disappeared almost completely, and the amplitudes of P4 and P5 were reduced by up to one-half. (**a**) ABR before midline transection of brainstem, (**b**) ABR after midline transection of brainstem, (**c**) Superimposed illustration of ABRs before (**a**) and after (**b**) midline transection of brainstem

lateral lemniscus nucleus) and then send these signals to the bilateral MGBs which then radiate these signals to the auditory cortex.

Field potentials, generated by acoustic clicks, were recorded by bipolar and monopolar electrodes from within the cat inferior colliculi at varying depths and these recordings are shown in Fig. 2.10. Large potentials, which correspond in latency of onset and amplitude to P4 and P5 of the simultaneously recorded click evoked ABR, were recorded and are shown for comparison. Contralaterally recorded large field potentials correspond to waves P4 and P5 of the ABR waveform and ipsilaterally recorded field potentials also correspond to P4 and P5 of the ABR waveform (Fig. 2.10). Perhaps P4 of the ABR waveform arises from the bilateral lateral lemniscus nuclei and contributes to the P4–P5 complex wave.

The bilateral inferior colliculi of the cat were then aspirated (ablated) and the click evoked ABR waveform changes before and after this aspiration are shown in Fig. 2.11. The major change in the waveform is that the amplitude of the ABR wave P5 was significantly reduced. There was slight effect on the ABR waveform following aspiration of the bilateral colliculi up to and including wave P4, but the amplitude of P5 is markedly reduced. The ABRs from this aspirated cat were obtained on three occasions over the following year and are shown to be unchanged Fig. 2.12. The P5 wave amplitude decreased immediately after aspiration of bilateral inferior colliculus and this decrease persisted over the following year.

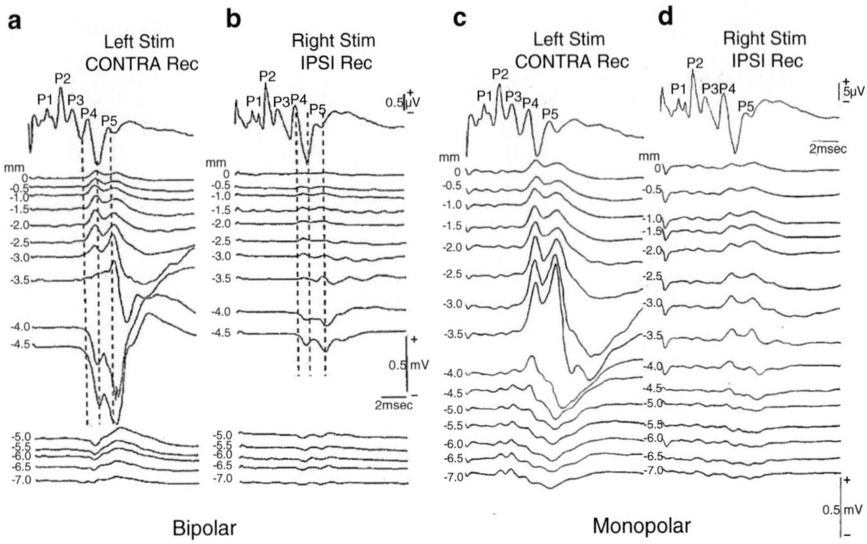

Fig. 2.10 (**a** and **c**) Left ear stimulation (contralateral recording) and (**b** and **d**) **r**ight ear stimulation (ipsilateral recording). Field potentials recorded from the right inferior colliculus in the cat, (**a** and **b**) Bipolar recording, (**c**) and (**d**) monopolar recordings

Fig. 2.11 ABR of a cat to monoaural stimulation before and after aspiration of both inferior colliculus (ICs). There is slight effect up to and including P4, but the amplitude of P5 was markedly reduced after aspiration

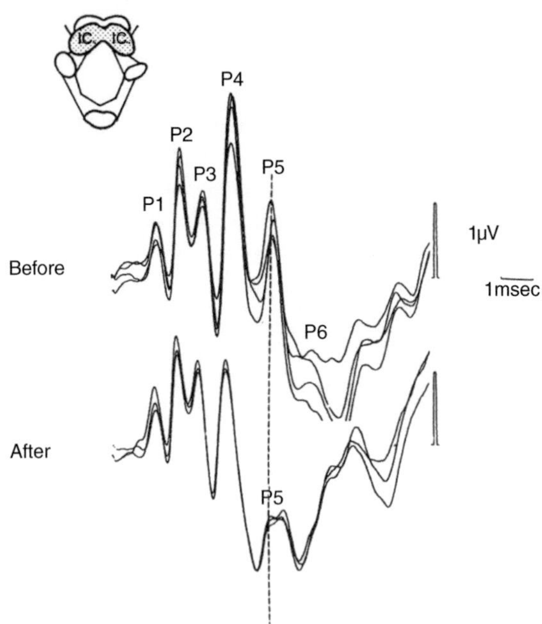

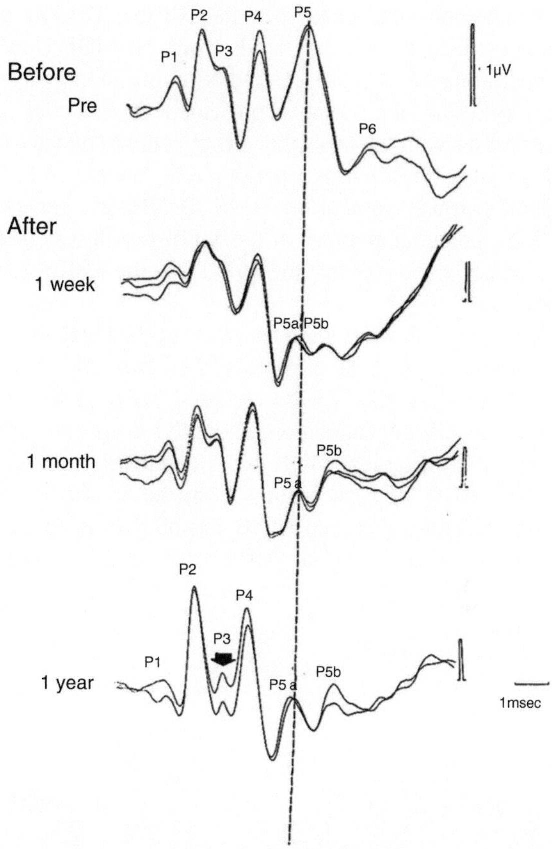

Fig. 2.12 ABRs changes in the cat one year after aspiration of the bilateral inferior colliculus. Note that the amplitude of P5 decreased remarkably immediately following aspiration and this decline of P5 amplitude persisted over the one year of follow-up ABR recordings. P3 amplitude decreased after one year (↓)

These studies comparing the ABR waveform potentials to those of depth recordings before and after aspiration of the inferior colliculi and midline transection of the brainstem suggest that wave P5 of the ABR could originate from the bilateral inferior colliculi.

2.2.5 *Medial Geniculate Body: ABR Wave P6*

The medial geniculate bodies (MGBs) are auditory nuclei along the ascending auditory pathway and are located between the inferior colliculi and the auditory cortecies. In Figs. 2.3 and 2.4, recordings of whole field MGB potentials from the cat are shown. The peak latency of the MGB response closely matches that of wave P6 in the waveform of the simultaneously recorded ABR.

The upper tracing of (a.) and (b.) in Fig. 2.13 shows the ABR-MLC waveform as recorded from the vertex of an intraperitoneally anesthetized cat by chrorarose. The middle latency components (MLCs) following the overall ABR waveform are considered to be waves Na, Pa, Nb (a). This figure also shows simultaneously recorded depth field potentials from the MGB (lower tracings) (b). The stimulus repetition rate of the presented stimuli (clicks) was increased over subsequent trials (a). The click stimuli presented at one click per second resulted in MGB responses with latencies that closely corresponded to P5 and P6 of the ABRs. Upon increasing the stimulus repetition rate, Na, Pa, and Nb of the vertex response disappeared around a repetition rate of 20–30 clicks per second (a) whereas the amplitude of the potential changes of the MGB responses changes was small (b). This lends credence to the idea that the P6 wave of the ABR waveform originates in the MGB in the cat.

In addition, we studied the effect of the local ablation of the MGB on ABR-MLC to further explore the origins of P6 of the ABR.

ABRs and MLCs were recorded before and after the destruction of unilateral MGB by electrocoagulation. In Fig. 2.14a, this lesion in the left MGB is shown histologically (the large obvious white area in the thalamus). Figure 2.14b shows the ipsilateral ABR-MLC recordings from the left or lesion side (upper tracing) and the contralaterally recorded MGB response (second tracing). Both of these recorded waveforms have normal ABR waves and a normal NA, PA of the ABR-MLC

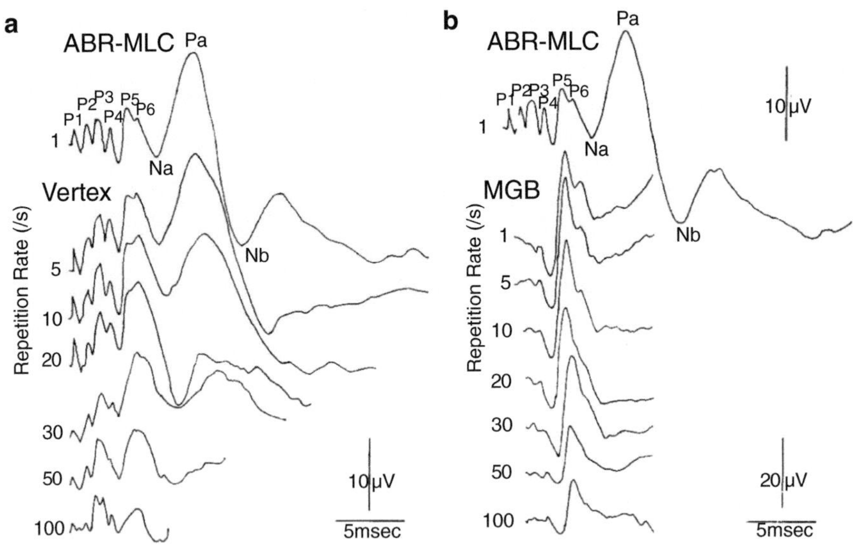

Fig. 2.13 (**a**) Effect of click stimulus repetition rate on vertex recorded ABR-MLC recordings. With increasing repetition rate, Na, Pa, and Nb of the ABR-MLC component disappeared around a 20–30 per second repetition rate but P1–P6 of ABR were preserved. (**b**) Effect of repetition rate on field potentials recorded from the MGB. These latencies were close to P5, P6, and Na. With increased repetition rate, field potentials recorded from the MGB were preserved

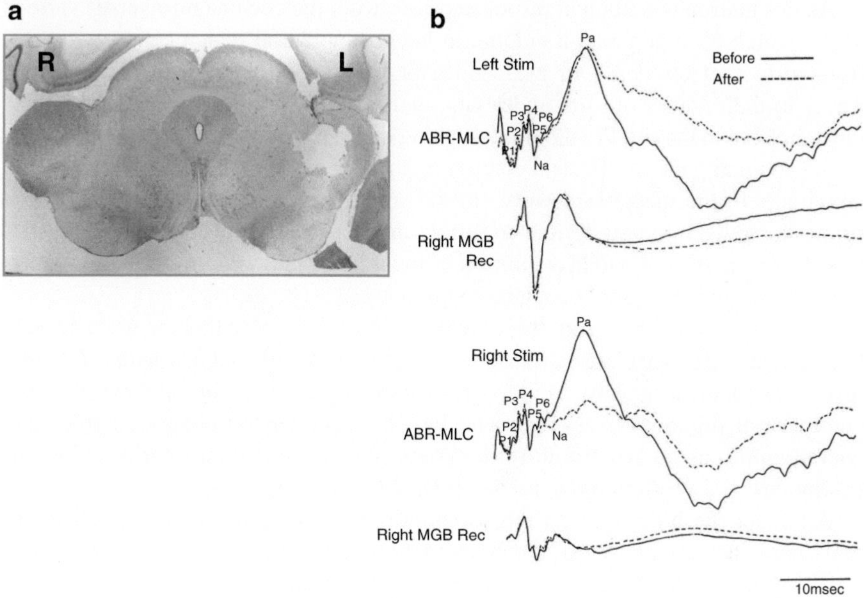

Fig. 2.14 (**a**) Histology of electrocoagulated lesion in the left MGB of a cat. (**b**) Effect of this lesion of the left MGB on the ABR-MLC waves (Na, Pa, and Nb). Right MGB shows a field potential recording from an electrode in the right, contralateral, MGB. This right MGB response is preserved after ablation of the contralateral MGB. Note the loss of the MGB response from the side contralateral to the stimulated ear

waveforms. However, simultaneously recorded, contralaterally evoked, ABR-MLC recordings indicate a near-total loss of the ABR wave P6 and the Na and Pa waves (the MLCs).

These experimental studies of the MGB in cats lead us to decisively conclude that the P6 wave of the ipsilaterally recorded ABR waveform originates from the contralateral auditory pathway, specifically the contralateral MGB in the thalamus.

2.2.6 *Comments*

The aim of the first experiment was to map out the auditory pathways within the brainstem, up to and including the MGBs, by recording and analyzing the latencies and amplitudes of the various waves evoked from click evoked ABRs in cats. Once a sharp acoustic click is presented to the ear, the neurological response to this click travels rapidly (within 9 msec) to the MGB.

As this neurophysiological response passes from the cochlea it traverses various nuclei which each generate a unique, in latency, potential which can be recorded from surface electrodes. Our next endeavor was to correlate these various ABR waves to their sources in the underlying auditory neurophysiological substrate of the brainstem in the cat. We did this by taking depth recordings of various brainstem nuclei, including the MGBs, and comparing these responses, in terms of latency and amplitude, to the recognized waves in the simultaneously recorded ABRs. These studies included inflicting lesions to further investigate specific changes to the ABR waveform and they included aspiration of the inferior colliculi, midline transection of the brainstem, and electrocoagulation of a MGB.

Based on our findings from these experiments, we propose that the main generators of each ABR wave are as follows: P1—the ipsilateral cochlear nerve; P2—the ipsilateral cochlear nucleus and the superior olivary complex in the pons; P3—the contralateral superior olivary complex; P4—the contralateral olivary complex and lateral lemniscus nucleus (both in the pons); P5—contralateral inferior colliculus (midbrain); and P6—contralateral MGB (in the thalamus).

Although the brainstem differs structurally between humans and small mammals, animal experiments are valuable for investigating the generators of the various ABR waves. The possible generators of each ABR peak in cats have been identified (Table 2.1) [1–11]. On the other hand, the determination of the generators of each ABR waveform peak or potential in human subjects has only been based on ABR recordings of known localized neurological lesions (Table 2.2) [12–15].

Table 2.1 Possible generators of the ABR waveform peaks in cats, historically

Study	Year	P1	P2	P3	P4	P5	P6
Jewett	1970	Ipsi. AN	Near CN	Near SOC	In and on either side	IC	
Buchwald et al.	1975	Ipsi. AN	Ipsi. CN	Contra. SOC	Both ICs	Contra. IC	
Achor and Starr	1980	Ipsi. AN	Ipsi. CN Ipsi, CN	SO trapezoid body			
Caird et al.	1985				SOC		
Fullerton and Kiang	1990				LL		
Melcher and Kiang	1996	Spiral ganglion	Ipsi. CN	CN	Both medial SOCs	LL, IC	
Kaga, Shinoda,	1997	Ipsi. AN	Ipsi. CN Ipsi. SOC	Contra. SOC	Contra. SOC. LL	Contra. IC	Contra MGB

Ipsi. ipsilateral; *Contra.* contralateral; *AN* auditory nerve; *CN* cochlear nucleus; *SOC* superior olivary complex; *IC* inferior colliculus; *LL* lateral lemniscus nucleus; *MGB* medial geniculate body

Table 2.2 Proposed generators of the ABR waveform peaks in human subjects, historically

	I	II	III	IV	V	VI	VII
Starr A & Hamilton (1976)	AN	CN	SOC	LL	IC	Unknown	Unknown
Stockard J, et al. (1977)	AN	Pontomedullary Junction	Caudal pons	Rostral pons or Midbrain	Midbrain	Thalamus	Thalamus or Auditory radiation
Hashimoto I (1986)	AN	CN	SOC	Pons	Contra JC	MGB	Unknown
Møller A.R. (1999)	AN	AN	CN or SOC	LL	LL	IC	IC

AN auditory nerve; *CN* cochlear nucleus; *SOC* superior olivary complex; *LL* lateral lemniscus nucleus; *IC* interior colliculus; *MGB* medial geniculate body

References

1. Buchwald JS, Huang C. Far-field acoustics response: origins in the cat. Science. 1975;189:382–4.
2. Jewett DL. Volume-conducted potentials in response to auditory stimuli as detected by averaging in the cat. Electroencephalogr Clin Neurophysiol. 1970;28:609–18.
3. Achor LJ, Starr A. Auditory brains stem responses in the cat. I. Intracranial and extra-cranial recordings. Electroencephalogr Clin Neurophysiol. 1980;48:154–73.
4. Achor LJ, Starr A. Auditory brain stem responses in the cat. II. Effects of lesions. Electroencephalogr Clin Neurophysiol. 1980;48:174–90.
5. Caird D, Sontheimer D, Klinkc R. Intra-and extracranially recorded auditory evoked potentials in the cat. I. Source location and binaural interaction. Electroencephalogr Clin Neurophysiol. 1985;61:50–60.
6. Fullerton BF, Kiang NYS. The effect of brain stem lesions on brain stem auditory evoked potentials in the cat. Hear Res. 1990;49:363–90.
7. Melcher JR, Knudson IM, Fullerton BC, et al. Generators of the brain stem auditory evoked potentials in cat. I. an experimental approach to their identification. Hear Res. 1996;93:1–27.
8. Melcher JR, Guinan JJ, Knudson IM, et al. Generators of the brain stem auditory evoked potentials in cat. II. Correlating lesions sites with waveform change. Hear Res. 1996;93:28–51.
9. Melcher JR, Kiang NYS. Generators of the brain stem auditory evoked potential in cat. III. Identified cell populations. Hear Res. 1996;93:52–71.
10. Kaga K, Shinoda Y, Suzuki J-I. Origin of auditory brainstem responses in cats: whole brainstem mapping, and a lesion and HRP study of the inferior colliculus. Acta Otolaryngol. 1997;117(2):197–201.
11. Kaga K, editor. Central auditory pathway disorders. Tokyo, Berlin, NY: Springer; 2009.
12. Starr A, Hamilton AE. Correlation between confirmed sites of neurological lesions and abnormalities of far-field auditory brainstem responses. Electroencephalogr Clin Neurophysiol. 1976;41:595–608.
13. Stockard JJ, Rossiter VS. Clinical and pathologic correlates of brain stem auditory response abnormalities. Neurol. 1977;27:316–25.
14. Hasimoto I. Neural generators of early auditory evoked potential components in man. In: Kunze K, et al., editors. Clinical problems of brain stem disorders. NY: Georg Thime; 1986. p. 111–20.
15. Møller AR. Neural mechanisms of BAEP. Functional Neuroscience: Evoked Potentials and Magnetic Fields (EEG Suppl, 49) 1997:27–35.

Chapter 3
Gestational Development of the Human Auditory System Including the Cochlea and the Central Auditory Pathways

Kimitaka Kaga

Abstract Embryologically, in the human, the cochlea and its auditory sensory cells (inner and outer hair cells) begin to develop just after the fourth week of pregnancy and both are completely developed at the end of gestation whereas the vestibular organs and their sensory cells begin development much earlier. The neuronal myelination of both systems begins around the fourth month of pregnancy. Phylogenetically, the auditory system is a more recent development than the older vestibular system. Compared across species, the overall neuronal development and myelination of these systems begin later in human embryos than in other species. In human, complete development of both systems continues after birth and progresses through infancy and into puberty. In the central auditory pathways, the developmental rate of axonal myelination does not proceed uniformly across the different auditory relay nuclei. The neuronal axonal tracts only become fully functional after they are completely myelinated. Myelination and function are closely related. Because the gestational onset of the vestibular neurons (axons) precedes that of the auditory organs, complete myelination of the vestibular neurons and relay nuclei tends to occur sooner in the vestibular system versus the auditory system. This supports the concept that the auditory system and its' central neuronal pathways is, phylogenetically, a more recent development compared to the older vestibular system.

Keywords Cochlea · Cochlear nerve · Myelination · Brainstem auditory pathway · Auditory cortex

---

K. Kaga (✉)
National Institute of Sensory Organs, National Hospital Organization, Tokyo Medical Center, Audiology Clinic, Kamio Memorial Hospital, Tokyo, Japan
e-mail: kimitaka.kaga@kankakuki.jp

© Springer Japan KK, part of Springer Nature 2022

K. Kaga (ed.), *ABRs and Electrically Evoked ABRs in Children*, Modern Otology and Neurotology, https://doi.org/10.1007/978-4-431-54189-9_3

3.1 Gestational Development of Inner Ear

In Table 3.1, a timeline of the major embryologically developmental events of the human inner ear is illustrated [1].

Embryologically, the cochlea and its sensory cells complete their development at a relatively late stage of fetal development compared to the vestibular organs (Fig. 3.1) [2]. The vestibular otocysts separate from the neural crest around the fourth week of pregnancy and the endolymphatic duct develops around the fifth week [3]. The entire membranous labyrinth develops almost into the physical shape and size of an adult at around the 12th gestational week. The entire cochlea, and the Organs of Corti within, are completely developed by approximately the 24th week of gestation (Fig. 3.2) and neither significantly change their shape or function through adulthood (Fig. 3.3). In other words, the cochlea of a newborn is morphologically and functionally intact [1, 3]. This developmental sequence of the cochlea suggests that inner ear malformations can be caused by a disruption of cochlear development at a very early stage of pregnancy. In that there are many types of inner ear malformations then they each probably occur at various times of disruption during the development of the fetus.

Table 3.1 Timetable of major events in the human inner ear development

Fetal week	Inner ear
3rd	Auditory placode; auditory pit
4th	Auditory vesicle (otocyst); vestibular-cochlear division
6th	Utricle and saccule present; semicircular canal begins
7th	One cochlear coil present; sensory cells in utricle and saccule
8th	Ductus reuniens present; sensory cells in semicircular canals
11th	Two and one-half cochlear coils present
12th	Sensory cells in the cochlea; membranous labyrinth complete; otic capsule begins to ossify
20th	Maturation of internal ear; internal ear adult size

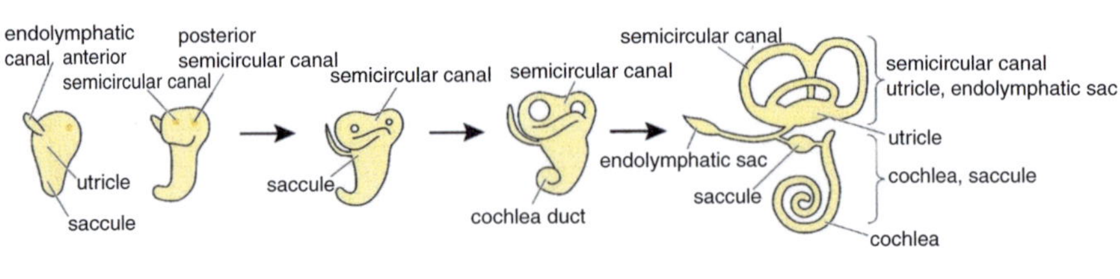

Fig. 3.1 Illustration showing the fetal development of the inner ear during gestation [2]

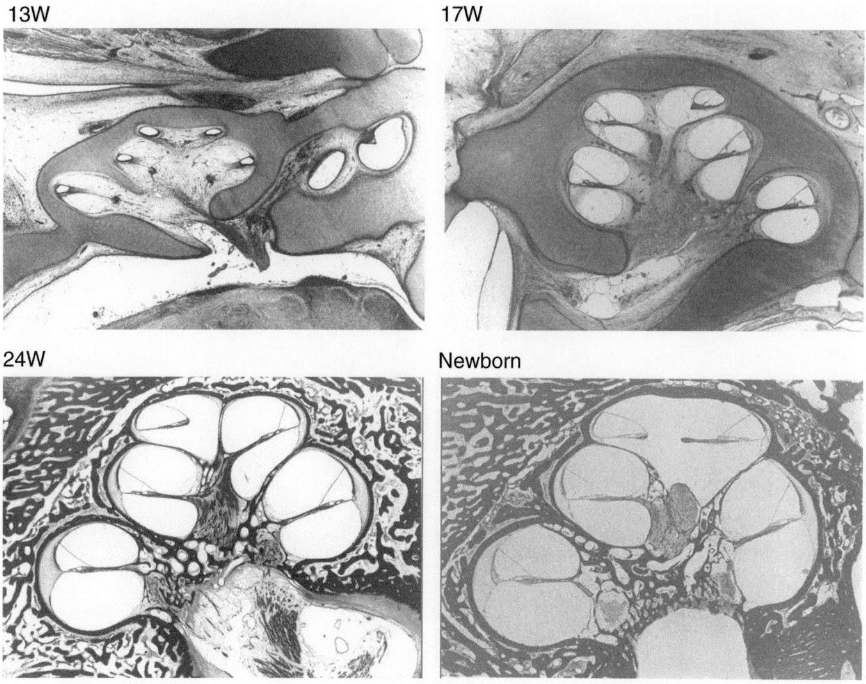

Fig. 3.2 Mid-modiolar section of the temporal bone showing the development of the fetal cochlea at different times during gestation from the 13th week of pregnancy to birth

3.2 Development of the Inner Ear Hair Cells and the Ganglion Cells

The development of the inner ear hair cells, its ganglion cells and the central ascending auditory pathway is summarized below from the classical study by Rubel [4].

3.2.1 Formation of the Otic Vesicle and the Development of the Inner Ear During Gestation

6–16 weeks: Cavitation of the otic cavity involves chondrolysis by histocyte cells.

3–20 weeks: Onset of otocyst formation and duct division and expansion.

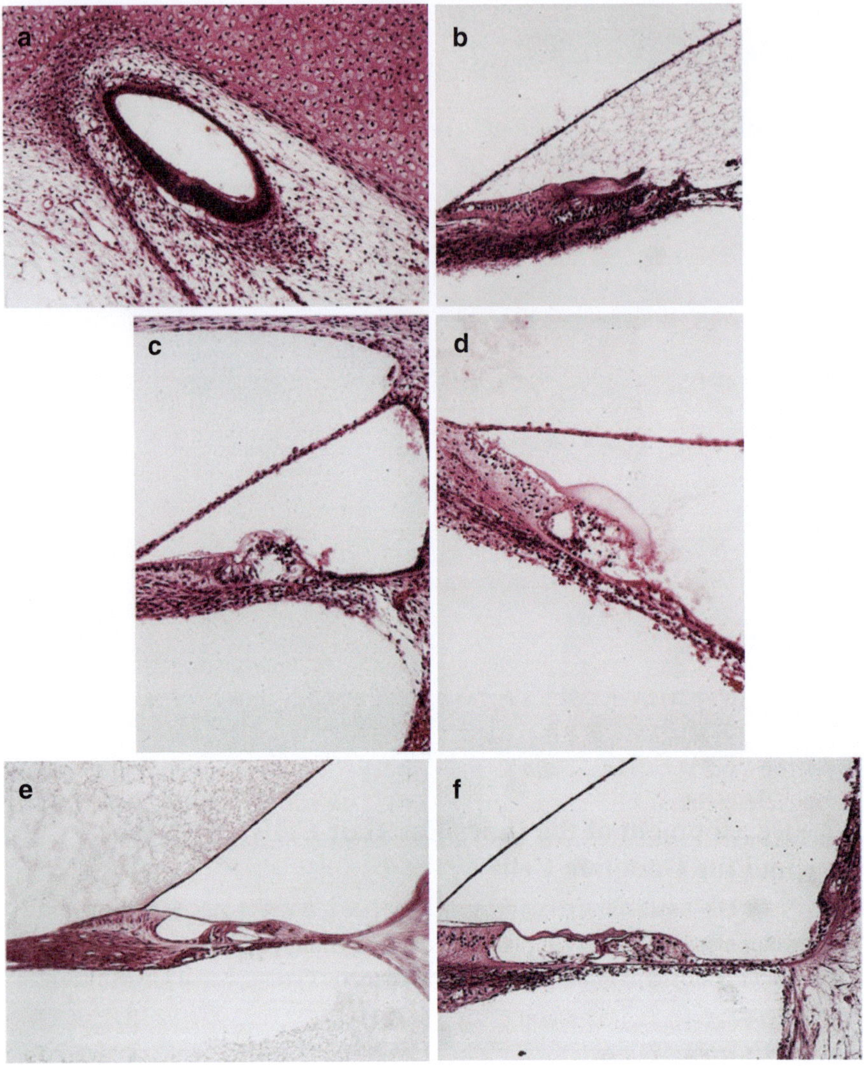

Fig. 3.3 Temporal bone histology showing the development of the Organ of Corti from the 13th week of pregnancy to birth. The Organ of Corti is completely developed by the 24th week of gestation. (**a**) week 13, (**b**) week 17, (**c**) week 19, (**d**) week 21, (**e**) week 24, (**f**) newborn

3.2.2 Differentiation of Inner Ear Hair Cells within the Organ of Corti

10–25 weeks: Histogenesis of cochlear hair cells follows a timeline wherein there is a basal-to-apical temporal developmental difference indicating that the inner hair cells develop prior to the outer hair cells.

12–27 weeks: The earliest differentiation of hair cells occurs in the middle section of the basal turn of the cochlea and which proceeds from there in both directions. The inner hair cells can be recognized prior to the appearance of the outer hair cells. A quantification of hair cell population is shown in Rubels' article [4], at 3–6 months.

3.2.3 *Differentiation of the Spiral Ganglion Cells within the Cochlea*

Opinions are divided regarding the origin of these cells, placodal vs. the neural crest. Cells of the spiral ganglion can be recognized at the 2.8–4 mm size of the fetus.

3.2.4 *Innervation of the Inner Ear Hair Cells*

At 4.5 weeks of gestation, neural fibers from the spiral ganglion appear to enter the cochlear vesicle. At 6 weeks there is an increased fiber outgrowth from these ganglion cells. At 7.5 weeks these neural fibers from the ganglion then enter the sensory epithelium (hair cells) of the cochlea. The basal-to-apical timing sequence of this innervation differs. The inner hair cells become innervated before the outer hair cells. At the fourth gestational month, ganglionic nerve fibers can be identified throughout all turns of the cochlea.

3.3 Development of the Central Ascending Auditory Pathway

Table 3.2 is a timeline of the major developmental events in the central auditory ascending pathway of the fetus.

Myelination of developing neuronal axonal tracts in human brains starts around the fourth month of pregnancy but complete myelination continues through infancy

Table 3.2 Timeline of the onset of myelination in the central auditory system of the human fetus

1. Brainstem auditory nuclei	2. Appearance of neuronal cells	3. Start age of myelinations
Cochlear nerve (spiral ganglion)	8 weeks	6 months
Cochlear nucleus	6–7 weeks	6 months
Superior olivary complex	6–7 weeks	6 months
Nucleus of lateral lemniscus	6–7 weeks	6 months
Inferior colliculus	6–7 weeks	6 months
Medial geniculate body	10 weeks	7 months
Primary auditory cortex	8 months	10 months
* acoustic radiation	Postnatal 1 month - 3 years	
** cerebral commissures	Postnatal 2 months - 7 years	

and into puberty. However, myelination of each neuronal system does not occur at the same time. Myelination is completed sooner or later depending on the specific division of the brain and it follows a certain order. A rule applies here, in principle, that the phylogenetically older specific divisions of the brain are myelinated sooner during an individual's development. Flechsig [5] concluded that the different neuronal tracts become completely functional only after completion of myelination. In fact, the function of the brain and the myelination of each neuronal system are closely related and myelination tends to be completed sooner in the specific divisions of the brain which exhibit an earlier gestational onset of function.

Yakovlev et al. [6], also reported, in their study of the embryological development of myelination, that the duration required for completion of the myelin sheath differs across the various neuronal fiber bundles. Each fiber bundle starts to develop a myelin sheath at a unique time following a predetermined cycle of myelination which they called the "myelogenetic cycle." They indicated that the myelination of motor neurons has a short cycle (developing between the fifth and tenth gestational months) whereas development of myelination of sensory neurons begins at a later stage and takes longer to complete (onset at the sixth month of gestation) and continues until age 4. Myelination of the statoacoustic tectum and its sensory cells has a short cycle and occurs in the sixth month of fetal development.

Phylogenetically, the human central auditory system is a recent development and both its development, and its myelination, occur at a later gestation time relative to other species [4].

3.3.1 Gestational Development of Myelination of the Human Cochlear Nerve

The myelination of the cochlear nerve begins in the sixth month of development of the fetus. Both the growth of the axons and their myelination begin at the basal turn of the cochlea and proceed apically innervating subsequent cochlear nerve fibers. The spiral ganglion cell growth follows closely to the prolonged cochlear nerve myelination. The proximal nerve roots of the cochlear nerve are present in the medulla oblongata at 8 weeks of embryonic development.

3.3.2 Development of the Rhombencephalon (Medulla Oblongata)

3.3.2.1 The Developmental Origin of the Cochlear Nucleus and Its Neural Proliferation

The cochlear nuclei arise from the third of the primary otic vesicles to develop, the lip of the rhombencephalon being at its mid rostral and caudal level. The site of the origin of other auditory nuclei may be the ventral brainstem.

3.3.2.2 Migration of the Cochlear Nucleus During Fetal Development

The incoming acoustic fibers from various ganglia influence the migration of cochlear nuclei innervation and the ordered "streaming" of the cells from the rhombencephalon is also influential. Interestingly, removal of the otocysts has little influence on this migration sequence [4].

3.3.2.3 Differentiation Between the Development of the Primary and Secondary Cochlear Nuclei

The differentiation of the primary and secondary nuclei of the CN (cochlear nuclei) appears to occur simultaneously. The ultimate cell count of each nucleus is determined by afferents that regulate cell death. Human brainstem cochlear nuclei can be identified at about the sixth or seventh week of gestation.

3.3.2.4 Myelination of the Auditory Neural Substrate

Myelination of auditory neurons begins around the sixth month of pregnancy. It starts slowly, rapidly increases, and then tapers off over time. The rate and extensiveness of myelination are probably regulated by external neuronal activity (Fig. 3.4).

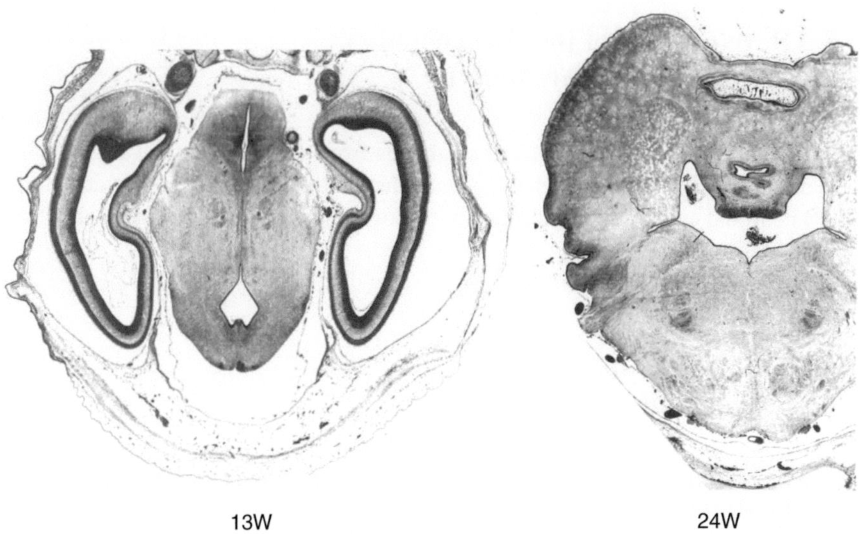

Fig. 3.4 Histological view of the development of a human brainstem over a gestation period of 13 weeks to 24 weeks

3.4 Development of the Mesencephalon (Inferior Colliculus)

Neuronal cells in the inferior colliculus [IC] appear at the sixth or seventh gestational week and begin myelination at the sixth month of gestation.

3.4.1 Differentiation of the Inferior Colliculus in the Midbrain

Dendrites and axons from the IC appear in the midbrain well before the onset of any functionality. The development of dendrites in the central IC precedes that of those in the superficial layers. The extracellular space around this nucleus decreases with the onset of hearing.

3.4.2 Myelination of the Inferior Colliculus

Neuronal axonal myelination of the IC begins around the sixth gestational month and is only complete after the first year of life, as revealed by the evocation of wave V of the ABR from neonates [7].

3.5 Development of the Diencephalon (Medial Geniculate Body)

The medial geniculate body (MGB) originates from the region of the dorsal thalamus and it migrates along the same path as the ventral thalamus. Newly developed MGB neuronal cells can be identified in the dorsal thalamus of the fetus at about the tenth gestational week.

3.5.1 Differentiation of the Medial Geniculate Body

At 6 months of in utero development most embryonic cells are small and multipolar. Axonal development of the MBG continues through gestation and is only completed by the end of the second postpartum week. The larger part of the MGB, its ventral division, differentiates prior to the dorsal division.

3.5.2 Myelination of the Medial Geniculate Body

Myelination of the MGB begins during the seventh month of gestation and its fibers are among the earliest to become myelinated.

3.5.3 Development of the Telencephalon (the Auditory Cortex)

In the telencephalon (the auditory cortex), the neuronal density decreases at about the eighth month of gestation, but it then rapidly increases in density just before term and continues to increase for up to 4 years post-partum.

3.5.4 Neuronal Differentiation within the Auditory Cortex

In humans, massive dendritic development begins to occur only after the eighth gestational month.

3.5.5 Myelination of the Auditory Radiation

Complete myelination of the thalami-cortical fibers (its auditory radiation) occurs gradually during the postnatal period (Figs. 3.5 and 3.6) [5] and correlates with the peak latency decreases and amplitude increases as recorded by auditory evoked potentials from neonates [7].

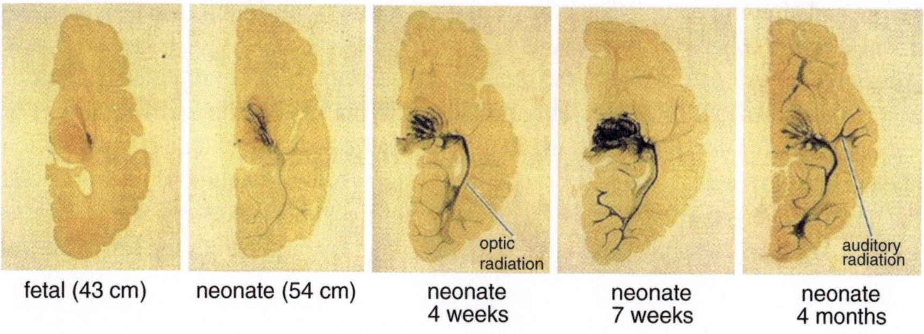

Fig. 3.5 Flechsig's histological study of the developing brain and its myelination of the auditory radiation (horizontal sections) [5]

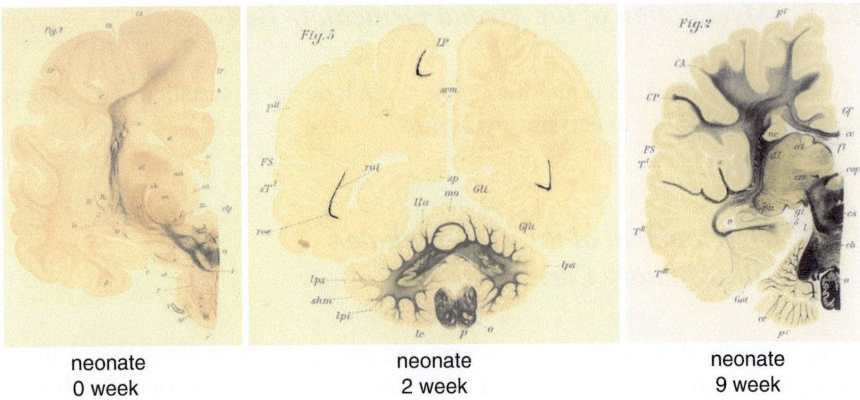

Fig. 3.6 Flechsig's histological study of the developing brain and its myelination of the auditory radiation (coronary sections) [5]

3.5.6 Cytoarchitectural and Axonal Maturation of the Human Auditory Cortex

Moor, JK, and Guan, Y [8] followed the histological and immunohistochemical maturation of the human auditory cortex from the beginning of the second trimester of pregnancy through young childhood. They noted that between the 22nd week of gestation and the fourth postnatal month a two-tiered band of neurofilament-immunoreactive axons developed in layer I of the auditory cortex. Between the middle of the first year of life and at age 3, a laminar pattern of cytoarchitecture becomes fully mature and a network of immune-stained axons develops in layers VI, V, IV, and in layer IIIa. Beginning at age 5, another network of neurofilament-positive axons develops in the superficial cortical layers IIIb, IIIa, and II and by 11 or 12 years of age the overall axonal density is equivalent to that seen in young adulthood (Fig. 3.7).

Of note, it is instructive to be aware of the conductive velocity of nerve impulses before and after the completion of myelination. Prior to myelination, nerve impulses travel through otherwise bare axons with a conductive velocity of less than 2 m/s. After myelination is complete, the conductive velocity of nerve impulses increases to a maximum of 120 m/s [9]. This difference in the neural conductive velocity at various stages of development suggests that knowledge of the extent of myelination at each stage of development is crucial in the study of brain neuronal networks and the postnatal staged appearance of various cerebral and peripheral functions such as audition, balance, speech, language, learning, memory, and mentation [10].

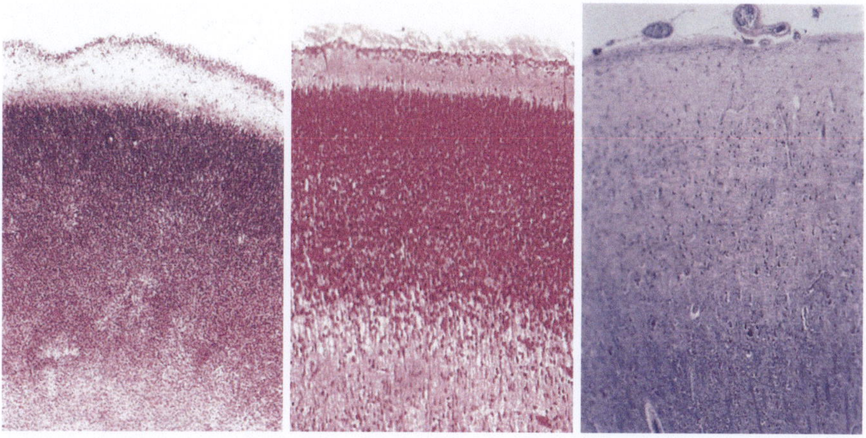

Fig. 3.7 Histology of the cerebral cortex during the 13th and 21st weeks of fetal development and at adulthood

References

1. Northern J, Downs MP. Hearing in children. Baltimore: Lippincott William & Wilkins; 1974.
2. Nomura Y, Harada Y, Hiraide F, Kobayashi H, Kimura Y. Atlas of otology. 4th ed. Japan: Maruzenn; 2017.
3. Kaga K, Sakurai H, Ogawa Y, Mizutani T, Toriyama M. Morphological changes of vestibular ganglion cells in human fetuses and in pediatric patients. Int J Pediatr Otorhinolaryngol. 2001;60(1):11–20.
4. Rubel EW. Chapter 5. Ontogeny of structure and function in the vertebrate auditory system. In: Jacobson M, editor. Handbook of sensory physiology, Vol.IX. Development of sensory systems. Springer-Verlag; 1978. p. 135–237.
5. Flechsig P. Anatomie des menschichen Gehims und Rückenmarks auf myelogenetischer Grundlage. Leipzig: G. Thieme; 1920.
6. Yakovlev P, Lecours AR. The myelogenetic cycles of regional maturation of the brain. In: Regional development of the brain in early life. Oxford: Blackwell Scientific Publications; 1967.
7. Kaga K, Tanaka Y. Auditory brainstem response and behavioral audiometry. Developmental Correlates Arch Otolaryngol. 1980;106(9):564–6.
8. Moore JK, Guan YL. Cytoarchitectural and axonal maturation in human auditory cortex. J Assoc Res Otolaryngol. 2001;2(4):297–311.
9. Luo L. Principle of neurobiology. New York: Garland Science; 2015.
10. Tanji jin. Five years of integrated brain study. Grant-in-aid for scientific on priority areas. The 5th area. Research Bulletin, p. 1–32.

Chapter 4
ABR Recording Technique and the Evaluation of Peripheral Hearing Loss

Kimitaka Kaga and Dominic W. Hughes

Abstract The ABR is the neurological activity, evoked by an auditory stimulus, which is generated along the neural pathway as it travels from the cochlea on its way to the medial geniculate body (MGB) in the brain. This response, which can be recorded from external electrodes applied to the skull and mastoid process of the subject, is therefore called a "far-field recording," which means that the electrodes recording this response are externally placed on the skull, quite distant from the actual neurologic activity within the brainstem. The auditory stimulus, which is used to generate this response and is usually presented by earphones, is a short duration (<1 msec) click presented at various acoustic intensity (loudness) levels. The time required for the ABR to this click to travel from the cochlea to the MGB is approximately 9 msec. Seven distinct waves are evoked, from a subject with normal hearing, within this time span when the click stimulus intensity is set at a high level (100 dBHL). As the initial acoustic intensity of the click stimulus is decreased, usually in 10 dBHL increments, the peak latency of each evoked wave increases and the various wave amplitudes decrease and ultimately disappear at lower click intensities (threshold of detection). Of these initially recorded seven waves, wave V often persists as low as 10 dBHL in a normal hearing subject.

A major impediment to recording this response is the simultaneous, large amplitude, and random, ongoing background brain activity, and noise, which totally obscures the much smaller ABR. The solution to extracting the buried ABR from within the "noise" of this brain activity has been computer technology (circa 1970) and advances in amplifier technology wherein the summed and averaged ABR signal can be discerned. The ABR is clinically useful for both objective audiometry and neurological local diagnosis in brainstem.

Keywords ABR · Click · Conductive hearing loss · Sensory/neural hearing loss

K. Kaga (✉)
National Institute of Sensory Organs, National Hospital Organization, Tokyo Medical Center, Audiology Clinic, Kamio Memorial Hospital, Tokyo, Japan
e-mail: kimitaka.kaga@kankakuki.jp

D. W. Hughes
Neurotology, West Linn, OR, USA

© Springer Japan KK, part of Springer Nature 2022

K. Kaga (ed.), *ABRs and Electrically Evoked ABRs in Children*, Modern Otology and Neurotology, https://doi.org/10.1007/978-4-431-54189-9_4

4.1 Requirements Necessary to Obtain ABR Recordings

There are two requirements to obtain and analyze ABR recordings. The first requires the determination and preparation of the sites on the subjects' heads where the electrodes will be placed. The second is, of course, the availability of the equipment to do so which consists of computer-generated auditory stimuli and averaging capability to extract the ABR from the background EEG activity as mentioned in the abstract.

4.1.1 Location (Montage) and Application of ABR Electrodes

Three small (1 cm in diameter) saucer-like metal electrodes are most commonly used for obtaining human ABR recordings. The positive electrode is placed on the forehead near the hairline. The negative electrode is placed on the promontory of the mastoid bone ipsilateral to the acoustically stimulated ear. The earth (ground) electrode is placed on the mastoid promontory of the contralaterally stimulated ear (Fig. 4.1). Prior to placing the saucer electrodes, they are filled with a conductive electrolytic paste. To reduce the electrode contact impedance with the skin to below 5 KΩ, the electrode site should be vigorously scrubbed with an alcohol swab. Figure 4.2 shows an ABR recording setup from a neonate during sleep [1].

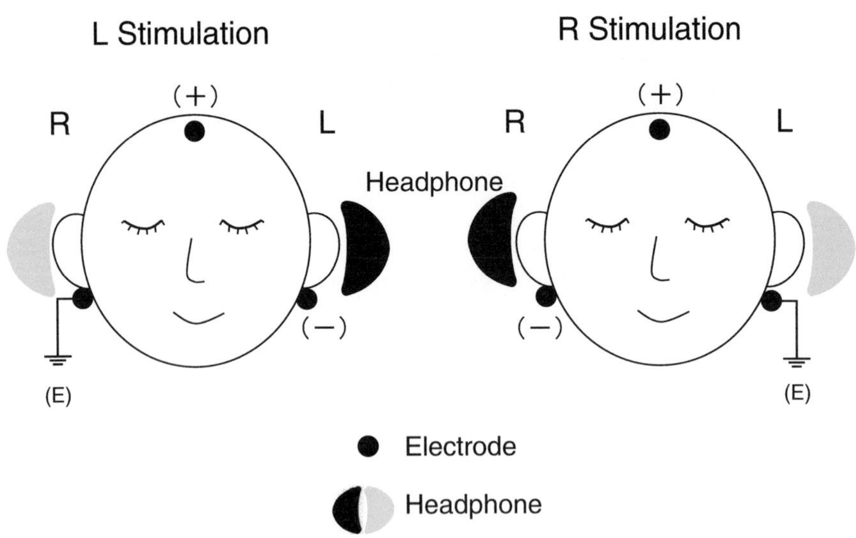

Fig. 4.1 Schematic showing the location of the ABR recording electrodes and the placement of headphones

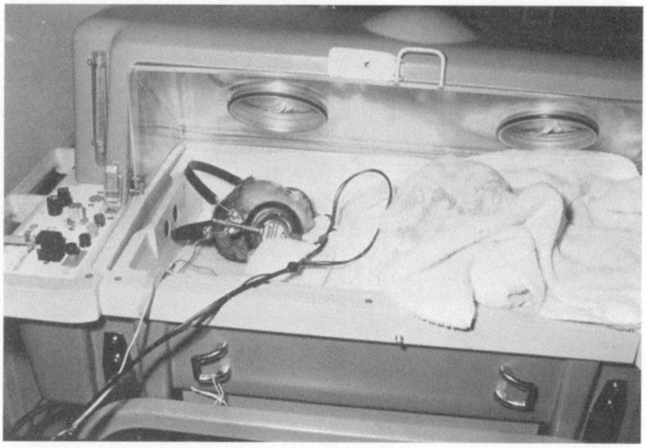

Fig. 4.2 ABR recording setup in a neonate

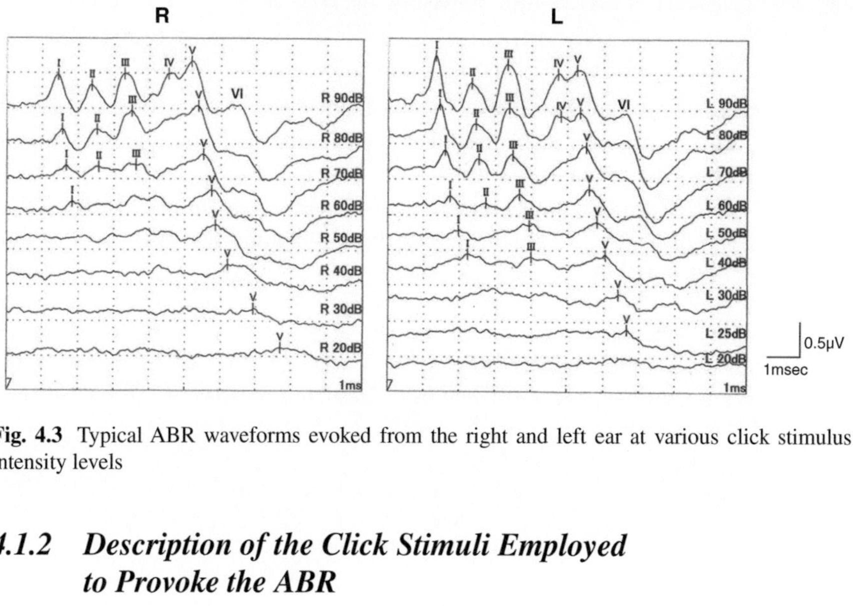

Fig. 4.3 Typical ABR waveforms evoked from the right and left ear at various click stimulus intensity levels

4.1.2 Description of the Click Stimuli Employed to Provoke the ABR

Discreet, short-duration clicks, generated by a computer, are presented unilaterally. White noise masking of the contralaterally stimulated ear is often applied. These clicks have a pulse width of approximately 100 microseconds. Clicks are presented, generally via TDH49 headphones, with an alternating polarity, condensating or refracting (plus or minus), this to prevent stimulus artifacts. ABR recordings, obtained from a normal hearing subject, are shown in Fig. 4.3 wherein the responses to click stimuli starting at the intensity level of 100dBHL and decreasing in intensity by 10dBHL increments until no ABR waves can be discerned. Clicks are presented at a repetition rate of between 10 and 20 per second and the average number of collected click responses to obtain discernible ABRs, during each test session and at each stimulus intensity, is between 500 and 1000. The analysis time, the time

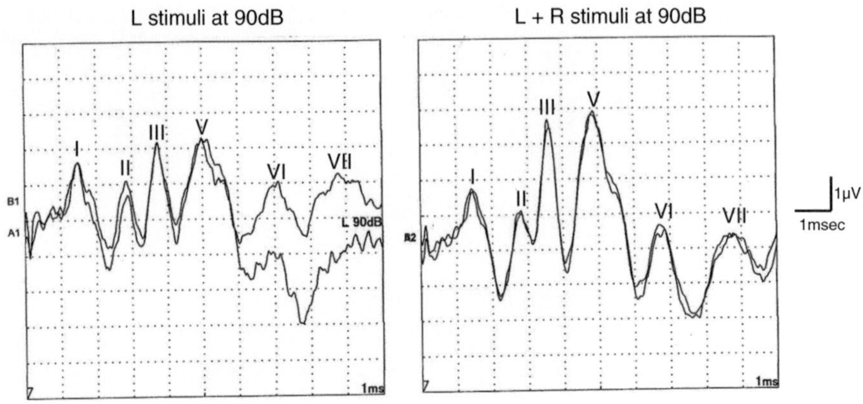

Fig. 4.4 Comparison of typical ABR waveforms following unilateral or bilateral stimulus presentation

window, necessary to capture the short-duration time span of the ABR is usually set at 10 msec and occasionally at 20 msec. The filter settings of the amplifier recording the ABR are set with the high pass filter at 30 Hz and the low pass filter at 3 KHz, each with a 3 dB-down set point [1]. The amplifier gain setting should be at least 105.

A comparison of ABRs recorded following unilaterally and bilaterally stimulated ears is illustrated in Fig. 4.4. The amplitudes of waves III and V are considerably more robust following *bilateral* stimulation versus *unilateral* stimulation because of the bilateral integration of the neural response from both ears at the superior olivary complex, which is the origin of wave III. The origin of each of the seven waves comprising the ABR has been localized to arise from the cochlear nerve and from each brainstem auditory nucleus as described elsewhere.

4.2 ABR Wave V Peak Latency-Intensity Curves

A graphic plot of the various latencies of each of the seven ABR waves as a function of the stimulus intensity, especially for wave V, is routinely used to evaluate the extent of hearing loss and the characteristics of this hearing loss (Fig. 4.5b).

4.2.1 ABRs from Normal Hearing Subjects

The ABR latency-intensity curves of waves I, II, III, IV, V, VI, and VII, evoked at various stimulus intensity levels, are presented in Fig. 4.5 and illustrate the various waveform changes at these different stimulus intensity levels. For audiological use, the latency-intensity curve of wave V is routinely plotted because the lowest

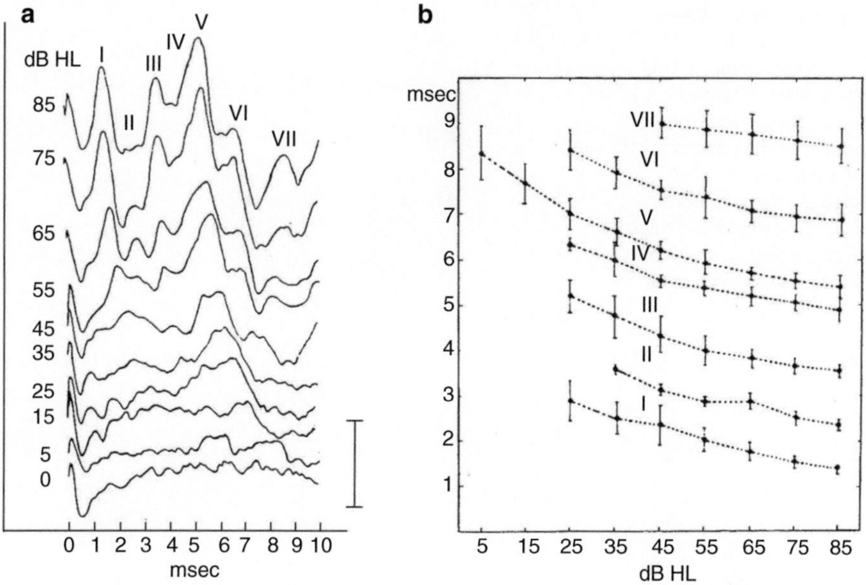

Fig. 4.5 Waveform changes of all of the ABR evoked waves at decreasing stimulus intensities (**a**) from a normal hearing subject. (**b**) illustrates the intensity-latency curves derived from each of these waves. Each black dot (in b.) is the peak latency of each wave at each of the different stimulus intensity levels and the bars indicate ± one standard deviation from the normal distribution

stimulus intensity level evoking a wave V, and its' latency, is closely related to the pure tone audiogram of the individual being tested. In other words, the ABR can be used as an objective evaluation of hearing loss.

In Fig. 4.6, the shadowed area represents the latency-intensity function (mean ± one standard deviation) of wave V from twenty normal hearing adults. In this population, there is a gradual increase in latency of wave V with decreasing stimulus intensity. The ABR wave V responses from a normal hearing subject are superimposed on this normal range (O indicates the right ear and X indicates the left) and are shown as an example.

4.3 Peripheral Hearing Loss

The concept of designing latency-intensity curves derived from the ABR was initially described by Hecox and Galambos (1974) [2]. In normal hearing subjects, the range of the individual variation of wave V peak latency-intensity curves is narrow and it has an upward concave configuration. This normal range of the wave V peak latency-intensity curve provides the basis for evaluating changes in these curves to determine the presence of a conductive versus a sensory/neural hearing loss.

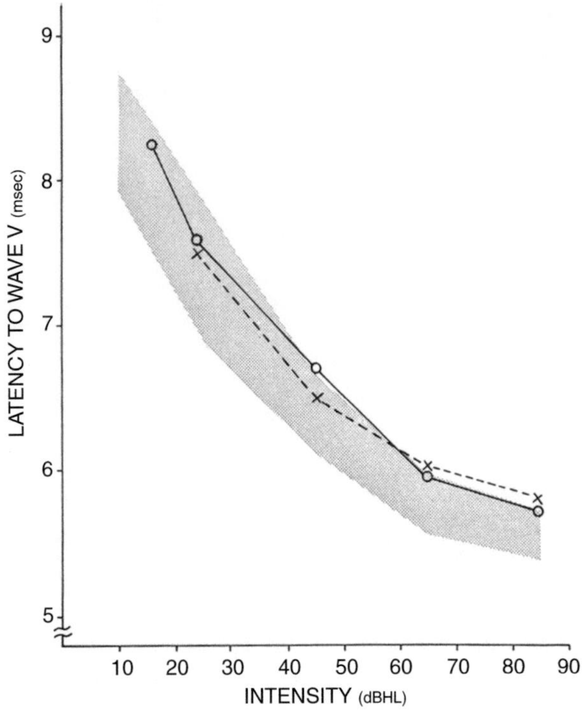

Fig. 4.6 The shadowed area indicates the distribution (mean ± 1SD) of the wave V latency-intensity function from normal hearing adults ($n = 20$). The overlaid tracing is from a normal hearing adult (O indicates right ear responses, X for left ear) and shown as an example

4.3.1 Conductive Hearing Loss as it Effects the ABR

In subjects with a conductive hearing loss, which occurs when the external auditory meatus is occluded or the middle ear is impaired, there is a parallel shift, in latency, of the wave V latency-intensity curve which gives a fair estimate of the degree of the subjects' hearing loss. ABRs show a parallel latency-intensity shift of both waves I and V which have been found to be characteristic of a conductive hearing loss. Figure 4.7 illustrates the ABR and latency-intensity curve of wave V from an infant with a conductive hearing loss as determined by this parallel latency shift of wave V (the shaded area represents the wave V peak latency-intensity range for normal listeners). The latency shift produced by a conductive hearing loss could be misinterpreted as a central abnormality, particularly if wave I is misidentified. A differential diagnosis of a conductive hearing loss versus a sensory/neural hearing loss can be determined by measuring the inter-wave latencies between wave I and wave V. If this interval shows an equal shift, then the hearing loss is probably conductive. If the shift only involves wave V, then the hearing loss is most likely sensory/neural [3].

The wave V peak latency-intensity curves for twelve adult patients are shown in Fig. 4.8. Conductive hearing losses yield wave V latency-intensity curves which closely parallel, visually, normal curves with varying degrees of horizontal displacement to the right [4].

Infants and children with bilateral congenital atresia of the ear suffer from bilateral conductive hearing loss. Therefore, it is very important for infants and children

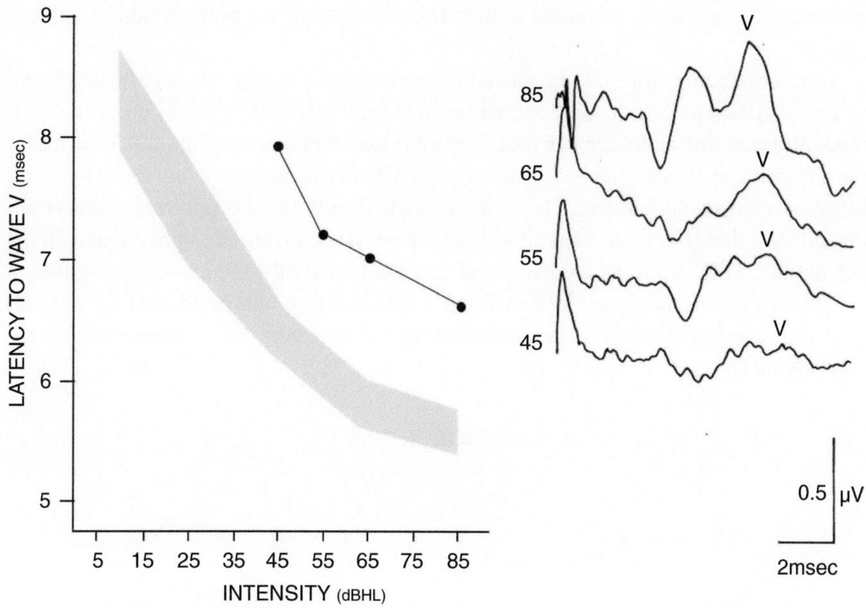

Fig. 4.7 ABR and latency-intensity curves of wave V from an infant with a conductive hearing loss as indicated by the parallel shifts of wave V latencies (shaded area is the distribution of the wave V peak latency-intensity curves from normal listeners)

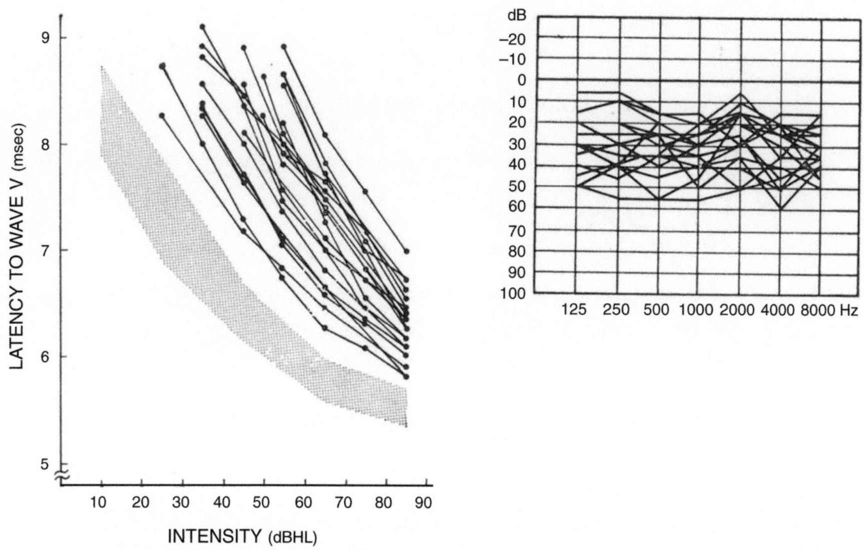

Fig. 4.8 ABR wave V peak latency-intensity curves from twenty patients with a conductive hearing loss (the shaded area is the wave V peak latency-intensity curve from normal listeners)

with such atresia to be provided with sufficient hearing via bone conduction hearing aids.

Bone conduction stimulators, placed on the mastoid process, can also be employed to obtain ABRs as well as air conduction stimulators (headphones) in order to determine air-bone threshold gaps as found by pure tone audiometry. Figure 4.9 illustrates the air conducted versus the bone conducted ABRs of a neonate at 2 months of age with bilateral microtia and atresia. The air-bone ABR threshold gaps (air versus bone conducted) at 2 months of age were 55 dB (65 minus 10 dB) from the right ear and 70 dB (85 minus 15 dB) from the left ear, consistent with bilateral conductive hearing loss.

This young female patient was fitted with a bone conduction hearing aid and later she acquired normal speech and hearing and was enrolled in a normal elementary school [5].

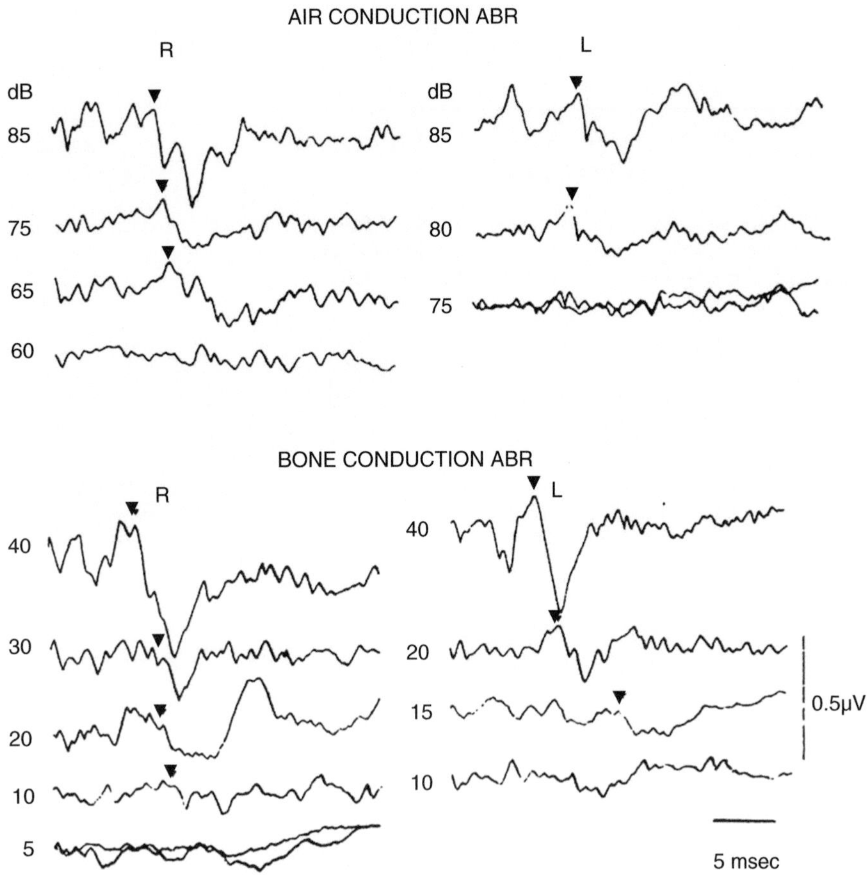

Fig. 4.9 A comparison of the air-conducted ABR (65dBHL stimulus intensity in the right ear and 80dbHL in the left at threshold) versus the bone-conducted ABR (10dBHL stimulus in the right ear and 15dBHL in the left at threshold) in a 2-month-old neonate with bilateral congenital aural atresia. The air-bone threshold gaps of these ABRs are 45 dB for both ears, consistent with bilateral conductive hearing loss

4.3.2 Sensorineural Hearing Loss as Manifest by the ABR

A sensory/neural hearing loss occurs when the hair cells within the cochlea or the cochlear nerve are damaged. The latency-intensity curve of wave V from patients with mild or moderate sensory/neural hearing loss differs from that of conductive hearing loss because of the phenomenon of recruitment which is common in a sensory/neural hearing loss [4]. Recruitment, which occurs at the level of hair cell loss in the cochlea, is an abnormal increase in the perception of loudness as the intensity of the sound stimulus increases.

In Meniere's disease, as in presbycusis, loud click stimulation evokes an ABR which shows an entirely normal waveform configuration, with normal peak latencies of each wave, as the intensity level of the stimulus is decreased. However, the peak latency of wave V remarkably increases near the threshold of the response.

Eventually, the slope of the latency-intensity function of wave V increases sharply approaching the threshold of this response. This has been referred to as the ABRs' recruitment phenomenon due to the abnormal growth of perceived loudness [3]. Yamada et al. demonstrated this ABR recruitment phenomenon in patients with Meniere disease (Fig. 4.10) [4] and Yokokoji and Kaga also demonstrated this phenomenon in 85% of patients with presbycusis (Fig. 4.11) [6]. Parallel

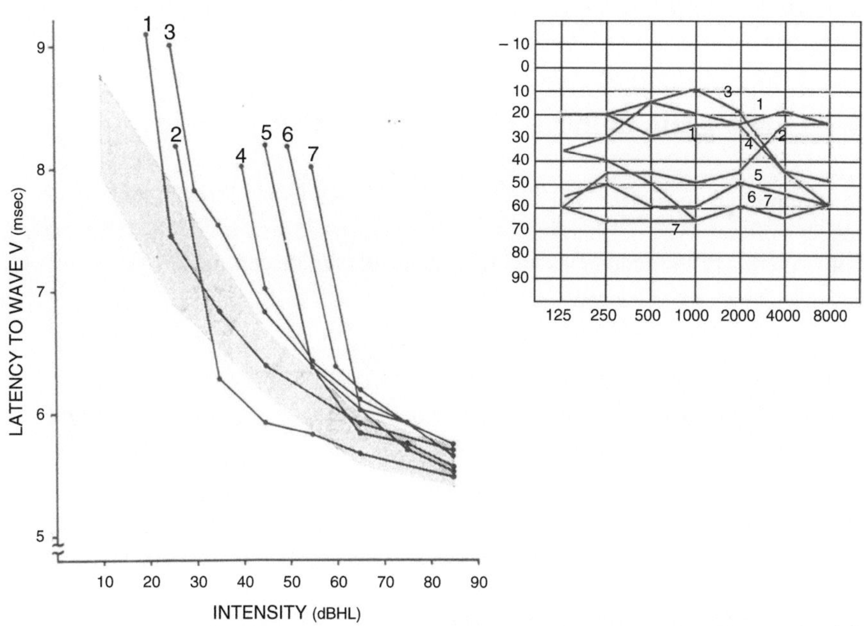

Fig. 4.10 In patients with Meniere's disease, the plotted ABR wave V latency-intensity curves reveal this loudness recruitment phenomenon in that the wave V latencies evoked by loud click stimulus intensities are usually within normal limits whereas the wave V latencies evoked by low click stimulus intensities at near threshold are significantly delayed relative to the normal hearing population

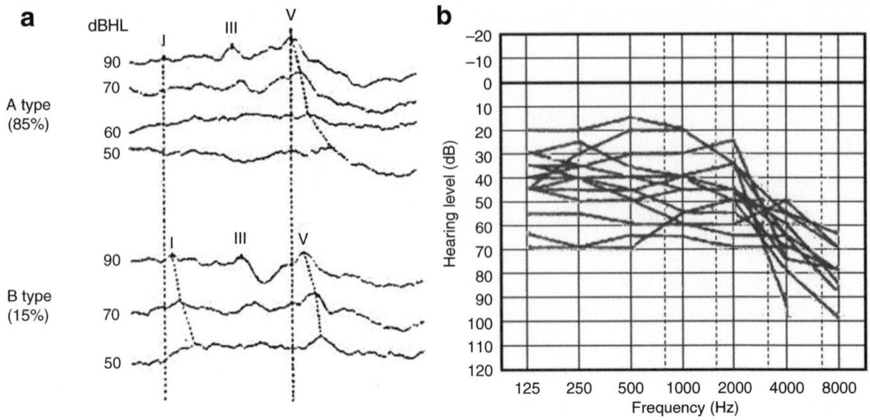

Fig. 4.11 In presbycusis, 85% of such patients (A type), who have a moderate sensory normal hearing loss, produce a wave V latency-intensity curve (**a**) which illustrates this loudness recruitment phenomenon. The wave V latencies at a loud click intensity are normal, yet 15% of these patients (B type) show a parallel shift of wave V latencies at any lower intensity (**b**)

latency-intensity shifts of the ABR latencies, as seen in patients with conductive hearing losses, do not occur with increasing levels of click stimulation in patients with a sensory/neural hearing loss.

4.4 Audiogram Patterns Compared to ABR Findings

It is important to realize that different audiometric patterns (audiograms) which reflect different types of hearing loss, can be mirrored in the various ABR waves, both in terms of their latencies and their thresholds of discernment.

4.4.1 ABR Findings of Patients with a Low-Frequency Hearing Loss but with Normal High-Frequency Hearing

In patients with this type of audiometric hearing loss, click evoked ABRs are apt to show normal wave configurations and wave V thresholds of detection throughout the stimulus intensity range. Figure 4.12 illustrates a patients' low-frequency audiometric pattern (a.) but with normal ABR wave latencies and detection thresholds as low as 20dBHL from both ears (b. and c.).

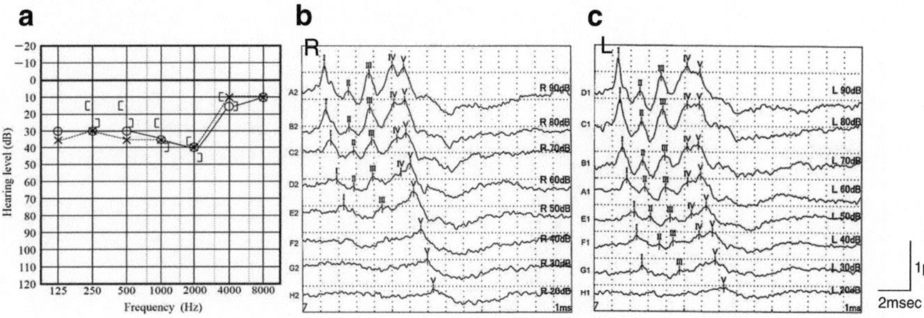

Fig. 4.12 ABR recordings (**b**. and **c**.) from a patient presenting with a low-frequency audiometric hearing loss (**a**.)

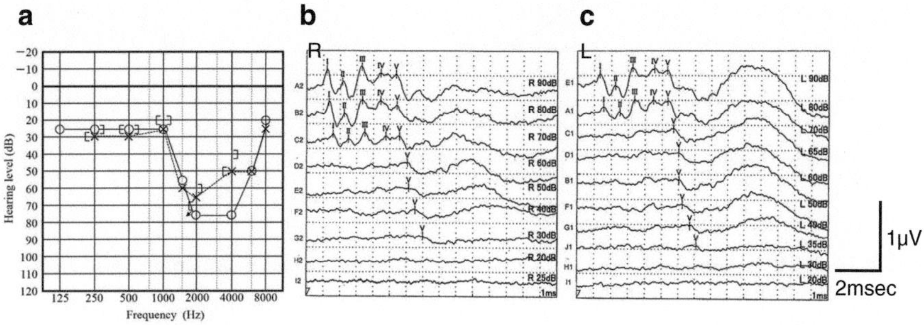

Fig. 4.13 A concave audiometric frequency loss pattern (**a**.) and the ABR recordings from each ear of the same patient (**b**. and **c**.)

4.4.2 ABR Recordings from Each Ear of a Patient with a Typical Noise-Induced Hearing Loss (an Audiometric Concave Frequency Loss Pattern)

In patients with such audiograms, click evoked ABRs are apt to show a normal wave configuration with a slight increase in the threshold of detection of wave V. Figure 4.13 shows a concave frequency loss pattern in this patients' audiogram (a.) but normal ABR wave configurations (b. and c.) to loud click stimuli and a slight elevation of wave V detection at 30dBHL. Also, the threshold of the detection of waves I through IV is considerably elevated at stimulus intensities below 70dBHL, relative to normal hearing patients.

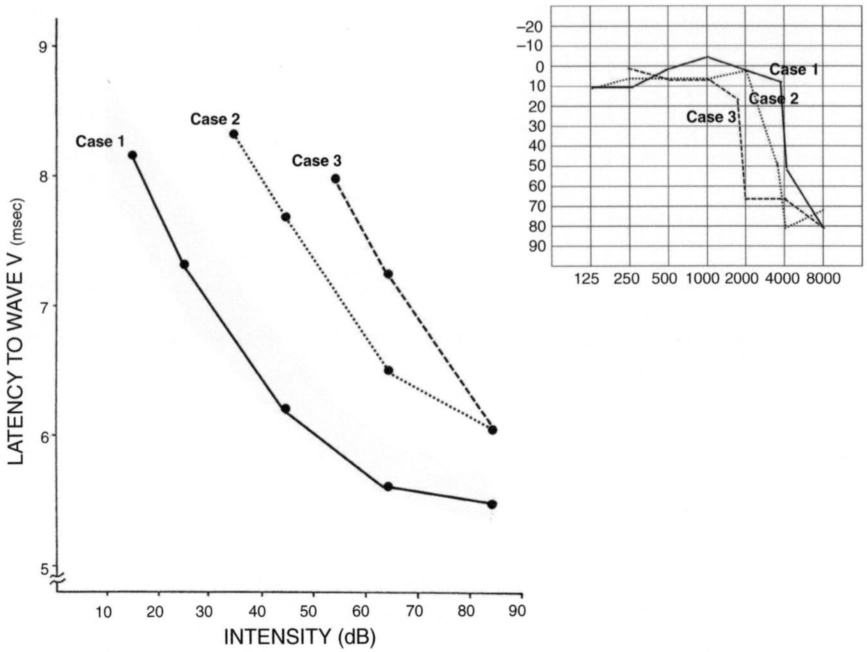

Fig. 4.14 ABR latency-intensity curves recorded from three patients presenting with varying degrees of sudden onset high-frequency hearing loss

4.5 ABR Recordings from Patients with High-Frequency Hearing Loss with Otherwise Normal Hearing Thresholds, Audiometrically, at the Low and Middle Frequencies

In patients with such audiograms, the wave V detection threshold is elevated relative to the extent of high-frequency hearing loss. However, exceptional cases do exist. Figure 4.14 illustrates the audiograms of three patients with varying degrees of high-frequency hearing loss and the effect of this hearing loss on the ABR wave V latency-intensity curve from each patient. Case 1 presented a normal wave V latency-intensity curve whereas the wave V curves of Case 2 and Case 3 were significantly delayed, and the detection level of Wave V was elevated both as a function of the degree and frequency of the audiometrically determined sensory/neural hearing loss.

4.6 Unusual ABR Findings

The entire acquired ABR wave configuration should be carefully examined due to the possibility of unusual variations in the appearance of each evoked wave and its latencies. An example of this is the case presented below.

4.6.1 *A "Bump" in the ABR Appearing within the Expected Latency Range of Wave I (~ 1 Msec) with no Subsequently Evoked ABR Waves*

There are exceptional ABRs that are characterized by the absence of wave I through wave V but yet reveal a small "bump" within the expected latency range of wave I (~1 msec) but with normal DPOAEs (Distortion Product Oto-Acoustic Emissions) from both ears. The DPOAE is a test of the integrity of the inner ear outer hair cells. This "bump" on the ABR is thought to be the summating potential (SP), which triggers the auditory nerve compound action potential (N1), and which "bump" is frequently observed in patients with auditory neuropathy who present with normal DPOAEs, i.e., their outer hair cells are intact. Electrophysiologically, the SP is usually recorded, as a separate evaluation (electrocochleography or ECoG), by means of an electrode placed on or near the tympanic membrane and using the same click stimuli and computer averaging technique as with the ABR but recorded over a shorter time span. Auditory neuropathy electrophysiological findings are characterized by the evocation of clear SPs but with no evoked compound action potentials (N1) and no subsequent ABR waves (Fig. 4.15). The interpretation of this is that auditory neuropathy is a pathology which involves the neural substrate of the auditory system but does not affect the outer hair cells within the cochlea [7, 8].

4.6.2 *Unusual ABR Findings Wherein Only Wave I or Waves I and II Are Evoked*

There are some specific neurological disorders in children in which only the ABR wave I or waves I and II can be evoked and waves III through V are absent, but yet these children can hear well. Chapter 8 lists and discusses these disorders.

4.6.3 *The Influence of Incomplete Brainstem Maturation in Preterm Infants and the Progression of Their ABRs with Development*

In preterm infants, their ABRs show overall prolonged latencies and elevation of wave V thresholds because of their incomplete brainstem maturation. If only the elevated threshold of the ABR wave V threshold is considered, then a preterm

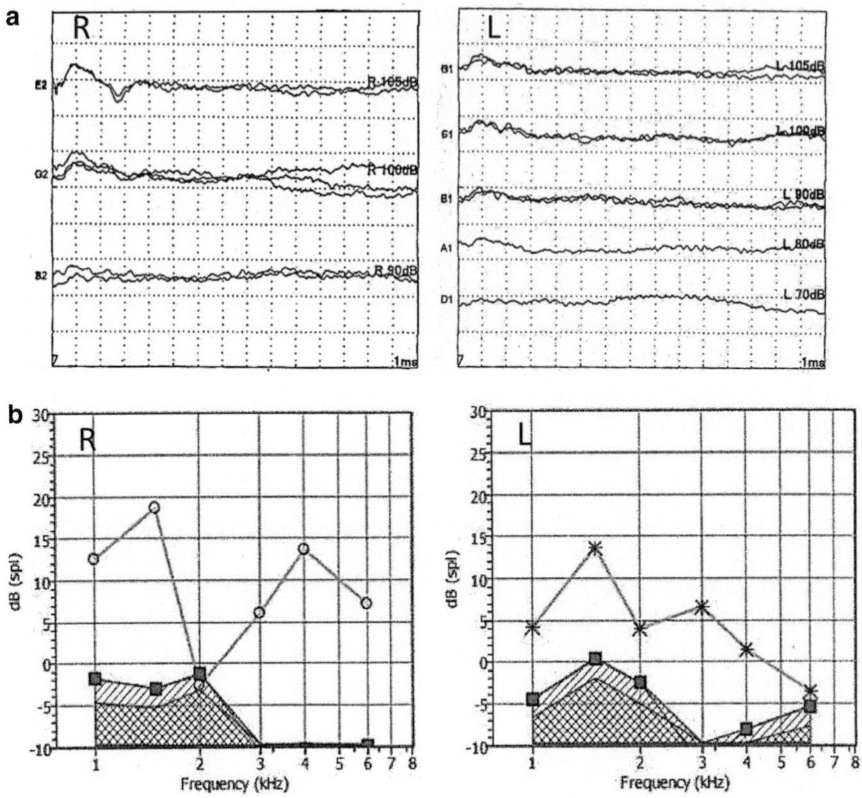

Fig. 4.15 Unusual ABR and DPOAE findings in a three-year-old patient with auditory neuropathy (**a**) ABRs; absence of waves I through V at a stimulus level of 90dBHL but with a small "bump" within the latency range of wave I, Rt and Lt ears. (**b**) DPOAEs; there are good responses from both ears. These are inconsistent findings indicating that each cochlea is functional, but the neural auditory substrate is not

hearing loss is suspect. However, the influence of incomplete brainstem maturation should be considered as a possible differential diagnosis rather than as a peripheral hearing loss.

Figure 4.16 shows the developmental changes of the ABRs from a preterm child taken over a developmental time span of twelve months. The ABRs only fell into the normal at this child's age of twelve months. This phenomenon has been called "normalization" of the ABR [4].

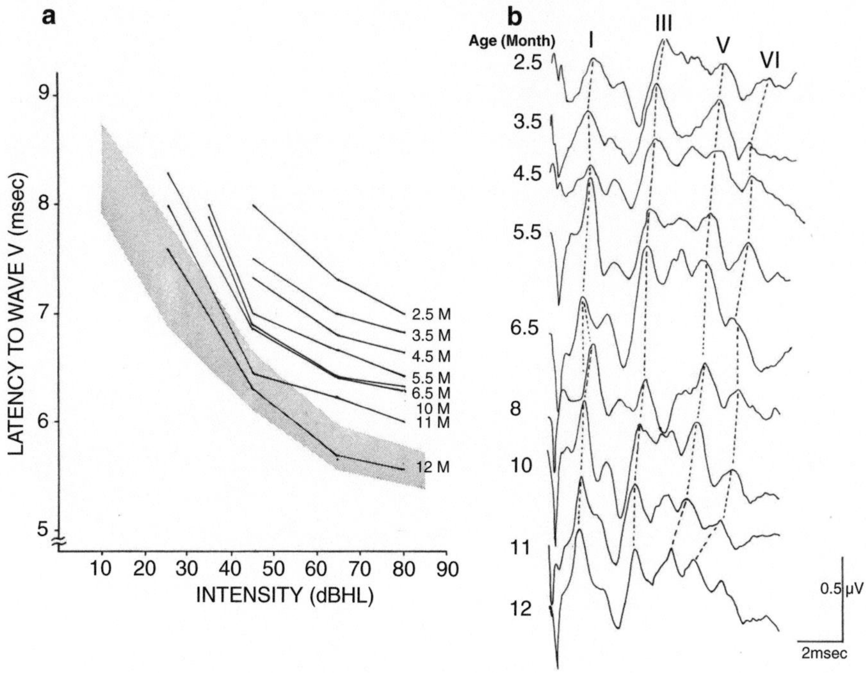

Fig. 4.16 Developmental changes of the ABR over 12 months from a preterm baby at 2.5 months. (**a**) developmental changes of ABR wave V latency-intensity curves from 2.5 months to 12 months, (**b**) developmental changes of ABR waves from 2.5 months to 12 months

References

1. Kaga K, Tanaka Y. Auditory brainstem response and behavioral audiometry. Developmental correlates. Arch Otolaryngol. 1980;106:564–8.
2. Hecox K, Galambos R. Brainstem auditory evoked responses in human infants. Arch Otolaryngol. 1974;99:30–3.
3. Donohoe CD. Application of the brainstem auditory evoked response in clinical neurologic practice. In: Owen JH, Donohoe CD, editors. Clinical atlas of auditory evoked potentials. USA: Grune & Stratton; 1986. p. 29–38.
4. Yamada O, Yagi T, Yamane H, Suzuki J-I. Clinical evaluation of the auditory evoked brainstem response. ANL. 1975;2:97–105.
5. Kaga K, Tanaka Y. Auditory air and bone conduction brainstem responses and damped rotation test for young children with bilateral congenital atresia of the ears. Int J Ped ORL. 1995;32:13–21.
6. Yokokoji M, Kaga K. ABRs loudness recruitment in the elderly over seventies with presbycusis. Audiol Jpn. 1994;37:475–6.
7. Kaga K, Nakamura M, Shinogami M, et al. Auditory nerve disease of both ears revealed by auditory brainstem response, electrocochleography and otoacoustic emissions. Scand Audiol. 1996;25:233–8.
8. Kaga K. Auditory nerve disease and auditory neuropathy spectrum disorders. ANL. 2016;43:10–20.

Chapter 5
Auditory Neuropathy Spectrum Disorders

Kimitaka Kaga

Abstract In 1996, a new type of bilateral hearing disorder was discovered, and its characteristics and etiology were published almost simultaneously by Kaga et al. and Starr et al. Although the pathophysiology of this disorder as reported by each author was essentially the same, Kaga described it as "auditory nerve disease" and Starr used the term "auditory neuropathy (AN)."

In 2008, a comprehensive study of hearing in newborn infants by the Colorado Children's Hospital group prompted the use of ANSD (auditory neuropathy spectrum disorder) as the proper and more inclusive term to delineate this pathology and this term has been broadly accepted later.

The major basis for the use of this term (ANSD) was the finding that in certain cases during neonate screening, ABRs could not be evoked but DPOAEs could be clearly recorded. In 2016, our group at the National Tokyo Medical Center further classified ANSD into three types on the basis of finding changes in the ABRs and DPOAEs of these infants as they developed into adulthood. In Type I, there is normalization of hearing over time. Type II is a development of profound hearing loss over time. Type III is true auditory neuropathy always with the presence DPOAE and absence of ABR. ANSD in newborns, infants, and children manifests differently in AN compared to in adults.

Keywords Auditory neuropathy spectrum disorders · DPOAE · ABR · *OTOF* · Hearing aid · Cochlear implant

---

K. Kaga (✉)
National Institute of Sensory Organs, National Hospital Organization, Tokyo Medical Center, Audiology Clinic, Kamio Memorial Hospital, Tokyo, Japan
e-mail: kimitaka.kaga@kankakuki.jp

© Springer Japan KK, part of Springer Nature 2022

K. Kaga (ed.), *ABRs and Electrically Evoked ABRs in Children*, Modern Otology and Neurotology, https://doi.org/10.1007/978-4-431-54189-9_5

5.1 The First Report of Auditory Nerve Disease and Auditory Neuropathy in 1996

In 1996, a new type of bilateral sensory/neural hearing disorder was discovered and published almost simultaneously by Kaga et al. [1] and Starr et al. [2]. Although the pathophysiology of this disorder as reported by each author was essentially identical, Kaga used the term “auditory nerve disease” and Starr used the term “auditory neuropathy (AN).”

5.2 Auditory Neuropathy Spectrum Disorders (ANSD) in Newborns

ANSD is a new classification that was proposed by the Colorado Children’s Hospital Group in 2008. This newborn infant hearing disorder is characterized by normal DPOAEs but absent ABRs [3]. The term ANSD is derived from “autism spectrum disorder.”

Hearing screening of newborns by automated ABR (AABR) have been the norm in many countries since Itano’s paper in 1998 describing its use and value [4]. When AABRs are found to be absent in these newborns then DPOAEs are administrated as a second step. If DPAOEs are present with no evocable AABRs then these newborns are suspected of having ANSD [5]. In 2016, our group at the National Tokyo Medical Center in Japan, classified ANSD into three types (Table 5.1) [6]. However, we reiterate that AN in teens and adults does not manifest the same as ANSD in newborns, infants, and children because of normal speech and hearing.

Table 5.1 Classification of subtypes of ANSD by the National Tokyo Medical Center since 2016

Type I: Developmental changes to normalization of hearing	
I-a	Normalization from absent ABR
I-b	Normalization from waves I and II of ABR
Type II: Developmental changes of hearing to profound hearing loss	
	Later disappearance of DPOAE and change to profound hearing loss
	Cochlear implantation candidate
Type III: Congenital auditory neuropathy	
III-a	True auditory neuropathy
	Poor auditory perception. Cochlear implantation candidate
III-b	True auditory neuropathy
	Poor auditory perception. Hearing aids are indicated
III-c	Pseudo auditory neuropathy
	No indication of hearing aid and cochlear implant because of normal speech and hearing after development and growth

5.3 Our Classification of ANSD in Newborns, Infants, and Children

Our recent classification of typical cases of ANSD in infants and children is based on our post 2016 follow-up studies (Table 5.1).

- Type I: Developmental changes of the ABR leading to normalization of hearing.
- We can determine two subtypes:
  - Type I-a. At birth, DPOAEs are normal but ABRs are completely absent. Over time, DPOAEs remain normal but the ABR begins to appear and ultimately shows a normal wave configuration. These patients are eventually able to acquire normal speech and hearing (Fig. 5.1).
  - Type I-b. At birth, DPOAEs are normal but ABRs show only waves I and II. In this subtype, the ABR, over time, evolves to a normal wave configuration (which includes wave V) and patients can ultimately acquire normal speech and hearing (Fig. 5.2).
- Type II: Developmental changes of DPOAEs leading to profound hearing loss.
- As newborns, DPOAEs are normal but ABRs are completely absent. However, as infants develop, the DPOAE disappears, and these patients manifest profound

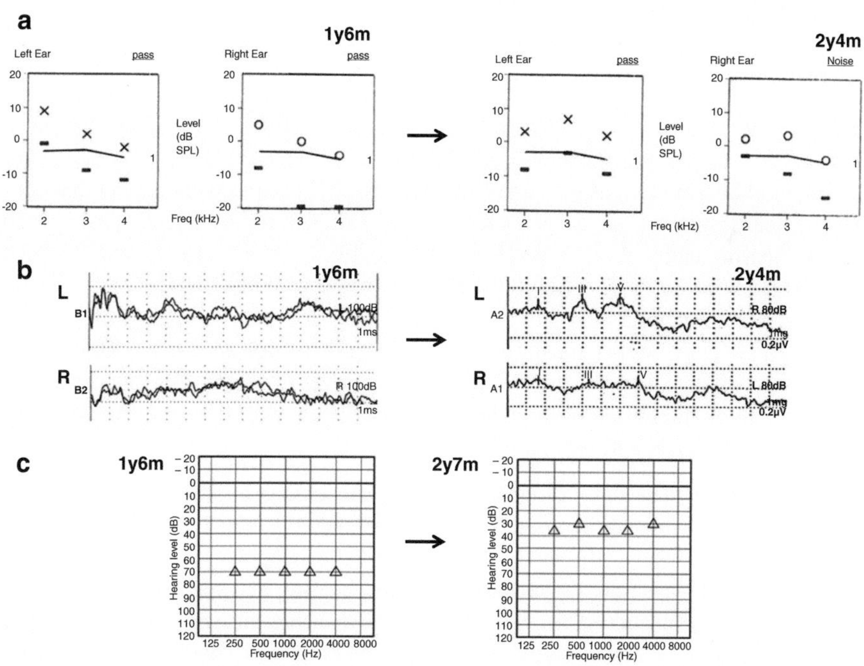

Fig. 5.1 Type I-a. Normalization of absent ABRs in a 700-g birth weight female. (**a**) DPOAE, (**b**) ABR, (**c**) VRA (visually reinforcement audiometry)

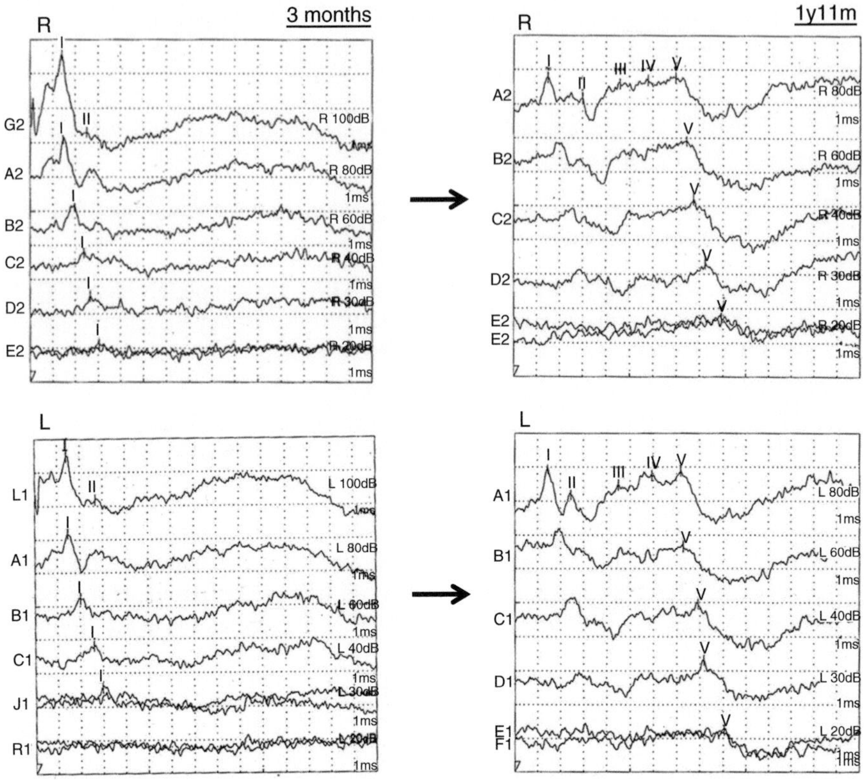

Fig. 5.2 Type I-b. Normalization of only waves I and II of the ABR in a 600-g birth weight male

bilateral hearing loss as they age (Fig. 5.3). Type II cases are good candidates for cochlear implantation. Early cochlear implantation is highly effective for speech and hearing acquisition. Type II may be thought of as a transient ANSD which changes because of a congenital severe sensory/neural hearing loss.

- Type III: Congenital AN
- In Type III, newborns have normal DPOAEs and no evocable ABRs. This profile does not change with the infants' development over time (true AN) and its occurrence rate is the lowest of the three types. However, within Type III there seems to exist a true AN and pseudo AN.
  - Type III-a (true AN). Good candidate for cochlear implantation because of poor ability to acquire speech and hearing even when aided.
  - Type III-b (true AN). Good candidate for hearing aid but not for cochlear implant because of good ability to acquire hearing and speech.
  - Type III-c (pseudo AN). No indication of hearing aid and cochlear implant because of a better ability to acquire hearing and speech naturally with development.

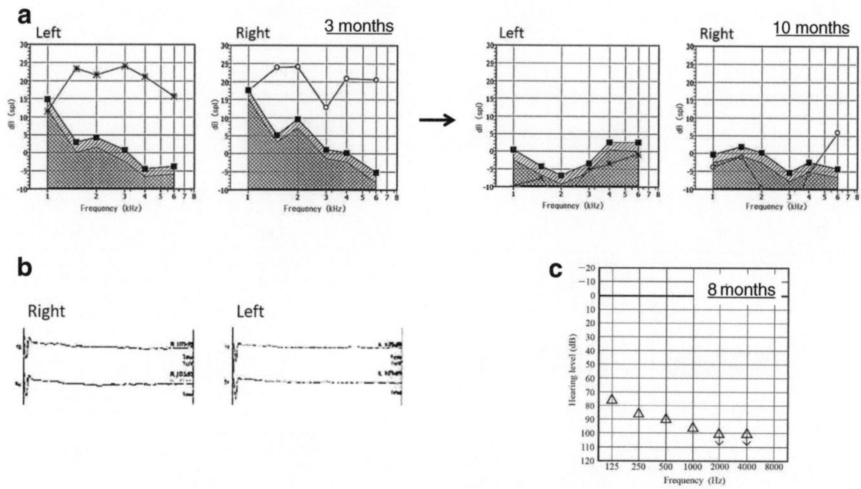

Fig. 5.3 Type II. Developmental change to profound hearing loss from ANSD. DPOAEs disappear with development (A well baby). (**a**) DPOAE, (**b**) ABR, (**c**) VRA

5.4 ANSD for Type III and Cochlear Implantation

Figure 5.4 shows a typical case of Type III-a. This type is a true congenital AN. This boy's speech and hearing did not develop even when aided prior to 1 year of age. He underwent a cochlear implantation at 3 years of age and he was then educated in an auditory oral school for the deaf. Twelve years after cochlear implantation he is now able to speak very well and his auditory speech perception test results are very good. Now he is being educated at an auditory oral high school for the deaf. Figure 5.5 shows a Type III-b. A 13-year-old Chinese girl was diagnosed as having congenital AN on the basis of *OTOF* gene mutation analysis. She manifests a mild sensory/neural hearing loss with a 50% maximum monosyllable speech discrimination rate, normal DPOAEs beyond ambient noise levels, only summating potentials (SPs) evoked during ECoG and absent ABRs bilaterally to clicks presented at 100 dBnHL. She was able to effectively communicate with others by speech reading owing to her mild hearing loss. Moreover, bilateral hearing aids helped her to communicate. Figure 5.6 shows a Type III-c (pseudo AN). In this type, children are able to hear and speak well naturally as they develop although their ABRs are persistently absent in the presence of normal DPOAEs. Most of these neonates are born with extremely low body weight, between 400 and 800 g. Cochlear implantation is contraindicated in Type III-c because as these children develop they can hear and speak well with improvement of their behavioral audiometry (VRA) thresholds although their DPOAEs and ABRs do not change over time.

ANSD cases should be carefully followed up by frequent evaluation of DPOAEs and ABRs to determine developmental changes. Therefore, the age of cochlear

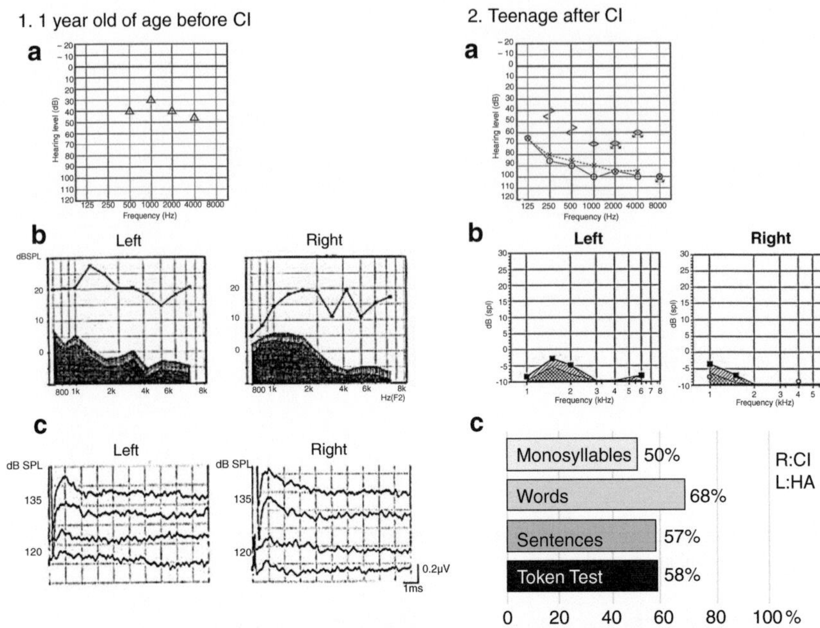

Fig. 5.4 Type III-a. Congenital AN with speech and hearing problems. Audiological findings of pre and post cochlear implantation in a (1) Preoperative: at 1 year, (**a**) VRA, (**b**) DPOAE, (**c**) ABR; (2) postoperative: teenage, (**a**) pure tone audiometry, (**b**) DPOAE, (**c**) perception of speech

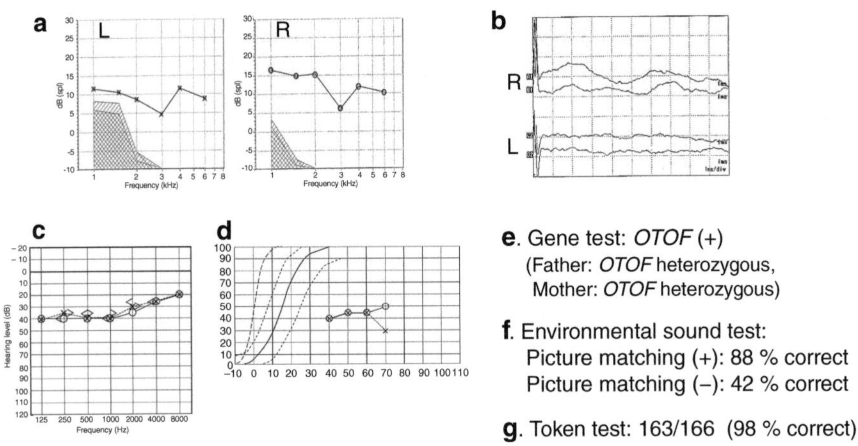

Fig. 5.5 Type III-b. True AN. Audiological findings of a junior high school female student. Hearing aids are indicated for both ears. (**a**) DPOAE, (**b**) ABR, (**c**) pure tone audiometry, (**d**) speech audiometry, (**e**) gene test, (**f**) environmental sound test, (**g**) Token test

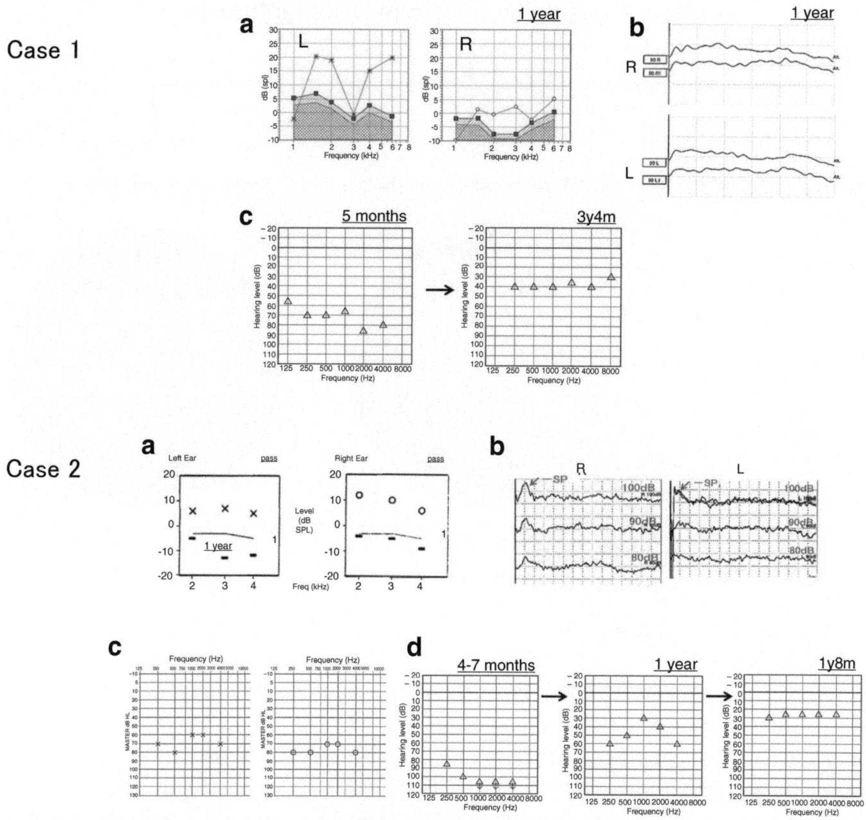

Fig. 5.6 Type III-c. Pseudo AN. Two cases. Case 1. Male. (**a**) DPOAE, (**b**) ABR, (**c**) VRA. Case 2. Female. (**a**) DPOAE, (**b**) ABR, (**c**) ASSR, and (**d**) VRA

implantation should be delayed until the age of 1 year, at least. It is important to follow the auditory and speech developmental changes in these patients.

5.5 Genetic Mutation

Matsunaga et al. [7] discerned the genes underlying deafness in Japanese infants who presented with ANSD. They found a high incidence of mutation in the *OTOF* gene and suggested that there may be a mixture of congenital deafness and true AN (Fig. 5.7). Hopefully, our classification of the subtypes of ANSD may shed light on this issue.

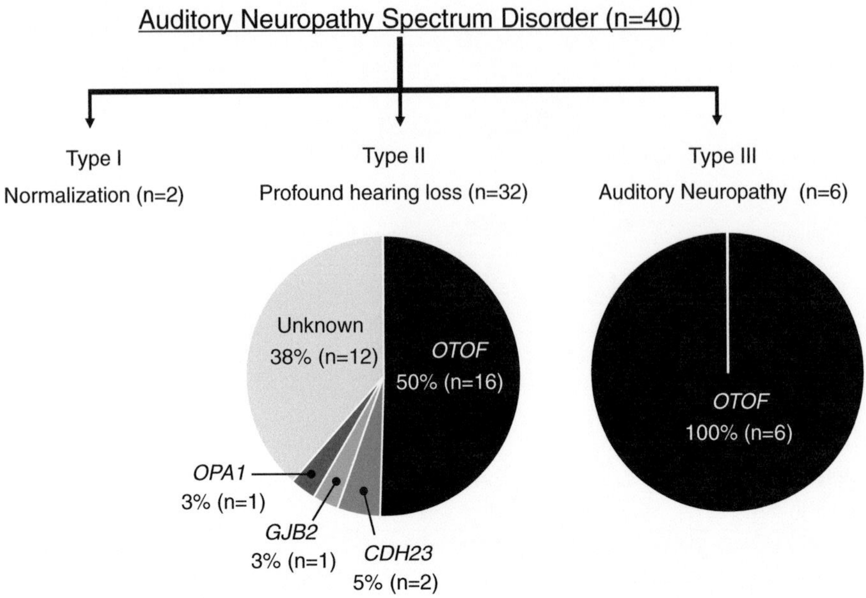

Fig. 5.7 Genetic mutation in Japan

We emphasize that ANSD infants should be carefully followed as they age and repeatedly examined by DPOAEs, ABRs, and VRA before considering a cochlear implant. Pediatric cochlear implantation, in the presence of profound hearing loss (Type II) and true congenital AN (Type III-a and III-b), very effectively aids in the development of speech and hearing [8–10]. Type I-a, Type I-b, and Type III-c are not good candidates for cochlear implantation because these children can develop good speech and hearing naturally over time. Type III-b cases are good candidates for hearing aids. In infants with detectable ANSD, one should very carefully serially monitor DPOAEs, ABRs, and VRA and look for the possible development of relatively normal speech and hearing. In Fig. 5.7, the types of gene mutations found in ANSD are illustrated graphically and indicate a high incidence of the *OTOF* gene mutation in Types II and III.

5.6 Adults AN and Newborns ANSD

ANSD in newborns is not the same as AN in adults. Various hypotheses of the pathophysiology of AN have been proposed: presynaptic or postsynaptic disorders of synapses between inner hair cells and the cochlear nerve; desynchronization within the cochlear nerve; demyelination or axonal atrophy of the cochlear nerve. Genetic mutations in AN involving *OTOF*, *OPA1*, and other genes have been reported [11, 12]. However, there is the possibility of unknown mutations because the reported gene mutations are not commonly detected.

Cochlear implantation in adult AN patients and in infants with ANSD, who progress into profound hearing loss or do not progress with development (true congenital AN) is very effective in the reacquisition of good speech and hearing. The essential pathophysiology of AN can be either pre- or postsynaptic and involve pathology between the inner ear hair cells and the cochlear nerve.

References

1. Kaga K, Nakamura M, Shinogami M, Tsuzuku T, Yamada K, Shindo M. Auditory nerve disease of both ears revealed by auditory brainstem response, electrocochleography and otoacousitc emissions. Scand Audiol. 1996;25:233–8.
2. Starr A, Picton TW, Sininger Y, Hood LJ, Berlin CI. Auditory neuropathy. Brain. 1996;119:741–53.
3. Northern J. Guidelines for identification and management of infants and young children with auditory neuropathy spectrum disorders. Aurora: The Children's Hospital Colorado; 2008.
4. Yoshinaga-Itano C, Sedey AN, Coulter DK, Mehl AL. Language of early- and later-identified children with hearing loss. Pediatrics. 1998;102:1161–71.
5. Berlin CI, Hood LJ, Morlet T, Wilensky D, Li L, Mattingly KR, Taylor-Jeanfrequ J, Keats BJB, John PS, Montgomery E, Shallop JK, Russell AB, Frisch SA. Multi-site diagnosis and management of 260 patients with auditory neuropathy/dis-synchrony (auditory neuropathy spectrum disorder). Int J Audiol. 2010;49:30–43.
6. Kaga K. Auditory nerve disease and auditory neuropathy spectrum disorders. Auris Nasus Larynx. 2016;43:10–20.
7. Matsunaga T, Mutai H, Kunishima S, Namba K, Morimoto N, Shinjo Y, Arimoto Y, Katoaka T, Shintani T, Morita N, Sugiuchi T, Masuda S, Nakano A, Taiji T, Kaga K. A prevalent founder mutation and genotype-phenotype VRA relations of OTOF in Japanese patients with auditory neuropathy. Clin Genet. 2012;82(5):425–32.
8. Miyamoto RT, Kirk KL, Renshaw J, Hussain D. Cochlear implantation in auditory neuropathy. Laryngoscope. 1999;109:181–5.
9. Busse E, Labadie RF, Brown CJ, Gross AJ, Grose JH, Pillsbury HC. Outcome of cochlear implantation in pediatric auditory neuropathy. Otol Neurotol. 2002;23:328–32.
10. Madden C, Hilbert L, Rutter M, Greinwald J, Choo D. Pediatric cochlear implantation in auditory neuropathy. Otol Neurotol. 2002;23(2):163–8.
11. Iwasa Y, Nishio SY, Yoshimura H, Kanda Y, Kumakawa K, Abe S, Naito Y, Nagai K, Usami S. OTOF mutation screening in Japanese severe to profound recessive hearing loss patients. BMC Med Genet. 2013;14:95.
12. Santarelli R, Rossi R, Scimemi P, Cama E, Valentino ML, Morgia C, Caporali L, Liguori R, Magnavita V, Monteleone A, Biscaro A, Arslan E, Carelli V. OPA1-related auditory neuropathy: site of lesion and outcome of cochlear implantation. Brain. 2015;138:563–76.

Chapter 6
Normalization and Deterioration of Auditory Brainstem Response (ABR) in Child Neurology

Makiko Kaga

Abstract The ABR can be recorded safely and repeatedly over time without pain and harm to the subjects being tested. Also, the origin of each of the seven ABR waves has been defined as the traverses along the auditory pathway. Since the clinical introduction of ABR, it has been an essential tool in the evaluation of children with high risk of hearing impairment and in those with possible or confirmed brainstem lesions. Normalization and deterioration of this ABR are known to occur but it can be only confirmed by the evaluation and comparison of successive ABRs. In this chapter, examples of normalization and deterioration of the ABR will be demonstrated and the usefulness and importance of ABR in neonatology, general pediatrics, and child neurology will be explained. Various cases of this phenomenon are presented along with their clinical evaluation.

Keywords Auditory brainstem response (ABR) · Child neurology · Neonatology Pediatrics · Normalization · Deterioration · Development · Serial recording

6.1 Normalization and Deterioration of ABR in Children

The ABR discovered by Jewett et al. and Sohmer et al. in 1970 [1, 2] is the recording of the neurophysiological response of the inner ear and its brainstem neural substrate to an auditory stimulus. A detailed description of this response is presented

M. Kaga (✉)
Tokyo Metropolitan Tobu Medical Center for Children with Developmental Disabilities, Tokyo, Japan

© Springer Japan KK, part of Springer Nature 2022

K. Kaga (ed.), *ABRs and Electrically Evoked ABRs in Children*, Modern Otology and Neurotology, https://doi.org/10.1007/978-4-431-54189-9_6

elsewhere in this text. Recordings of the ABR have been widely used clinically in the fields of child neurology, neonatology, and pediatrics since its clinical introduction.

In the clinical situation, the value of the ABR in these various fields lies in:

1. The ability to obtain objective audiometry to evaluate hearing threshold, especially of the high frequencies.
2. The availability of a tool to evaluate the severity of brainstem pathology.
3. A way to evaluate the growth and development of the auditory brainstem pathway.

The above three values and aims are very important objectives in child and neonatal neurology. In most clinical situations, the auditory stimuli which are employed to obtain ABR recordings are clicks and tone bursts/pips.

6.1.1 What Constitutes the Difference Between Normal and Abnormal ABR?

A normal ABR consists of the following elements:

1. The presence of normal wave configurations of waves I, II, III, IV, V, VI, and VII, especially I, III, and V, when provoked at a high-intensity stimulus level.
2. Each wave latency and their interpeak latencies are within the normal ranges compared with the healthy age matched controls (average ± 2 standard deviations (S.D.).
3. A normal threshold of wave V as a function of decreased stimulus intensity. In the clinical situation, wave V responds thresholds as low as 20 or 30 dB HL are usually considered to be normal. Thus, any ABR recording which does not fit into any one of the above criteria is considered, by definition, to be abnormal.

Standard configuration induced by click stimuli and its frequency change of stimuli, and a variety of configurations of ABR to high frequency and high sound pressure level stimuli are illustrated in the Figs. 6.1 and 6.2.

In infants and children, wave shape matures and interwave latency shortened. Acceleration of decrease in the later component of ABR (wave V) is clear. Shortening of the interwave latency are far marked in waves III and V than the earlier components of ABR (waves I and II). Developmental change in ABR reflects this finding (Fig. 6.3). ABR change depends on age by another researcher is also illustrated (Fig. 6.4).

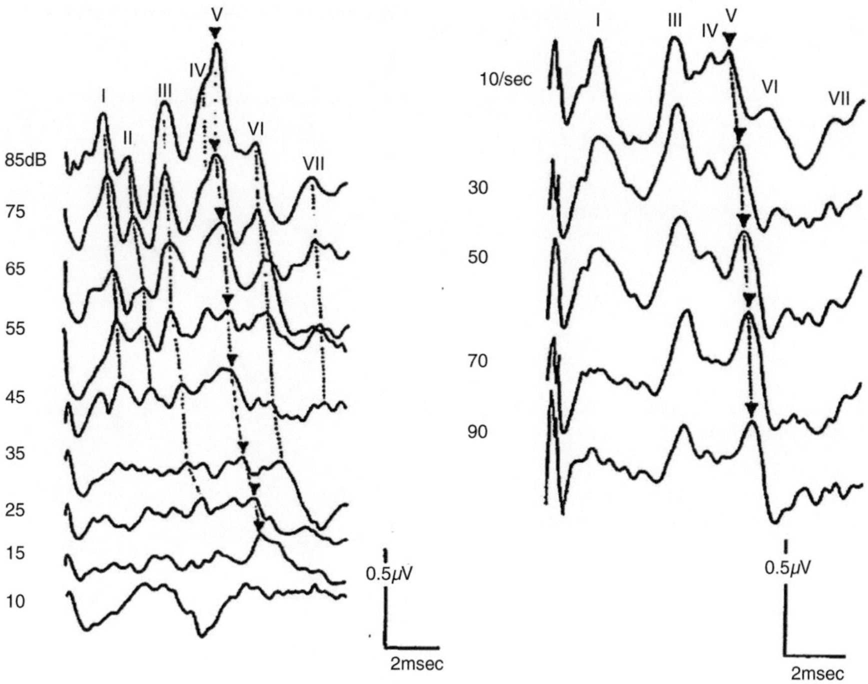

Fig. 6.1 Normal ABR. High-intensity click stimuli induce typical wave forms (waves I, II, III, IV, V, VI, and VII). Lowering the stimulus intensity, each wave latency is prolonged by lowering the wave amplitude. The lowest stimulus intensity which induces clear wave V is almost the hearing threshold of high-frequency stimuli (the left side). Frequency (10–90 s^{-1}) change of click stimuli changes each wave latency. High-frequency stimuli make prolonged latency of each wave (right side). In clinical situation, 10–20 s^{-1} frequency is used [3]

6.1.2 What Causes the Normalization and Deterioration of the ABR?

The normalization of the ABR occurs as a function of:

1. The overall development of the child.
2. Improvement in the child's hearing.
3. Recovery from organic or a functionally beneficial change of brainstem lesions.

The deterioration of the ABR is brought about by the early progression of hearing loss and aggravation of the auditory brainstem pathways. Of note, examinations of ABR recordings from childhood up to 20 years old, deterioration as a function of aging was not detected.

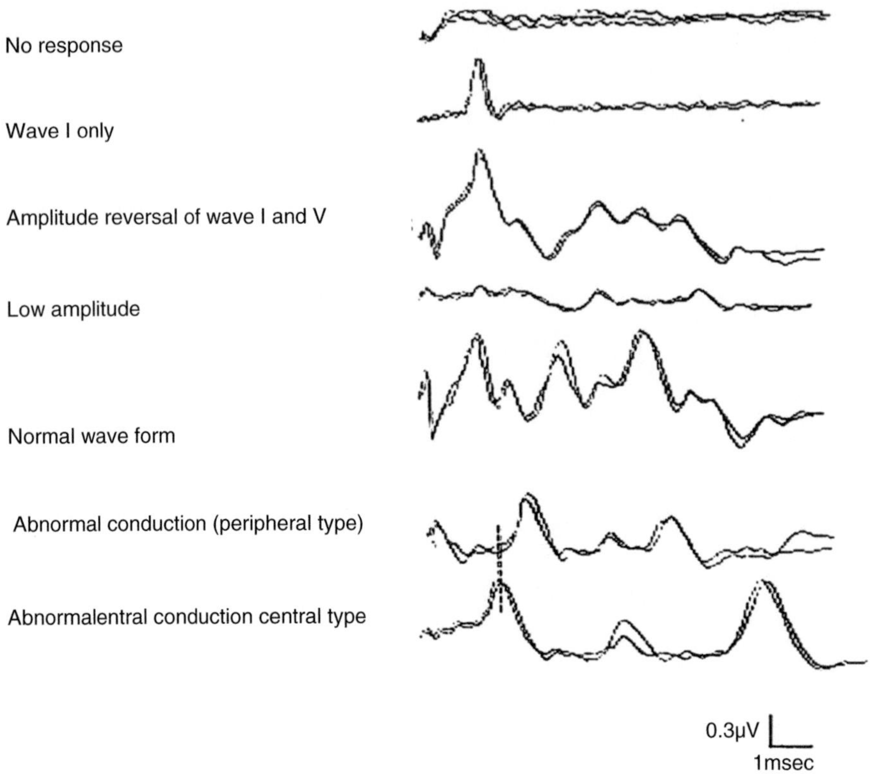

Fig. 6.2 Variety of configuration of ABR to high frequency and high sound pressure level stimuli. No response means hearing loss to high-intensity sounds or severe brainstem damage for any reason. Wave I only means severe pathology within the auditory pathway after auditory nerve. Amplitude reversal of waves I and V means nothing or anything. Usually, amplitude of wave V is higher than wave I, but it is not always. Low amplitude ABR suggests a highly elevated threshold of hearing level or overall brainstem pathology. Abnormal conduction means delayed interpeak latencies of each wave. Delayed wave I latency and preserved interpeak latency following wave I suggest conductive hearing loss as a principle

Among diseases known to induce premature aging (progeria) such as Hutchinson Gilford syndrome, Werner syndrome, and Cockayne syndrome, serial deterioration of the ABR in Cockayne syndrome could be detected only in Iwasaki et al.'s paper [6] possibly as a sequela of the progression of sensorineural hearing loss and possibly due to underlying brainstem pathology.

Worthington et al. in 1980 [7] and Kraus et al. in 1984 [8] both noted and reported their findings of a discrepancy between their patients' normal hearing in the presence of abnormal ABRs. This finding was noteworthy in that it led to the discovery of auditory neuropathy. However, these early studies did not evaluate nor consider the phenomenon of improvement (normalization) of the ABR as a natural course of development. Kaga et al. in 1993 [27] noted unexpected ABR normalization in some children with various possible neuropathology. On the

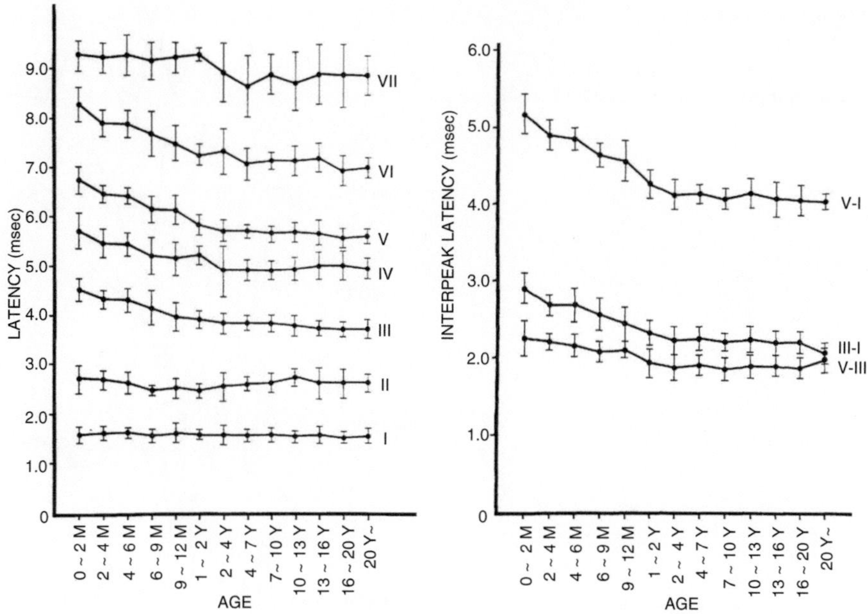

Fig. 6.3 Development of latency and interpeak latency of ABR. Acceleration of decrease in later component of ABR (waves III–V) compared with relatively stable interpeak latency in the earlier component of ABR (waves I and II). Decreased interwave latency reflects the above finding. $n = 202$ [4]

other hand, a deterioration of the ABR in a child should be considered as a medical emergency. The intent of this chapter is to further explain these phenomena, normalization and deterioration, and describe how they relate to various neuropathology in children and to provide an objective diagnostic basis as to refer the patient to a child neurologist.

6.2 Normalization

6.2.1 Normal Development of the ABR

Early on, when ABR recordings became available to the pediatric profession, a number of physicians began testing infants in NICUs (Neonatal Intensive Care Units) and reporting their findings in the literature [9, 10] (Fig. 6.4). Normative data from infants and children were published by Kaga in the early stage [11] (Fig. 6.5).

During the fetal developmental period, the Organ of Corti is known to physically mature by the 20th week of gestation, this is based on pathological studies of aborted fetuses. By the 30th week of gestation, primitive fetal hearing is thought to be attained.

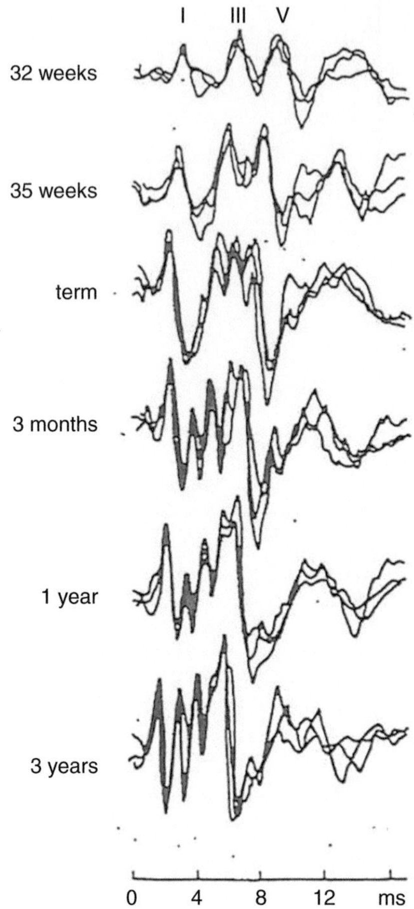

Fig. 6.4 Examples of ABR waveforms in infants from 32 weeks gestation to 3 years old [5]

The time line of the intrauterine development of human hearing has been vigorously investigated by a number of physicians/researchers. A common technique is to attempt observation by abdominal ultrasound, a blink-startle reaction of the fetus to a vibroacoustic stimulus applied to the abdomen. Birnholz and Benacerraf [12] reported that he could detect a blink-startle reaction at the 24th week of gestation. Ruben [13], using a similar technique, reported that fetal hearing begins at the 26th week of gestation. Hepper et al. [14] found in 1994 that the fetus initially responded to 500 Hz tones at the 19th week of gestation but then the frequency range eliciting a response gradually increased because of the maturation of the underlying auditory pathway. Fetal ABR recordings can only be obtained from experimental animals. Woods et al. [15] described their study of a pregnant lamb which has a gestation period of around 150 days. They found that prior to the 117th day of gestation an ABR could not be elicited but by the 126th day the ABR had matured to that of a 1-day-old lamb but with delayed peak latencies. Over this 9-day gestation period, the intensity of the stimulus necessary to elicit an ABR decreased as the fetus

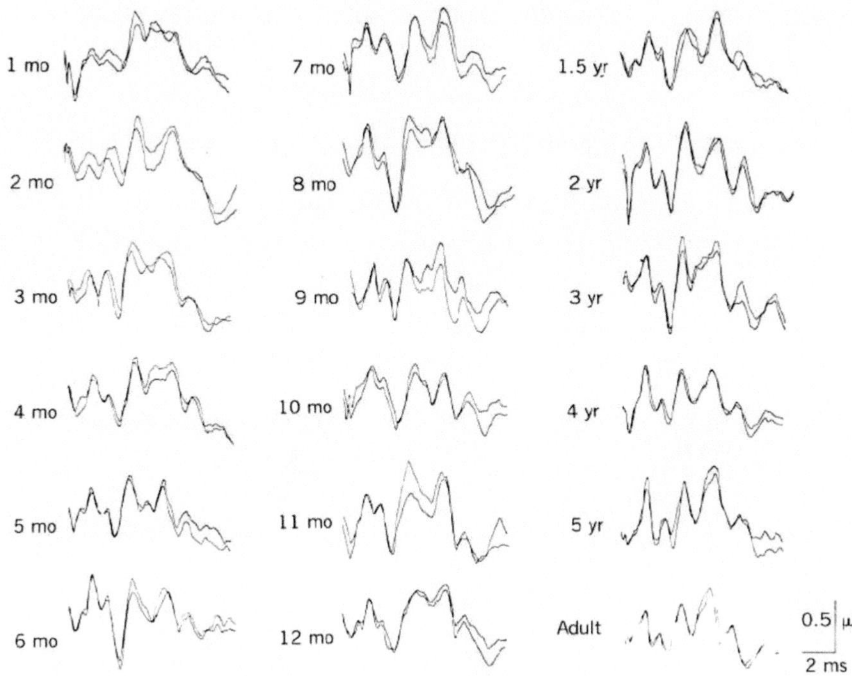

Fig. 6.5 Developmental change of ABR configuration [11]

matured. On this basis, the findings of premature and term infants [16] become more plausible.

In humans, at full term and at birth, the wave I latency of the ABR is almost as short as those of adults. The latter components of the ABR waveform develop and their interpeak latencies also become shortened as a function of overall age development. These latter developing ABR components, specifically wave V, attain the level of adult latencies at about 4–5 years of age. Interpeak latencies also show the same trend. Changes in waveform morphology during development (Fig. 6.5) and their latency and interpeak latency changes [4] are illustrated in the previous section (Fig. 6.3).

6.2.2 *Clinical Appreciation at NICU*

A very exciting article of just two pages in length was published [17] describing changes of serial ABRs during and recovery from neonatal jaundice and exchange transfusion treatment (Fig. 6.6). In fact, apparent ABR improvement could be recorded in a patient with neonatal jaundice. His ABR showed the improvement of waveform latency and threshold quickly from 8 days to 3 months of his age (Fig. 6.7). Wennberg's article literally changed the world of neonatology in that it

AGE (hrs)	TOTAL BILIRUBIN (mg/dl)	ALBUMIN (gm/dl)	AUBC (nmol/l)
24	(13.9)	(3.0)	(15)
27	–	–	–
33 (Pre–XT)	17.7 (15.7)	2.6	89
34	15.8 (14.7)	2.7	72
35.3	–	–	–
36 (Post–XT)	12.0 (13.3)	3.0	30
52	(5.2)	–	–

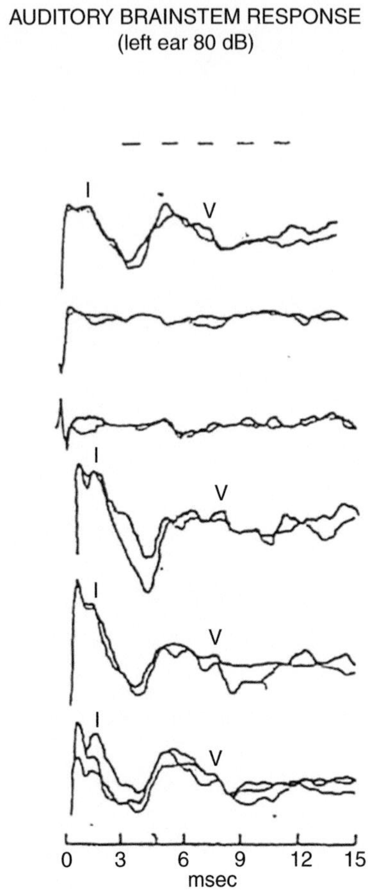

Fig. 6.6 ABR recovery in an infant with neonatal jaundice [17]

resulted in a revolution to include the ABR as a tool in the evaluation of neonates in the NICU. Many neonatologists have recorded ABRs in NICUs and many articles have been published [9, 10, 18]. As a result of these studies, they were able to diagnose a number of deaf suspected babies whose hearing improved, stable, or worsened on follow-up after their NICU experience. These studies led to the development and introduction of the automatic ABR (aABR) to be applied to all infants in the NICU and the graduates of such. This accelerated the use of universal hearing screening (UHS) programs in the NICU using the automated ABR (aABR) as a tool.

In some of these NICU patients an overdiagnosis of hearing impairment became apparent. In a certain percentage of abnormal ABRs found at the first examination and then followed by sequential ABR examinations revealed a recovery of the ABR concurrent with a change in the diagnosis or in the degree of severe impairment [19–22].

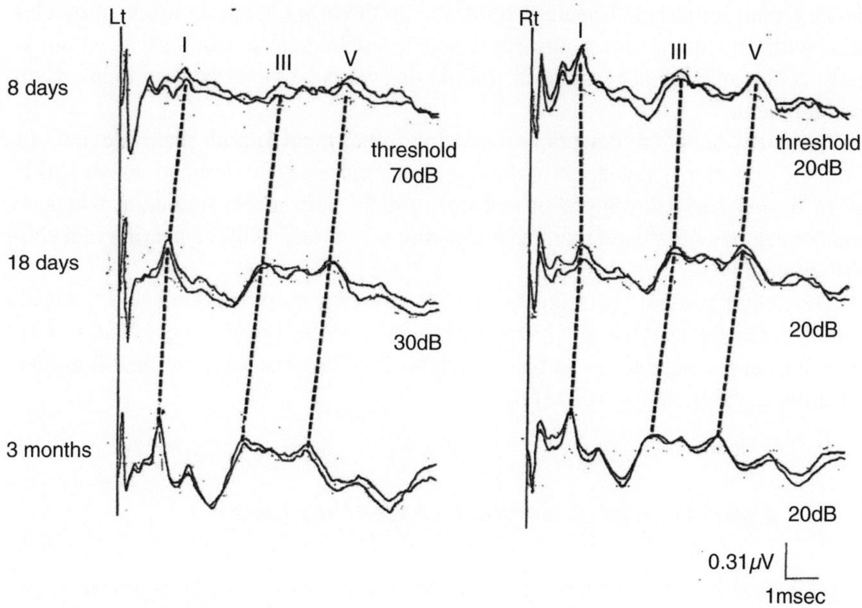

Fig. 6.7 Serial ABRs in a patient with neonatal jaundice. Male, born at 37 weeks gestation with 2450 g of birth weight. Maximum total bilirubin and unbound bilirubin were 24.1 and 1.26 mg/dL, respectively, at 5 days of his age

Specifically, Coenraad et al. noted that the ABRs of 21.2% of their NICU infant population, at high risk of hearing loss, significantly recovered from having no elicitable ABR to presenting a normal ABR over time.

Psarommatis et al. also noted the recovery of previously abnormal ABRs in neonates and infants who had graduated from their Greek NICU. They tested 2248 infants over a 22-year period from 1992 to 2014. Of these infants, 384 showed elevated thresholds of their ABRs on initial testing but 103 of these infants regained a full recovery of their ABRs after 4–6 months. Even amongst 168 of these patients, with an ABR threshold elevation of more than 80 dBsnl, 35 of these patients showed a full recovery of their ABRs and 10 showed a partial recovery. These findings point out the importance of obtaining serial recordings concurrent with a thorough clinical follow-up. This recovery phenomenon of the ABR can be explained by the delayed maturation of the auditory neural substrate. The author is aware of this recovery phenomenon, but more concise evidence is necessitated and further explored.

Recently, Universal Hearing Screening (UHS) is carried out by obtaining automatic ABRs (aABR) or Otoacoustic emissions (OAE). The OAE test is easier to perform in the nursery but it has the possibility of missing hearing impairment due to auditory neuropathy spectrum disorders or auditory nerve disease (Please refer Chap. 5). The early detection of significant hearing impairment has increased the use of early cochlear implantation (CI) with remarkably good results on language development in hearing impaired children. On the other hand, there are some children with autistic spectrum disorders and/or intellectual disabilities in whom an early cochlear implant resulted in limited or even adverse effects on their overall development.

The early, neonatal, detection of hearing impairment is both plausible and crucial. An important consideration is that serial successive examinations should be taken during early development and not hesitate with a reexamination whenever someone, a parent or caretaker, feels something is wrong with the hearing of a child in their care.

The author presents two figures to ABR recovery in two patients with neonatal jaundice. One is the ABR of a historical patient reported by Wennberg et al. in 1992 (Fig. 6.6) and a patient the author experienced whose maximum total and indirect bilirubin levels were recorded (Fig. 6.7).

6.2.3 Improvement of Conductive Hearing Loss

In peripheral hearing impairment, conductive hearing loss, the latencies of wave I and, consequently, the following waves of ABR are all delayed. The interpeak latencies typically remain unchanged. An example of an ABR recording of a conductive hearing loss which shows pre- and post-removal of cerumen during sleep is shown in Fig. 6.8. The shifts of ABR latency can be noted in children who suffer and recover from otitis media, although the ABR is not a part of the protocol in a routine examination of such children! However, to evaluate objective hearing acuity in uncooperative, malingering, or disabled patients, recordings of the ABR can be quite helpful to determine hearing thresholds.

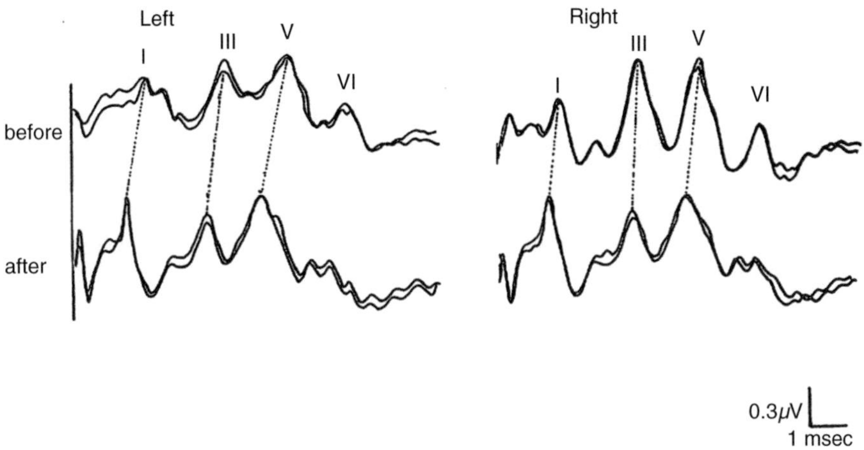

Fig. 6.8 Improvement of the ABR in a patient with conductive hearing impairment. Abnormal ABR suggests conductive hearing loss improved after removal of cerumen [23, 24]

6.2.4 *ABR Changes Pre- and Post-surgical Resection of Tumors on the Brainstem or Cerebellar*

Brainstem tumors, especially pontine gliomas, often result in abnormal ABRs [25, 26]. In this section, the case of a 10-year-old female with cerebellar astrocytoma is presented and discussed. The surgical removal of her tumor revealed that there was no direct invasion of the tumor to the brainstem and her ABR recordings markedly improved post-op.

The underlying cause of this post-op ABR change and, especially the recovery and origin of wave III are discussed.

A female10-year-old visited a children's hospital because of a progression of ataxic gait, dysmetria, discoordination, writing difficulty, and lateral gaze nystagmus predominantly to her right side (right beating).

Her CT scan revealed a cerebellar tumor and a subtotal resection of it was performed. Tumor was dominant in the right side. Thus, neurosurgeon had to resect larger portion of the right cerebellum. During the surgery, the relation with the tumor and brainstem was observed carefully and they found the tumor made no apparent compression to either side of brainstem. As stated, the tumor did not invade nor compress the brainstem. A pathological exam of the tumor confirmed it to be an astrocytoma located midline to both side extensions with right side dominancy. Serial ABRs and CT scan of pre- and post-surgery are presented in the Figs. 6.9 and 6.10.

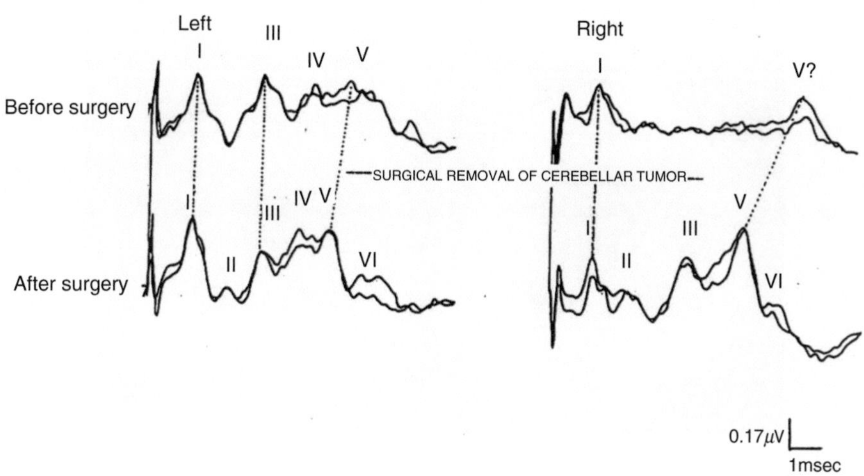

Fig. 6.9 Serial ABR recordings of pre-op (upper) and post-op (lower), elicited by 90 dBnHL clicks. Pre-op, the overall wave configurations from the left side were normal but showed a marked prolongation of waves V and the I–V interpeak latency (IPL). On the right side, only waves I and V were elicited but there was a marked prolongation of wave V. Post-surgery, the left ABR showed marked improvement of the latencies of waves V and VI. Also, the I–V IPL was also improved. On the right side, waves II, III, and IV were elicited and the latency of wave V approached normality as well as the I–V IPL. Wave VI was also elicited and well-formed. This post-op ABR configuration from both ears was considered as normal [27]

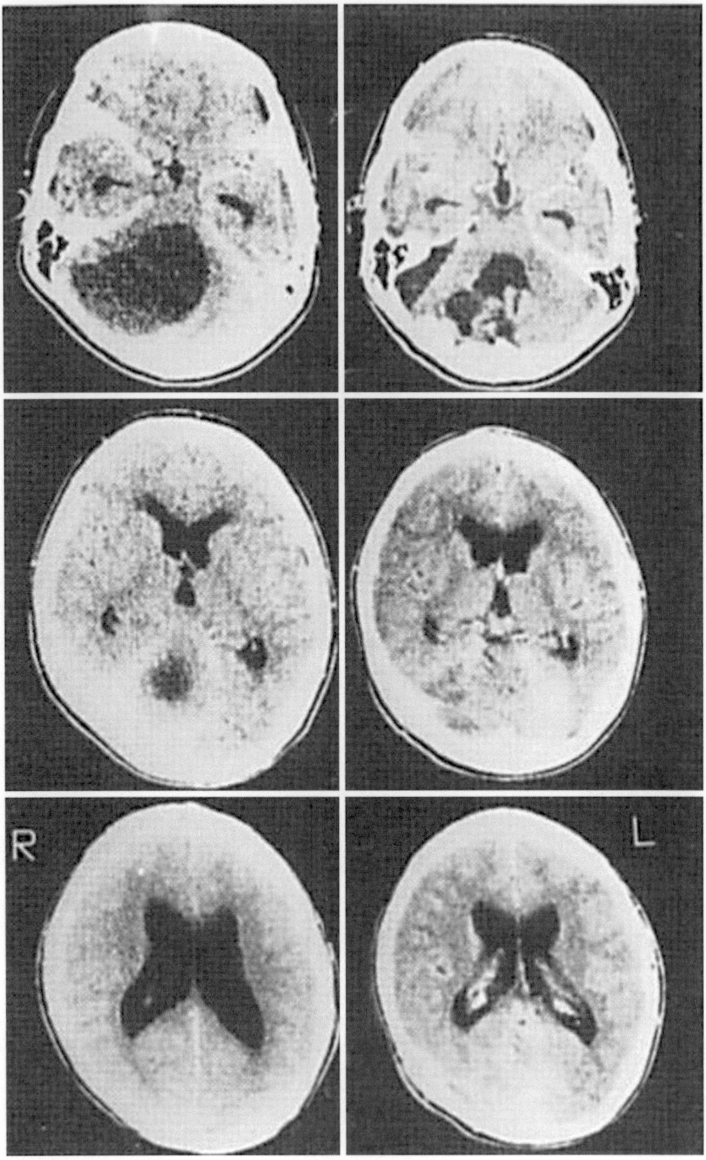

Fig. 6.10 Pre- and 13 days after surgical CT scan. This finding reveals the original tumor showed right side dominancy and wider resection of tumor was necessary in the right hemisphere [27]

Pre-surgical ABR recording (upper case) elicited by 90 dBnHL clicks showed left side ABR was normal in configuration with marked prolongation of wave V and the I–V interpeak latency (IPL). On the right side, only waves I and V were elicited with marked prolongation of wave V. Post-surgical left ABR showed marked shortening of the latencies of waves V and VI. Moreover, interpeak latency of waves I–V was improved. On the right side, waves II, III, and IV were elicited and the latency of wave V approached normality as well as the I–V IPL. Wave VI was also elicited and well formed. This post-op ABR configuration from both ears was considered as normal.

Pre- and post-surgical CT scans revealed the original tumor showed right side dominancy and wider resection of tumor was necessary in the right hemisphere. Based on the neurosurgeons, tumor did not seem to make apparent compression to the brainstem.

Explaining the phenomenon of post-op ABR recovery in this patient is twofold. One possibility is that the mechanical hydro-pressure may have caused a functional suppression of the auditory pathway which was resolved by the surgical removal of the tumor. The other possibility is that the tumor may have caused a bending of the auditory pathway by the tumor which altered the generator source of this far-field ABR potential.

These far-field potentials, the ABR, can be recorded when the evoked nerve impulses pass through the various nuclei (volume conductors) in the brainstem [28] or bend their direction of the nerve conduction of auditory pathway [29].

In this patient, since waves II and III were almost completely absent and appeared after surgery, the route of the brainstem auditory pathway might have been extended. Neither of these possibilities can be confirmed because of the lack of neuroradiological or neuropathological evidence. However, the findings in this patient provide a useful insight into the process and location of the generation of each ABR wave, especially of wave III as well as waves II and IV.

6.2.5 Normalization of the ABR as a Result of Effective Medical Treatment

Özmar reported this normalization following successful treatment of bacterial meningitis [30]. Spankovich also reported this normalization of the ABR following successful treatment of maple syrup urine disease [31]. Some exceptional cases, such as anoxic encephalopathy and various neurological diseases, are illustrated in a later section of this chapter.

6.2.6 Normalization of the ABR of Unknown Etiology

In 1984 Kaga et al. published an article entitled "Normalization of poor auditory brainstem response in infants and children" [32]. She presented nine patients who showed ABR improvement revealed by serial recordings.

The patients had an absent or difficult-to-detect ABR at the first examination but with subsequent normalization or marked improvement of ABR. Repeated otological examinations in some patients were normal in these patients. Four among nine patients had chromosomal aberration including Down syndrome. Other five patients had some neurological signs or symptoms such as delayed development of unknown origin, epilepsy, infantile convulsion, and intellectual disability with history of low birth weight.

Why the ABRs normalized in these patients was not clear and is yet to be fully determined. However, it is speculated but not confirmed that delayed maturation of the auditory pathway may underlie this normalization. This speculation is based on the high incidence in these patients of neurological abnormalities. In patients with major or minor chromosomal aberrations, neuropathological abnormalities occur throughout the brain, including the brainstem, and this has been precisely described in a famous neuropathology textbook [33]. MRI studies in Down's Syndrome also reveal brainstem abnormalities [34–36] but these studies did not obtain serial ABR recordings of supporting the possible sequential favorable ABR changes such as progressive myelination during development or morphological changes in their tissues or organs.

However, these diseases have basically static nature and not deteriorating nature. Thus under those conditions, living creatures can have power of remotely positive development.

6.2.6.1 Case Reports Showing Normalization of the ABR of Unknown Etiology

Serial ABRs of such patients are illustrated in figures with their short clinical summary in the text. Five patients without and nine patients with chromosomal abnormalities (including five patients with Down syndrome) are presented.

Five Patients Without Chromosomal Abnormalities

Patient 1—3-month-old female (Fig. 6.11).

Diagnosis: Delayed development.

This patient did not respond to auditory stimuli and ABR was absent during her neonatal period. Behavioral observation audiometry (BOA), during this early period of her development, revealed bilateral elevated auditory thresholds of more than 90 dBnHL. At 4 months of age her developmental quotient (DQ) was evaluated as 75. Bilateral ABRs were not evoked at high intensity sound stimuli. When she was 12 months old, her DQ increased to 90 and she gradually began to respond to sound stimuli. Her ABR recordings at 12 months of age became discernible with a traditional configuration but there was a bilateral prolonged latency of wave V. At 16 months of age her wave V latencies and thresholds were almost normal with a persistent prolongation of wave I. The short vertical lines in the figure are the average latencies of waves I and V of age matched healthy children. This study was completed prior to the advent of the Otoacoustic Emission test (OAE).

Patient 2—3-month-old female (Fig. 6.12).

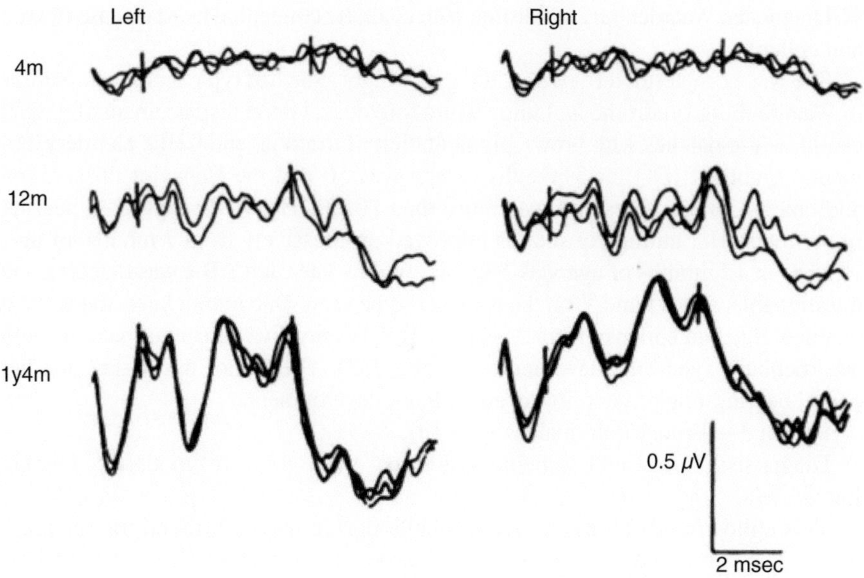

Fig. 6.11 Serial ABR of Patient #1—3 months old female. Delayed development [32]

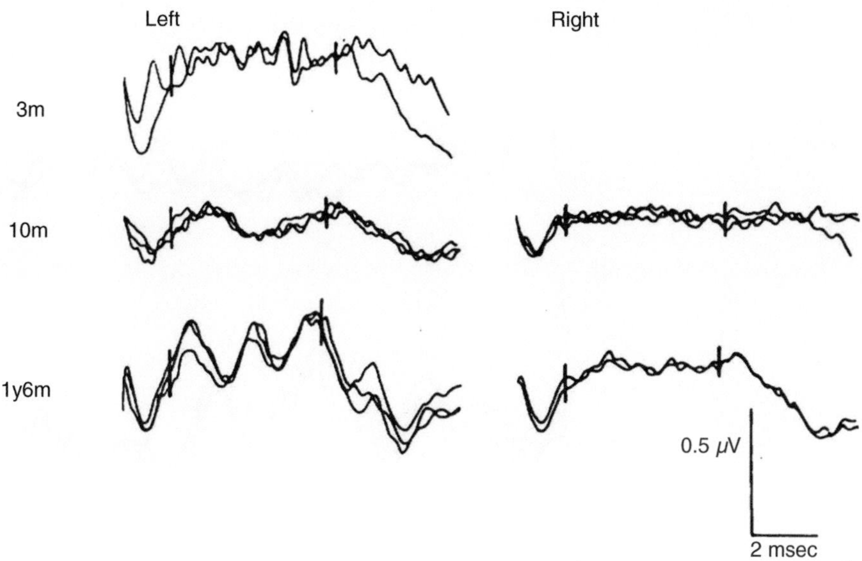

Fig. 6.12 Serial ABR of Patient #2—3 months old female. Waardenburg syndrome with cyanotic congenital heart disease (CHD) and epilepsy [32]

Diagnosis: Waardenburg syndrome with cyanotic congenital heart disease (CHD) and epilepsy.

She was born at full term with 2200 g of weight. She had typical clinical features of Waardenburg syndrome including white forelocks, lateral displacement of medial canthi, white patches with brown pigmentation of the skin, and CHD. Her developmental Quotient (DQ) at 3 months of age was 50 and the Behavior observation audiometry (BOA) threshold was more than 90 dB. Her ABR suggested hearing impairment. Her attitude to sounds improved progressively from 7 months of age. Her DQ at 12 months of age was 100. Six months later, left ABR was detected and questionable waves I and V on the right could be seen. One month later, she walked unaided. She had epilepsy from 2 years of age. Twenty-five percent of patients with Waardenburg syndrome have nerve deafness [38]. The author has to say that her neural hearing impairment improved with her development.

Patient 3—4-month-old male (Fig. 6.13).

Diagnosis: Congenital rubella syndrome with mild to moderate hearing impairment.

This child's mother suffered from rubella during the sixth month of her pregnancy. The child seemed to be hearing impaired at birth. His DQ was 100 and his BOA threshold was greater than 90 dBnHL. His ABR was difficult to elicit.

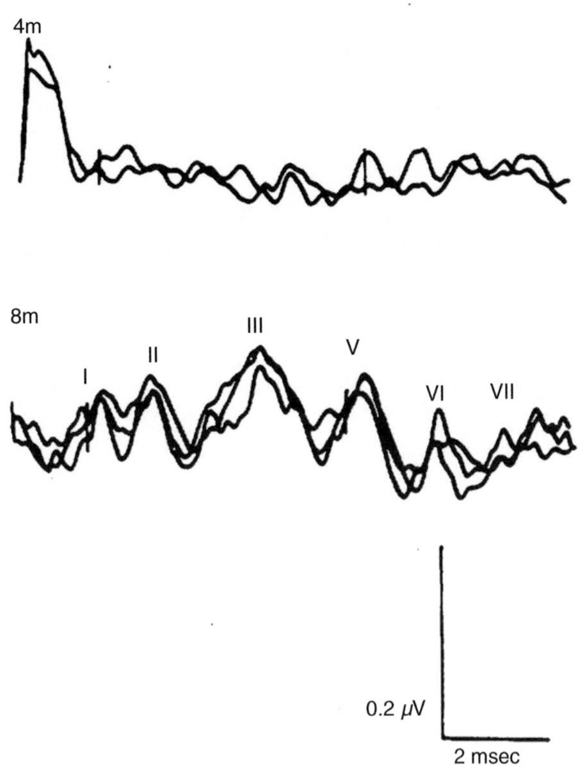

Fig. 6.13 Serial ABR of Patient #3—4 months old male. Congenital rubella syndrome with mild-to-moderate hearing impairment [32]

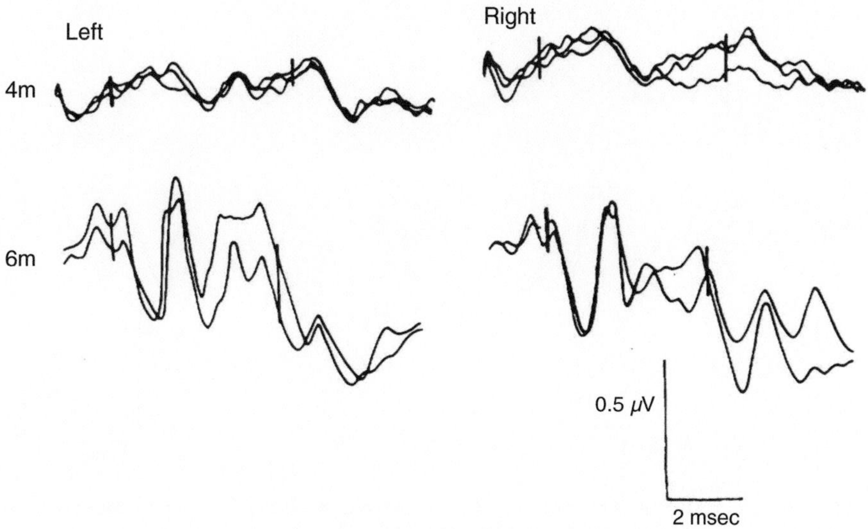

Fig. 6.14 Serial ABR of Patient #4—4 months old female. Infantile convulsion [32]

However, when he was 8 months of age, his ABR was much improved with prolonged latencies of all of the waves. His BOA threshold improved to 75 dBnHL. His development seems to have been normal other than his loss of auditory acuity. Unfortunately, we were not able to follow up with this case.

Patient 4—4-month-old female (Fig. 6.14).

Diagnosis: Infantile convulsion.

This child was born as a full-term healthy baby. Her mother noticed, early on, that her child did not respond to her voice. The child's DQ was 100. Her BOA threshold was 50 dBnHL. The amplitudes of her ABR recordings were quite low. Questionable waves I, III, and V could be discerned from stimulation of her left ear and questionable waves I and V were discerned from her right ear. At 6 months of age, she developed afebrile and generalized tonic-clonic (GTC) seizures, which persisted for only a few minutes. Her EEG was normal and her ABR ultimately attained a traditional configuration with normal wave latencies and thresholds bilaterally.

Patient 5—3-year-old female (Fig. 6.15).

Diagnosis: Intellectual disability with a low birth weight (1200 g) at her gestational age of 28 weeks.

This child suffered neonatal asphyxia. Her head control was attained at 5 months of age. Just prior to 3 years of age, she was able to walk unaided but she had febrile convulsions. Her DQ was 32 and the threshold of her BOA was 65 dBnHL. Low wave ABR amplitudes could be detected bilaterally. Three months after her third birthday, a definite ABR was evoked bilaterally but with prolonged latencies.

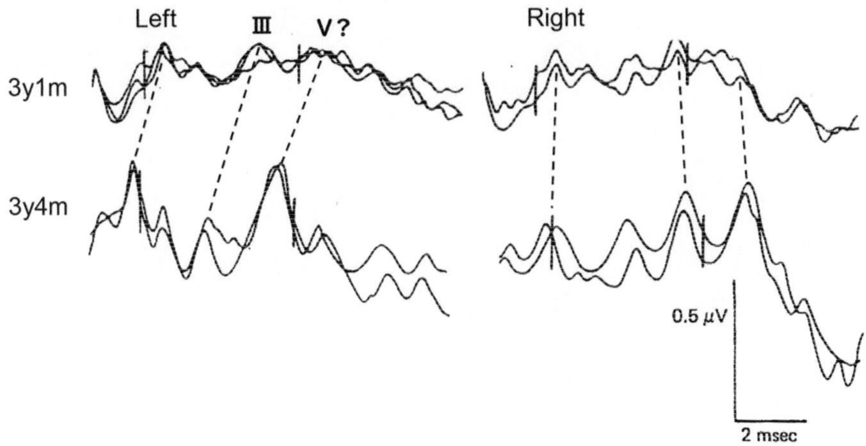

Fig. 6.15 Serial ABR of Patient #5—3 years old female. Intellectual disability with low birth weight (1200 g) at her gestational age of 28 weeks [32]

Nine Patients with Chromosomal Abnormalities Including Down Syndrome and ABR Improvement

Patients with a variety of chromosomal aberrations often suffer marked neurological abnormalities, hearing loss, and abnormal ABRs. Occasionally, and surprisingly, such patients may show a remarkable improvement of their ABR recordings during the course of their development. This normalization phenomenon has just an assumption of the severe neuropathological abnormalities can show slow development of the auditory pathway and later ABR improvement. The textbook by Friede, noted above, exquisitely identified the developmental neuropathology of the auditory organs, the brainstem and midbrain, the cerebellum, and the cerebrum. However, Friede did not discuss the development of these systems as a function of the maturation of the nervous system. Recent developments in molecular genetics and chromosomal analysis have revealed an overwhelming variety of chromosomal aberrations, and the severity of such, which have been associated with a multitude of clinical findings. Year by year, total number of post-mortem examination has decreased. Because most family members of the deceased do not want the body of a loved one caused hurt. Moreover, from medical side, shortage of qualified neuropathologists, technical persons, lack of fiscal resources and respect to time consuming secure work by general population, and public administration. High-resolution imaging has been introduced to clinical and post-mortem examination. However, it is yet deficient to fully recognize the anatomical and microscopic image. Thus, anatomical and neuroimaging measures cannot be explained the neurophysiological improvement demonstrated by ABR change. The exact reason underlying this normalization has as yet to be fully explained. These patients often had severe to profound neurological symptoms with a poor prognosis. Neither technique can explain

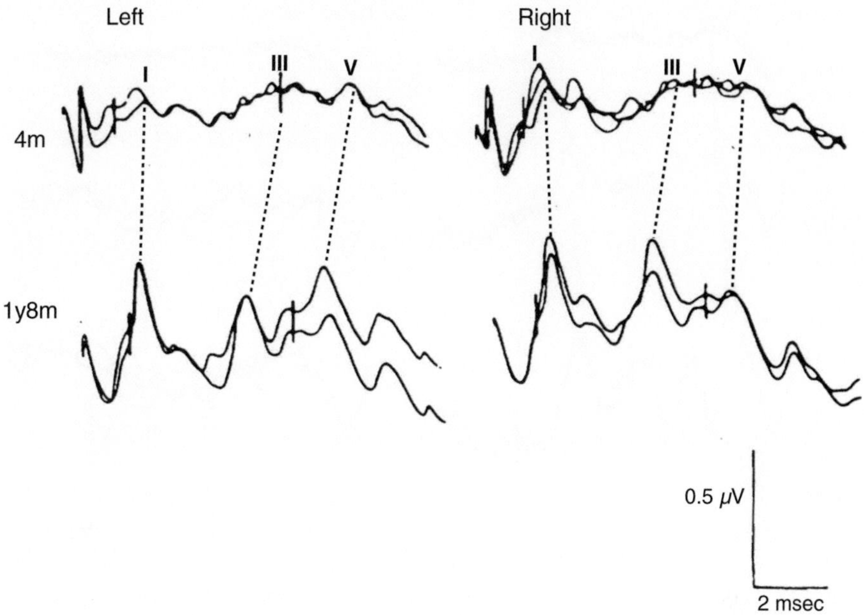

Fig. 6.16 Serial ABR of Patient #1 with chromosomal aberration—a 4-month-old male. Partial trisomy of chromosome 7 (46, XY, −9+der (9), t(7; 9)(q22; pter)mat) [32]

the neurophysiological improvement as demonstrated by normalization of the ABR. The ambiguous explanation of "brainstem maturation" demands further consideration.

Examples of the ABRs of such patients are shown below with a short clinical summary. The below examples are a few of 31 patients with chromosomal aberrations [37].

Patient 1—4-month-old male (Fig. 6.16).

Diagnosis: Partial trisomy of chromosome 7 (46, XY, −9+der (9), t(7; 9)(q22; pter)mat).

This child's birth weight was 2645 g (5.83 lb) at his GA of 39 weeks. He presented with a number of minor anomalies such as hypertelorism, anti-mongoloid slant, small mouth, micrognathia, high-arched palate, round ears, narrow external ear canals, hoarseness, a large anterior fontanel, and dilated scalp veins. At 4 months of age his DQ was lower than 20. An axial CT scan revealed external hydrocephalus. Radiograms of the ear revealed normal internal auditory meati and normal cochleas. The threshold of his BOA was greater than 90 dBnHL. His ABR showed questionable waves I and V on the left side, but on the right side definite waves I and II were elicited with prolonged latencies. The threshold of his wave V of ABR was 70 dBnHL. At 20 months of age, his ABR normalized with a threshold of 20 dBnHL but with persistent prolonged latencies. This child died at 2 years of age due to bronchopneumonia. An autopsy was not performed.

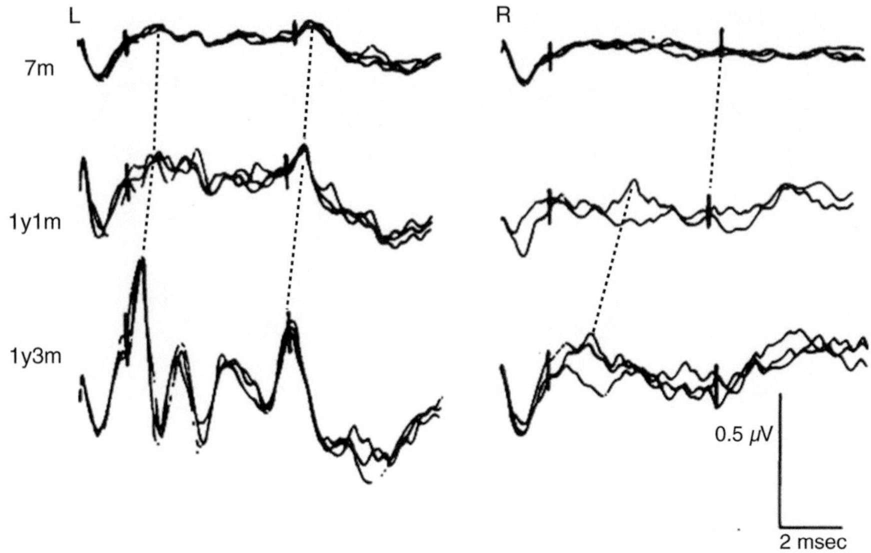

Fig. 6.17 Serial ABR of Patient #2 with chromosomal aberration. A 7-month-old female. Chromosomal aberration (46, XX, t(1; 4)(q32; q31)) [32]

Patient 2—7-month-old female (Fig. 6.17).

Diagnosis: Chromosomal aberration (46, XX, t(1; 4)(q32; q31)).

This infant was underweight at birth (1960 g) at her 36th week of gestation. She had minor anomalies such as blepharoptosis, micrognathia, upward nostrils, anti-mongoloid slant, umbilical hernia, and coloboma of the uvea. She did not respond to auditory stimuli. Her DQ was 75 and her BOA threshold was 90 dBnHL. Her left ABR showed questionable waves I, III, and V with very low amplitudes and prolonged latencies. Her right ABR was flat. When she was 15 months old, a definite ABR was detected on the left, but her right ABR could not be discerned with certainty.

Patient 3—1-year and 5-month-old male (Fig. 6.18).

Diagnosis: Partial trisomy of chromosome 15 (47, XY, +der(15), t(3; 15)(p25; q15)mat).

This child was born at the 42nd week of gestation with a low birthweight (2270 g, 5.8 lb). He had a cleft palate which involved the lip, a flat face with a broad nasal bridge, deep skin creases and pes cavus equinovarus (high-arched feet). He attained head control at 10 months. When he was 17 months old, he was able to respond to the nearby sound of paper crimping but he did not turn to localize other sounds. His DQ was 35 and his BOA threshold was 30 dBnHL. An ABR was difficult to elicit on his left side. On his right side, questionable waves I and V could be discerned at a stimulus level of 85 dBnHL with a threshold of 30 dBnHL. He could walk with support when he was 2 years and 2 months old. When he was 2 years and 4 months old, ABRs were confidently elicited bilaterally but showed prolonged latencies bilaterally. The stimulus thresholds evoking these ABRs were essentially identical to those when he was 17 months old.

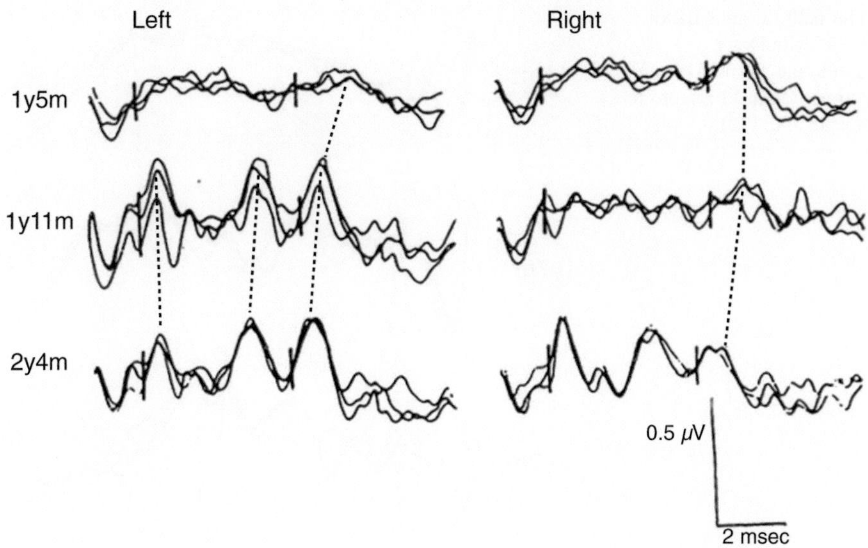

Fig. 6.18 Serial ABR of Patient #3 with chromosomal aberration other than Down syndrome. One year and 5 months old male. Partial trisomy of chromosome 15 (47, XY, +der(15), t(3; 15)(p25; q15)mat) [32]

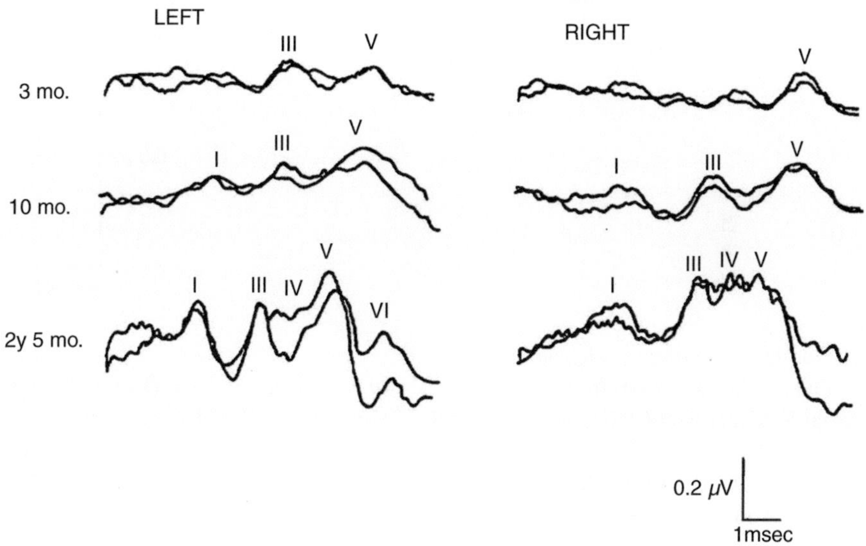

Fig. 6.19 Serial ABR of Patient #4 with chromosomal aberration. 9p+ syndrome [37]

Patient 4—(Fig. 6.19).
Diagnosis: 9p + syndrome. 3 months old, male.
ABR recorded at 3 months, 10 months, and 2 years 5 months of age are presented.

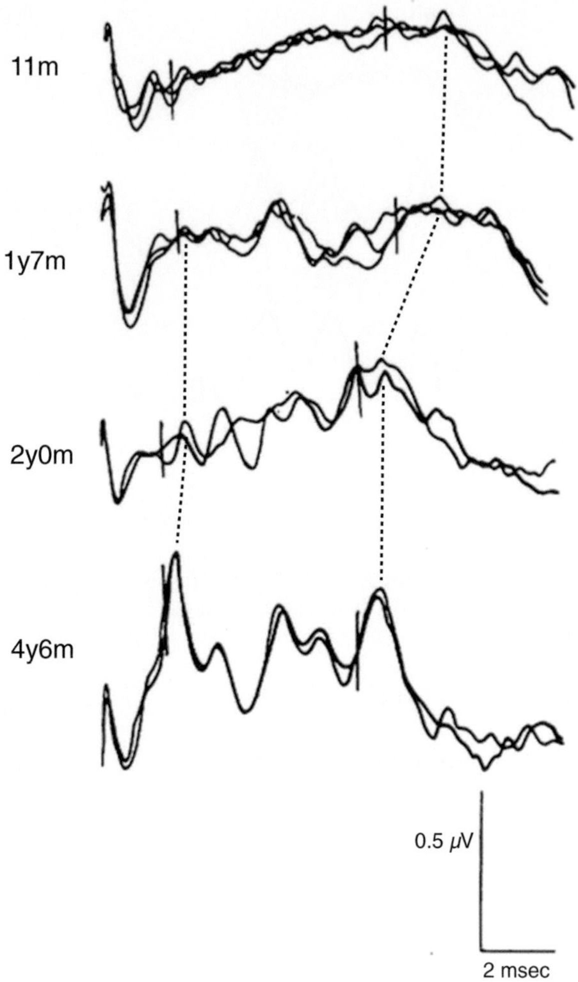

Fig. 6.20 Serial ABR of Pt. #5 with Down Syndrome. Serial ABRs for 4 times (from 11 months to 4 years old) [32]

Patient 5—11-month-old male (Fig. 6.20).

Diagnosis: Down syndrome (47, XY, +21) with Congenital Heart Disease (CHD, Atrial Septal Defect (ASD), and Ventricular Septal Defect (VSD)).

This child presented all of the typical clinical features of Down's Syndrome. His DQ was 50 and his BOA threshold was greater than 90 dBnHL. His ABR showed a questionable wave V. He was able to walk unaided at 26 months of age. When he was 4 years and 6 months old, his ABR had a normal configuration bilaterally with persistent prolonged latencies. He is now 6 years old and has near normal hearing.

Serial ABRs with or without audiometry in additional 4 patients with Down syndrome are presented (Figs. 6.21, 6.22, 6.23, 6.24, 6.25 and 6.26).

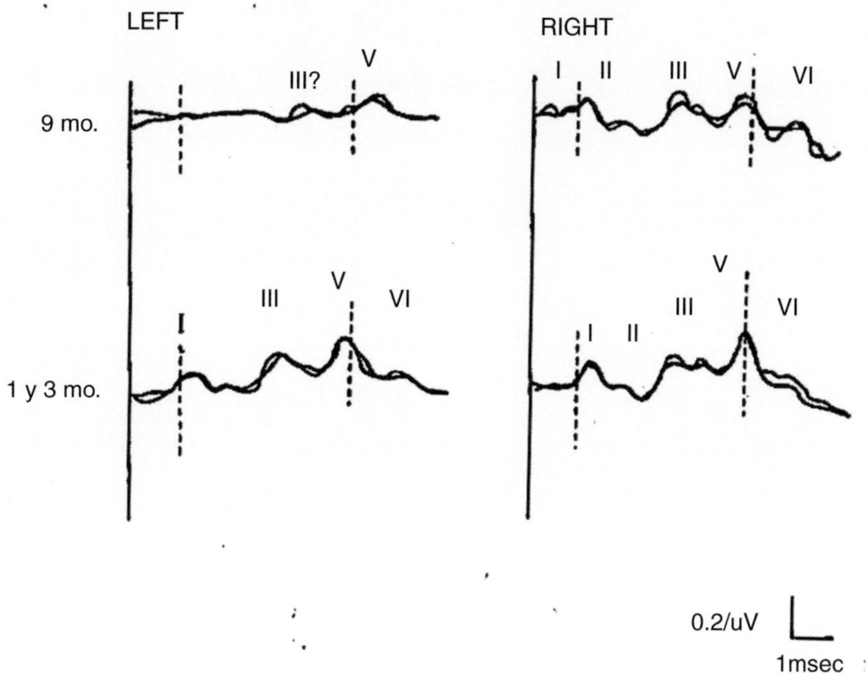

Fig. 6.21 Serial ABR of Pt #6 with Down Syndrome. ABRs at 9 months and 1 year 3 months [39]

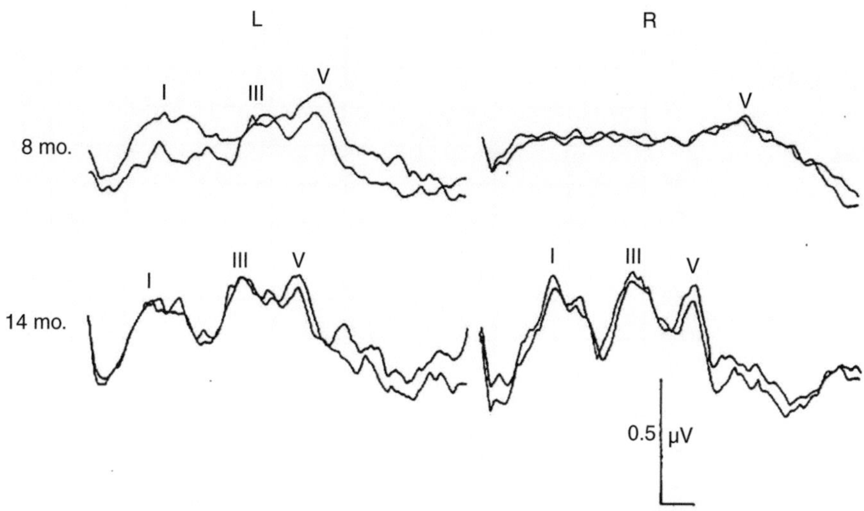

Fig. 6.22 Serial ABR of Pt #7 with Down Syndrome. ABRs at 8 and 14 months [37]

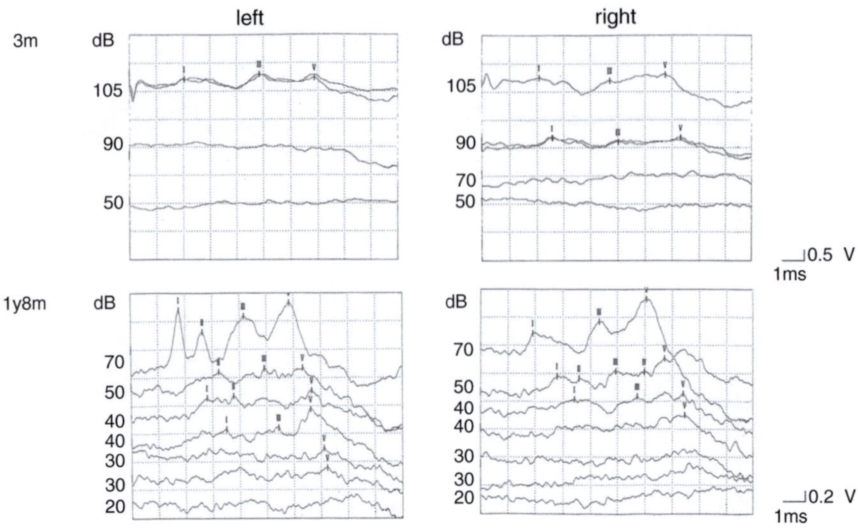

Fig. 6.23 Serial ABR of Pt #8 with Down Syndrome. ABRs at 3 months and 1 year 8 months

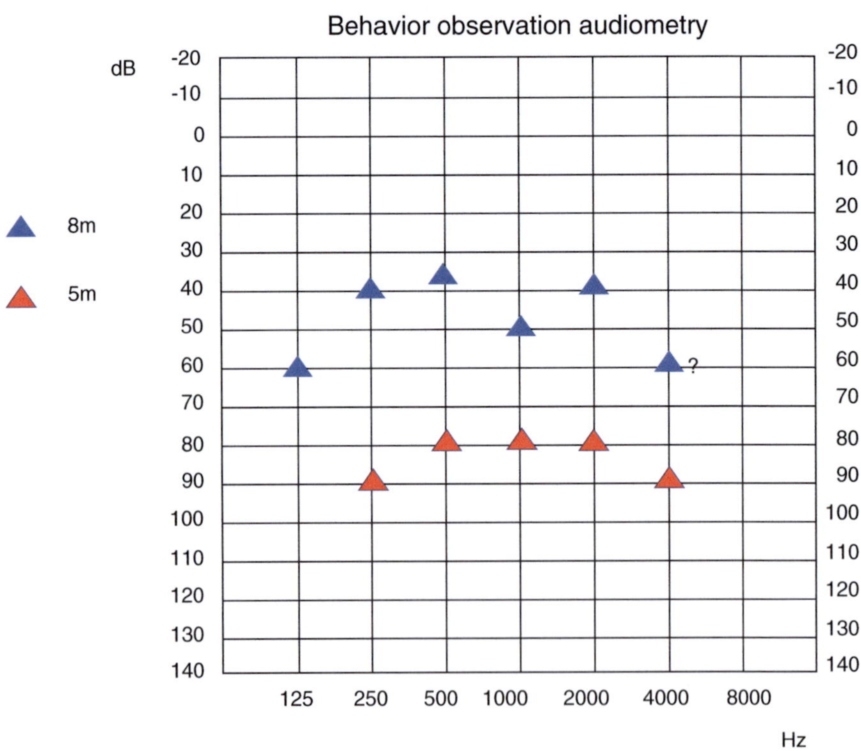

Fig. 6.24 Serial BOA of Pt #8 with Down Syndrome. BOA at 5 and 8 months

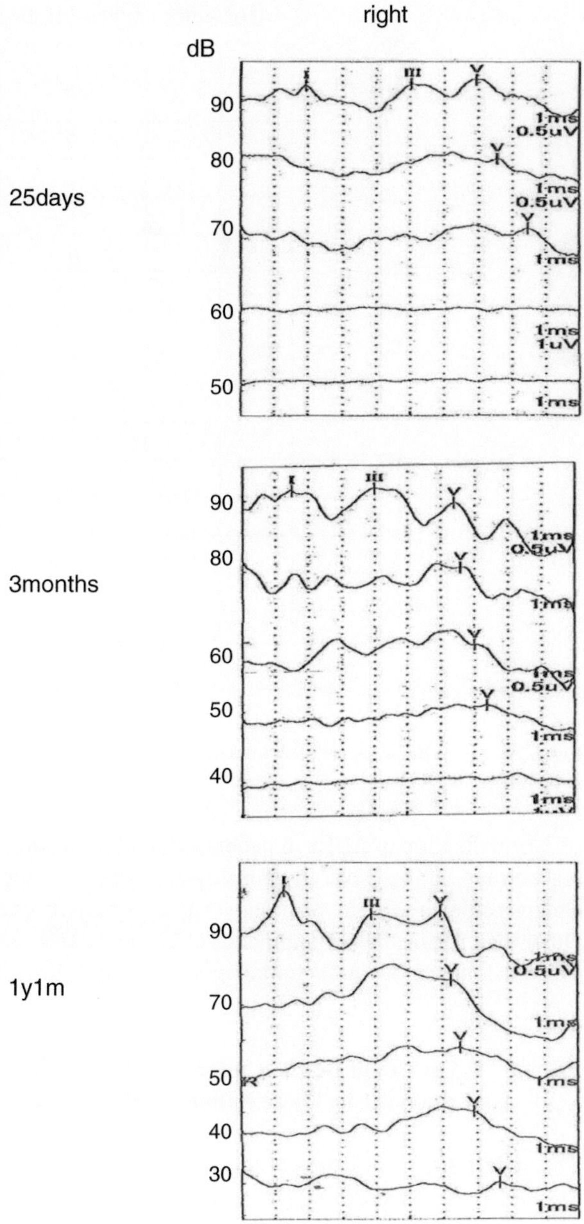

Fig. 6.25 Serial ABR of Pt #9 with Down Syndrome. ABRs at 25 days, 3 months and 1 year 1 month

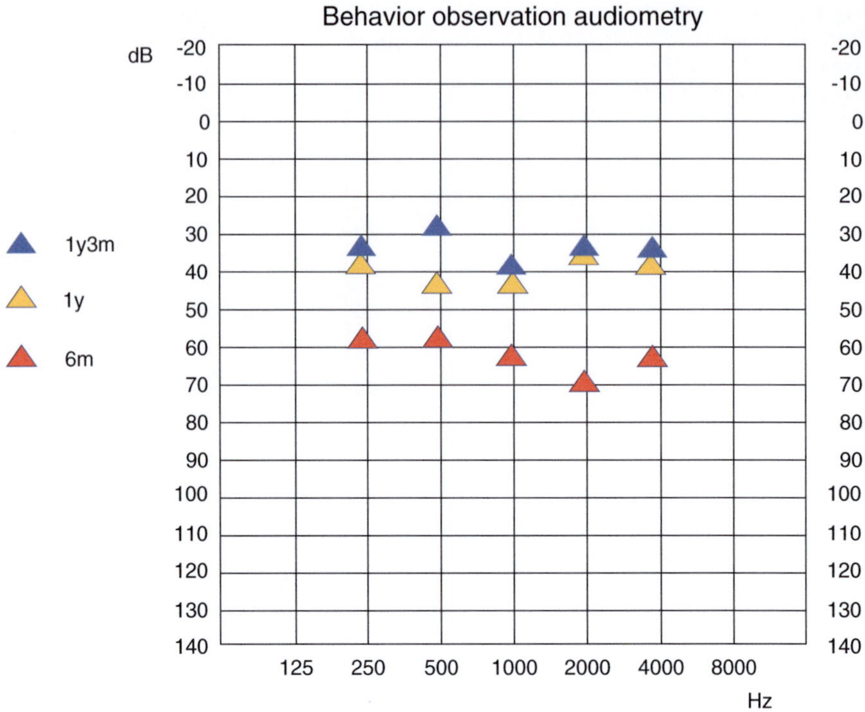

Fig. 6.26 Serial BOA results of Pt #9 with Down Syndrome. BOA at 6 months 1 year and 1 year 3 months are presented

Normalization of ABRs in patients with chromosomal aberration stands out. The reason may be their overall neurological symptoms including hearing impairment and possible brainstem pathology cause increased chance of ABR examination. Other than various minor anomalies of chromosome, patients with Down syndrome showed conspicuous ABR improvement during follow-up.

6.2.6.2 What Could Be the Underlying Cause/Causes of Normalization of the ABR in These Patients with Chromosomal Aberration?

The underlying pathologies of these patients were quite variable, but it is noteworthy that five of these nine patients had chromosomal aberrations. Chromosomal aberrations, in and of themselves, do not usually progress to a degenerative disease. Despite little evidence of this, there may be delayed myelinization or slow maturation of the brainstem auditory pathway in such patients as seen in Pelizaeus-Merzbacher disease (a leukodystrophy interfering with myelin growth). It seems, at this point, that normalization of the ABR depends on the maturation of the auditory neural substrate and its myelination [22].

6.2.7 *Recovery from Severe Anoxic Events with Normalization of the ABR*

In most comatose patients with undetectable ABRs, their prognoses are quite poor unless there is an underlying, transient metabolic disorder. The following five pediatric patients, while deeply comatose state due to episodes of acute cardiopulmonary arrest (CPA) and had no detectable ABRs. Their ABRs ultimately normalized at least tentatively and they all survived subsequent anoxic episodes which resulted in profound anoxic encephalopathy (AE).

6.2.7.1 ABRs in Anoxia

Generally, severe anoxia results in major destructive changes to the central nervous system, such changes dependent on the severity and the duration of the anoxia. There have been many reports showing the ABR after anoxia both in basic and in clinical research.

Severe to profound anoxia (hypoxia) is often fatal or, if not, it usually results in profound intellectual and motor abnormalities along with deterioration of the ABR. Sohmer [40] noted that during severe experimentally induced hypoxia in the cat, the ABR showed a deterioration of the ABR which occurred in two stages related to the extent the animal was able to maintain mean arterial blood pressure (MAP). If MAP was maintained, the other evoked potentials (somatosensory and visual evoked potentials, SEP and VEP) remained intact. But if MAP was not maintained, all of these potentials, SEP, VEP, including the ABR, were depressed. This suggests that there are different patterns of hypoxic depression of the ABR because of different underlying causes. In Sohmers' study, when the cats' MAP fell, ABR deterioration began with the later waves and sequentially progressed to the earlier waves. This suggests a hypoxic progression of central nervous function. This is probably due to the initial decrease in cerebral perfusion and blood flow. However, if MAP is maintained, severe hypoxia causes a depression of all of the ABR waves simultaneously. The cochlear microphonic potentials (ECoGs) were also depressed. This finding points to a peripheral cochlear effect as a result of hypoxia. Thus, the ABR abnormalities (prolonged interpeak latencies, loss of later waves and finally loss of all waves except wave I) seen in patients who have suffered a hypoxic or anoxic episode are always due to ischemia, even if the initial insult was hypoxic. The following is a discussion of patients who had shown both anoxic and hypoxic deteriorations of their ABRs and who had subsequent normalizations.

6.2.7.2 Case Reports of Anoxic Patients with Unexpected ABR Recovery

Five patients who survived serious anoxic events with normalization of their ABRs are presented (Table 6.1). All of these patients had severe underlying neurological diseases such as subacute sclerosing panencephalitis (SSPE), intractable epilepsy,

Table 6.1 Clinical summary of five patients with severe neurological diseases who survived serious anoxic events with ABR recovery

Pt	Age	Sex	Underlying disease	Time for resuscitation (min)
1	14	M	SSPE	15–20
2	13	M	IA, ID, EP	15–20
3	5	F	Leigh's encephalopathy	4–5 or more
4	2	M	Joubert syndrome	4–5
5	1	F	Brainstem encephalitis	4–5

SSPE subacute sclerosing panencephalitis (steadily progressive fatal disease related to measles infection), *IA* infantile autism, *ID* intellectual disability, *EP* epilepsy

autism with severe intellectual disabilities, Leigh syndrome (psychomotor regression), Joubert syndrome (cerebellar vermal hypoplasia with infantile spasms), and brainstem encephalitis. These patients all survived their anoxic episodes, but one patient died later. During their early post-anoxic episodes, no ABRs could be evoked and their clinical brainstem reflexes were absent. In three of these patients, their action potentials (APs) were absent and their extra-meatal electrocochleograms (ECoGs) were only minimally discerned.

A discrepancy in the time of recovery of the ABR, short latency somatosensory evoked potentials (SSEP) and the EEG was noted in one patient. This particular patient showed an initial burst suppression in his EEG and absent ABR followed by a normalization of the ABR and reappearance of the EEG.

Ordinarily, the prognosis for all of these patients would have been terminal. Nevertheless, it appears that some patients with very severe neurological diseases as a result of anoxia are able to survive. These five cases are probably exceptional but the findings in each case, presented below, are instructive.

Patient 1—14-year-old male (Fig. 6.27).

Diagnosis: Subacute sclerosing panencephalitis (SSPE).

This child contracted measles when he was 10 months old. At his age of 7 years, he began to demonstrate psychomotor deterioration and he was diagnosed with SSPE a few months later. When he was 13 years old, he had a non-specific upper respiratory infection with a high fever followed by a sudden cardiopulmonary arrest (CPA) which persisted for more than 15 min. He was successfully resuscitated but remained comatose for days. His ABRs pre and post this episode were recorded (Fig. 6.27). Forty-five days later of his CPA episode his EEG has lost its synchronicity, but multiple sporadic spikes were evident consistent with SSPE. His CT scan revealed significant cortical atrophy and ventricular dilations. Since then he had never gained his consciousness and had been on mechanical ventilation and he passed away 10 years later of this anoxic episode.

Patient 2—13-year-old male (Fig. 6.28).

Diagnosis: Autism with intellectual disability, and epilepsy.

This child walked unaided at 18 months but his speech was delayed. At 3 years of age he was diagnosed with autism and profound intellectual disability. He also had intractable epilepsy and had been on medication for this since his age of 7 years. At 14 years of age, he was hospitalized because of status epilepticus which was

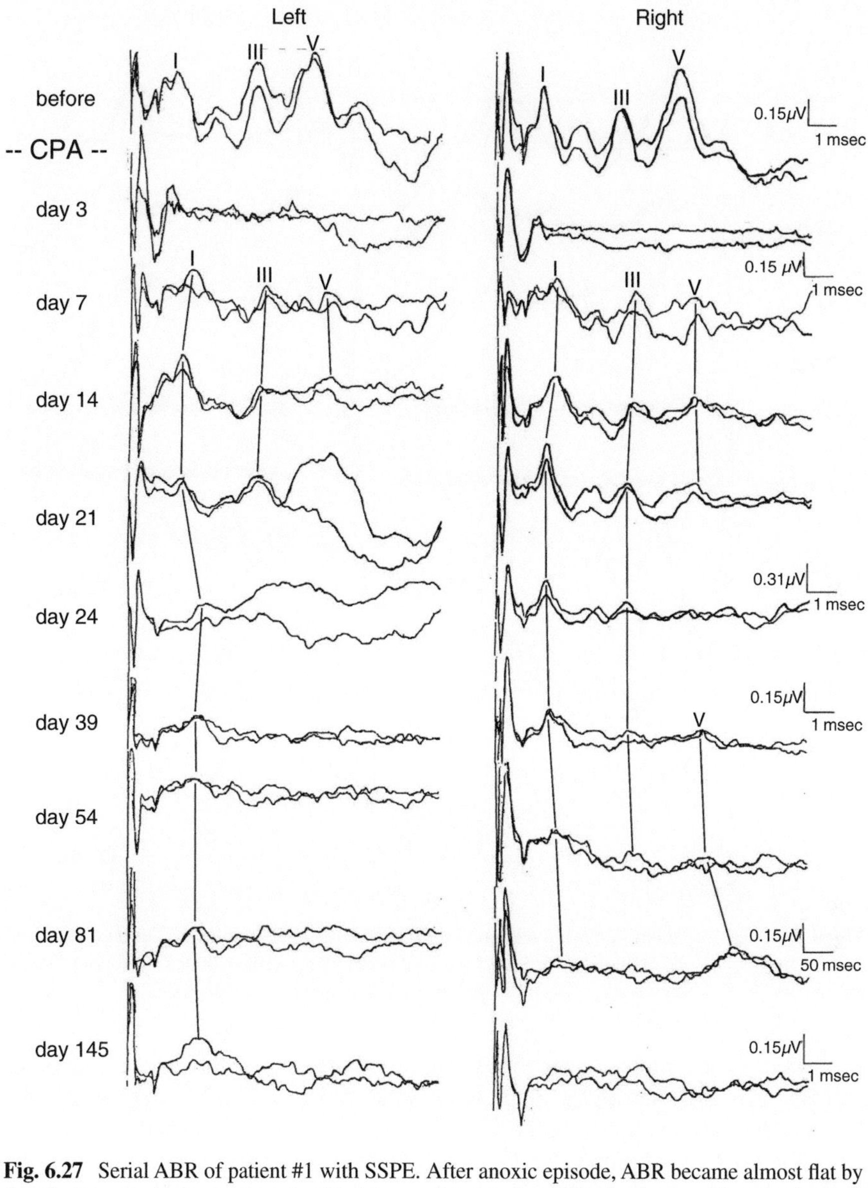

Fig. 6.27 Serial ABR of patient #1 with SSPE. After anoxic episode, ABR became almost flat by day 3, then gradually improved with later re-deterioration. His death was 10 years later of this episode

resolved by energetic treatment over 6 weeks, during which time he was comatose. However, 2 weeks after arousal from coma, he suffered a cardiopulmonary arrest (CPA) and he was anoxic for 15–20 min until he was successfully resuscitated. Following this episode, he remained deeply comatose with no clinically detectable brainstem function. Five days after his CPA, cilliar and corneal reflexes were detected. One week later, he recovered scarce spontaneous respiration assisted by

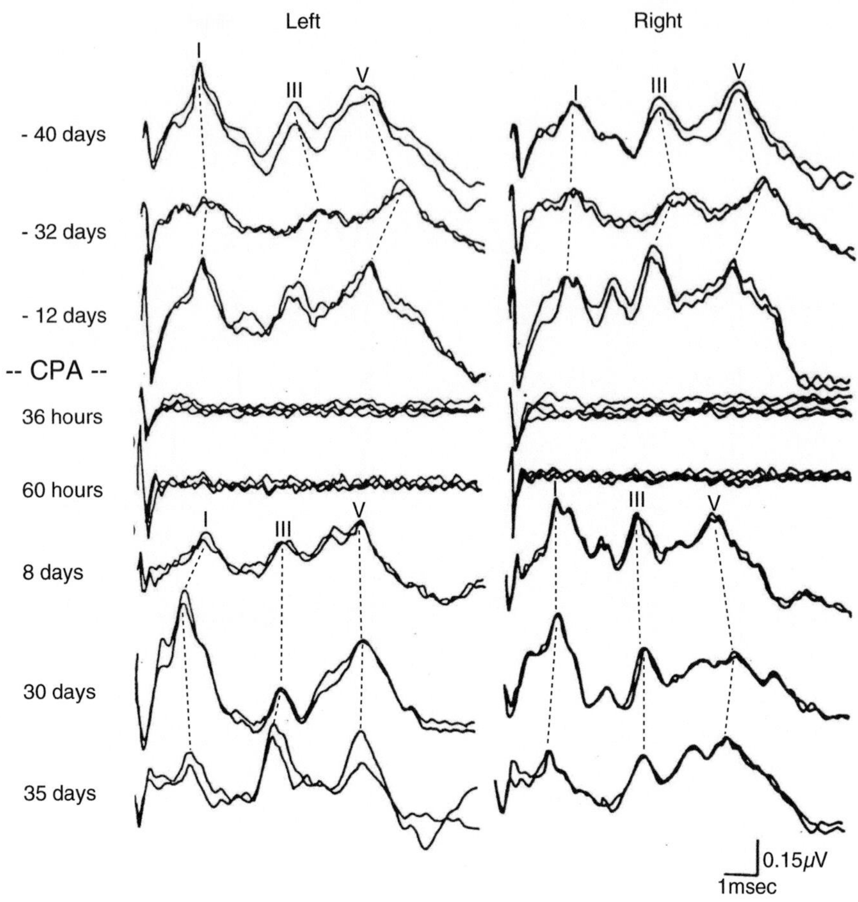

Fig. 6.28 ABR of patient #2 with intellectual disability, autism, and epilepsy. Thirteen years old male. After his episode of cardiopulmonary arrest followed by no ABR with no brainstem reflexes. After 1 week, partial recovery of his brainstem dysfunction associated with ABR

mechanical ventilation. Finger thrust (tactile stimulus) did not induce a physical reaction. His EEG showed a suppression burst pattern 2 h after CPA. Thirty-two hours later, a periodic synchronous EEG discharge was noted. On the third day post-CPA this discharge disappeared. On the sixth day his EEG was almost flat. On the ninth day post-CPA, a 50-μV theta wave appeared amongst an otherwise flat EEG. His ABR, to 90 dBnHL clicks, changed from normal at pre-CPA episode to a waves I and V amplitude reversal. Since his CVA and anoxic episode he had been in a vegetative state with a decorticated posture for more than 10 years.

Patient 3—5-year-old female (Fig. 6.29).

Diagnosis: Leigh's encephalopathy.

This child was essentially normal until she was 7 months old when she developed repeated episodes of unconsciousness following a minor infectious disease which was resolved by supportive therapy. During the intervals between these episodes, she

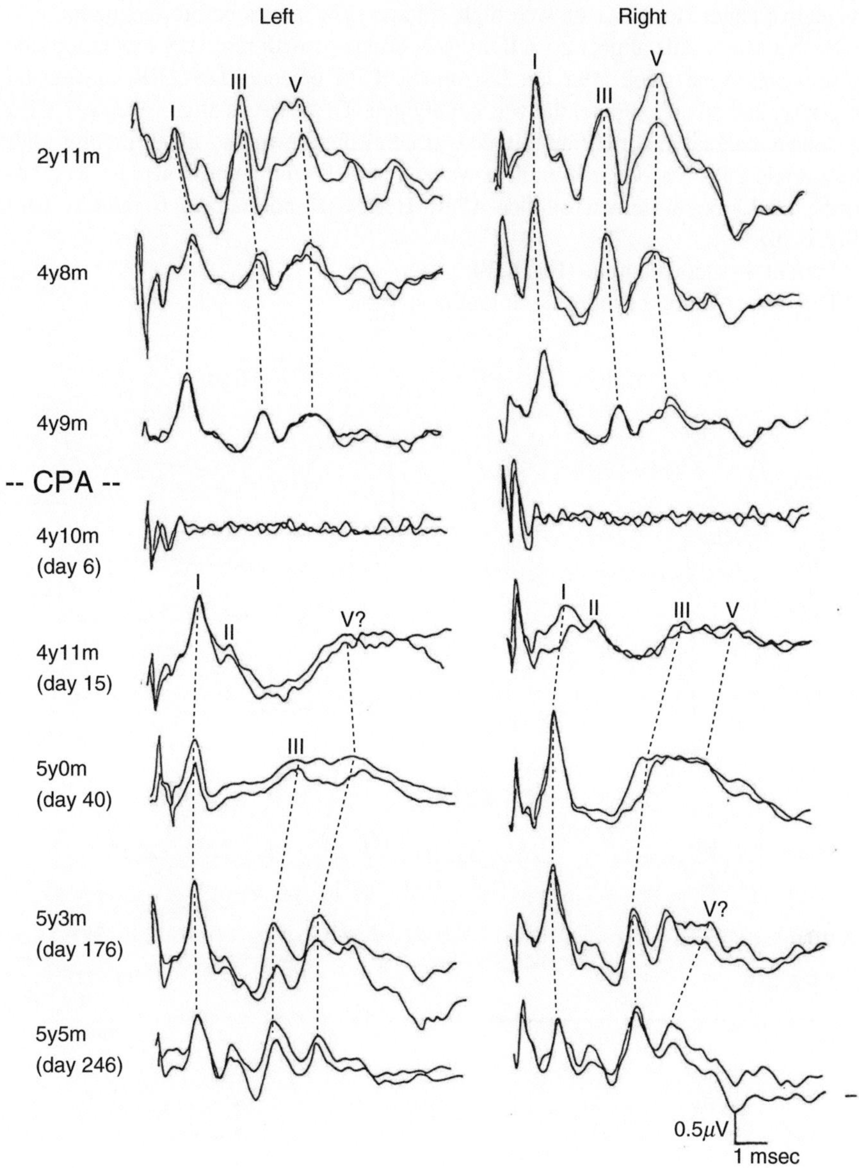

Fig. 6.29 Serial ABRs of patient #3 with Leigh's encephalopathy. After anoxic episode at 4 years 9 months of age, ABR disappeared but gradually recovered after 15 days of CPA

could walk unaided but she displayed a moderate intellectual disability. Repeated ABRs were almost normal except for a slight prolongation of the late, central waves. At age 4 she had not recovered from these unconscious episodes despite energetic therapy for such. She incurred frequent attacks of apnea and ultimately a CPA which lasted for more than a few minutes. She was successively resuscitated and mechanically ventilated. Upon resuscitation, she was flaccid, and she has thence been in a vegetative state. Her EEG showed high voltage slow waves before the anoxic episodes but afterwards almost no activity was observed with rare very low amplitude slow waves. One week after her last anoxic CPA episode, her ABR showed no response, and an action potential was not elicited. Three weeks after her anoxic CPA episode a reversal in her I/V amplitude was confirmed. Two-and-a-half months after this anoxic CPA episode, a definitive waves I and II, with amorphous later components, could be discerned on her ABR. Her ABR normalized 6 months later (Fig. 6.29).

Patient 4—neonate male (Fig. 6.30).

Diagnosis: Joubert syndrome, Infantile spasms.

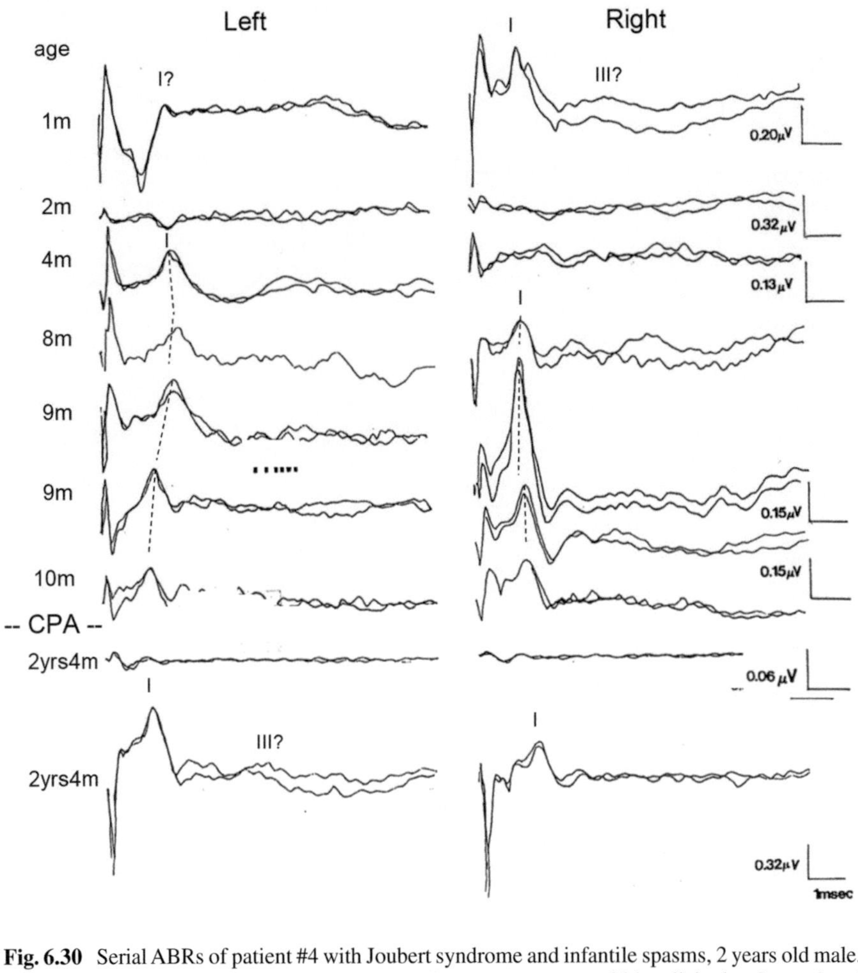

Fig. 6.30 Serial ABRs of patient #4 with Joubert syndrome and infantile spasms, 2 years old male. At 1 month of his age, only wave I was present but no response could be elicited at 2 months of age. Then his ABRs gradually improved. At 9 months of age an extremely high amplitude wave I was recorded from his right side. When he was 2 years and 4 months of age, no ABR could be elicited once again. He passed away due to respiratory failure at 3 years and 3 months of age

This child was large for his gestational age with his birth weight of 4400 g at 40 weeks of gestation. His Apgar score of 1 and 5 at 1 and 5 min, respectively. His infantile spasms began at 2 months of age and were successfully treated by ACTH therapy. Neuroimaging disclosed partial agenesis of his corpus callosum with cerebellar vermal hypoplasia. After birth, he was hypotonic, reluctant to search for a light source and he did not respond to sounds. Oculocephalic responses were elicited but his gag reflex was ambiguous. Abnormal respiration was noted which is one of the characteristic signs of Joubert syndrome. He passed away due to respiratory failure at 3 years and 3 months of age.

Patient 5—15-month-old female (Fig. 6.31).

Diagnosis: Brainstem encephalitis.

This child was normal until she was 12 months old at which time she began to experience falls. One month later, she developed seizures which occurred 7–8 times

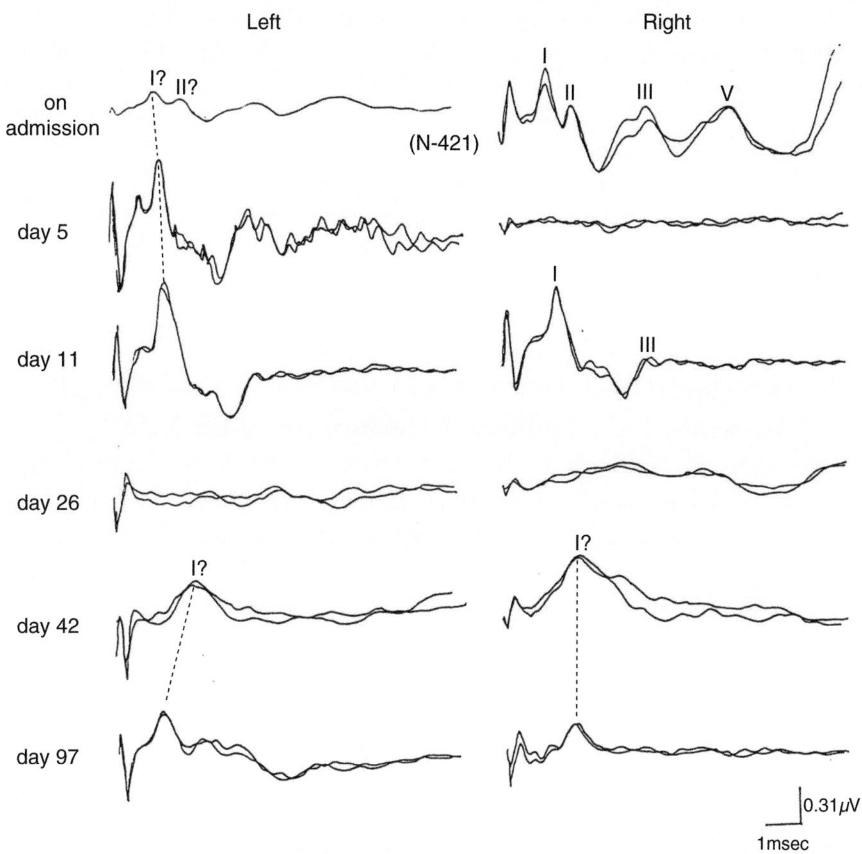

Fig. 6.31 Serial ABRs of patient #5 with brainstem encephalitis. Female, 15 months old. After the episode of coma followed by irregular respiration and apneic episode, ABR became marked deterioration but the early components are almost preserved

a day and she lost her ability to walk. Her EEG and CT scan had no particular abnormalities at the time. When she was 15 months of age, she was admitted to ICU on an emergency basis because of irregular respiration. She became deeply comatose but retained reactive pupils and gag reflexes. A spinal tap obtained clear CSF with normal cytology and biochemistry. Because of her frequent apnea and bradycardia, she was intubated and placed on mechanical ventilation. The sequential changes of her ABR are shown in Fig. 6.31.

In three of these patients, during the periods when no ABR was detected, brainstem reflexes were also absent and the action potentials (APs) of the ECoG were also not evoked.

6.2.7.3 Discussion of Anoxic Patients with Unexpected ABR Recovery

Despite their desperate conditions at birth or anoxic episodes of any age, all of these children survived for various lengths of time and their ABRs unexpectedly improved (normalized). Infants and children who are brain-dead have been known to survive for months and even years given respiratory support. This is usually not the case with school aged children to adults. These children in this chapter were not brain-dead but lesions with brainstem involvement. However, their clinical evaluations after a CPA surprisingly showed ABR responses with reversals, similar to children with basically intact neurological function. The lesson from all of this is that clinicians should be very cautious about discontinuing treatment prematurely during their management of children with severe to profound neurological disabilities.

6.3 Deterioration of ABR in Child Neurology: Neurological Assessment of Childhood Deterioration of the ABR

Early, sequential recordings of the ABR to determine any deterioration is helpful to determine its cause and the course. Candidates for serial ABRs are children showing a decline in hearing acuity or there are signs of progressive brainstem pathology, either organic or functional.

6.3.1 Loss or Decline of Hearing Acuity

The causes of hearing impairment are variable such as genetic, infectious, ototoxic, anoxic, traumatic, conductive, sporadic, and others. A genetic and severe sensory neural hearing loss occurs once in 1000–2000 births. More than 50% of these congenital hearing losses has been confirmed to be of genetic origin arising from a specific gene mutation. Some specific hearing losses have been found to begin and subsequently progress after birth.

6.3.1.1 Intrauterine Infections

Intrauterine infections of rubella, syphilis, cytomegalovirus (CMV), Herpes virus, toxoplasma, and others may induce what appears to be a congenital hearing loss. CMV infection as a fetus is notorious for the progressive deterioration of hearing along with the deterioration of ABRs. Hearing loss may also occur, at any age, as a sequela of a variety of bacterial or viral invasions, i.e., meningoencephalitis, often concurrent with severe-to-profound intellectual disability. Meningitis, as a result of mumps, could also result in unilateral or bilateral hearing loss. Congenital rubella syndrome may also result in decreased auditory acuity and is confirmed at birth. But in some patients, deterioration of hearing appears during their course of development (Figs. 6.32 and 6.33).

6.3.1.2 Neurocutaneous Syndrome as a Category of Genetically Determined Systemic Diseases with Central Nervous System Involvement

There are many diseases in this category. Examples are tuberous sclerosis, neurofibromatosis type I (NF I, Recklinghausen disease), neurofibromatosis type II (NF II), xeroderma pigmentosum, Sturge-Weber syndrome, linear nevus sebaceous syndrome, hypo-melanosis Ito syndrome, and as such.

In this section, NF II is presented as the representative of this category because of the acoustic neurinoma is the early and important symptom of which ABR is one of the most appropriate tool for diagnosis and follow-up measure. NF II shows

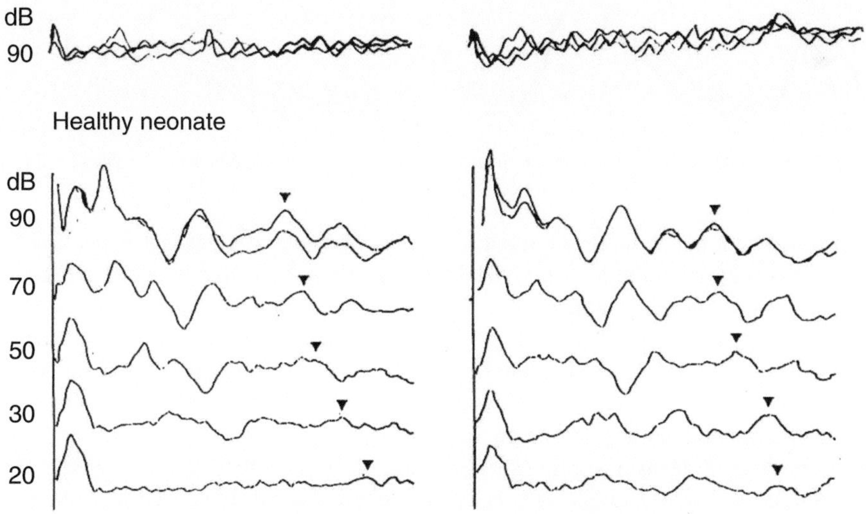

Fig. 6.32 ABR in a patient with congenital rubella syndrome. He had profound hearing loss from birth (upper diagram). Compare with the ABR of a healthy neonate (lower diagram)

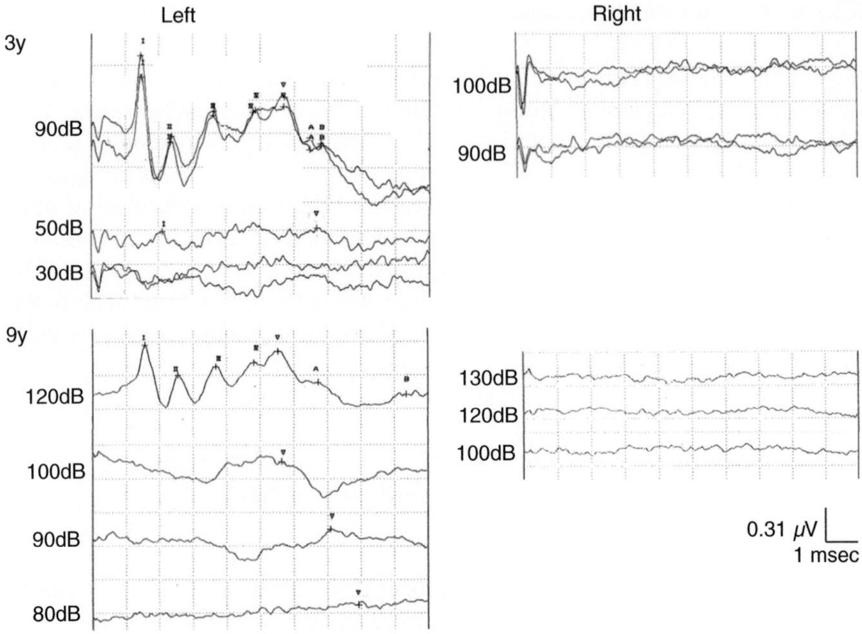

Fig. 6.33 ABR of another patient with congenital rubella syndrome. Deterioration of hearing and ABR was confirmed during his follow-up. This patient teaches us there are children with congenital rubella syndrome and progressive hearing impairment

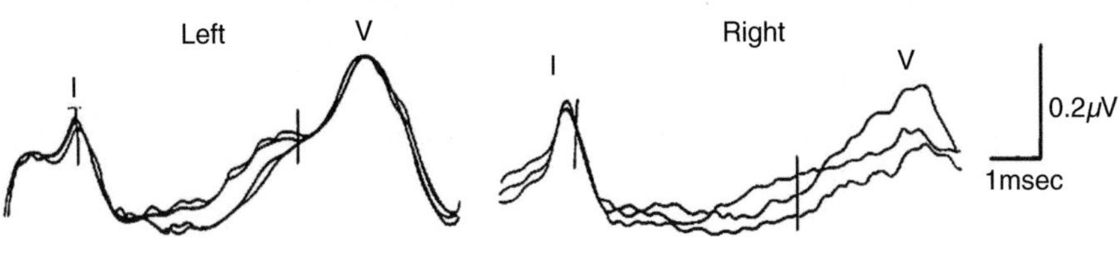

Fig. 6.34 Single ABR of a patient with neurofibromatosis type II. Nine years old, male [23, 24]

autosomal-dominant mode of inheritance. Responsible gene is *merlin* which is located on chromosome 22q12. *Merlin* has a function of tumor suppressor. Acoustic neurinoma is the most conspicuous clinical feature in this disease and usually becomes apparent in teens to twenties. It often appears as dermal neurofibromatosis, acoustic neurinoma-related hearing impairment and dermal pigmentation. Acoustic and vestibular neurinoma is a slowly growing tumor with gradual progress of hearing impairment and ataxia based on the slowly enlarging tumor.

It is often a devastating disease. Single and Serial ABRs of two patients are shown in Figs. 6.34 and 6.35. Resection of enlarged acoustic neurinoma is sometimes difficult because of the facial nerve with gustatory and vestibular nerve injury.

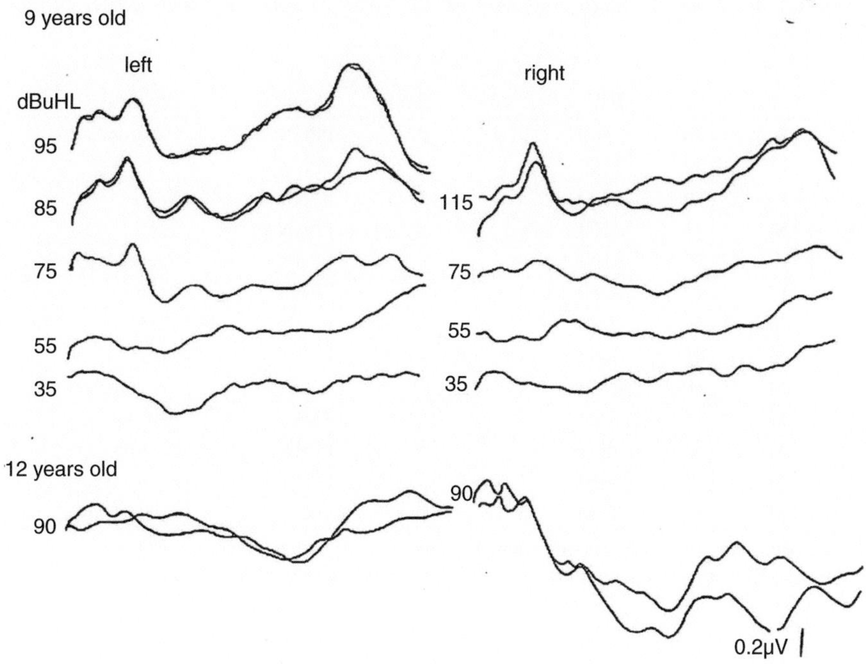

Fig. 6.35 Serial ABR of a patient with neurofibromatosis type II. Progressive hearing impairment caused by acoustic neurinoma are shown in the figure

6.3.1.3 Progressive Hearing Loss in NICU Patients and the Graduates from NICU

ABRs have been clinically employed in the pediatric wards and in neonatal intensive care unit (NICU). Patients who showed later hearing loss are shown in Table 6.2. Examples of their deterioration of hearing threshold are illustrated compared with their age.

Figure 6.36 illustrates the age and rate of hearing decline in the above 13 patients listed in Table 6.2. It is important to recognize that such patients exist, and they should be carefully followed-up, especially patients with persistent pulmonary hypertension in neonates (PPHN). The frequency of hearing loss in NICU graduates is higher than that of the general population [18], especially in patients with PPHN.

The author will write about PPHN in the following section.

Patients with Hearing Loss Discovered in NICUs and in NICU Graduates

In 1985, Sell et al. noted that 20% of their 40 patients in *NICU* with PPHN had impaired hearing [41]. Nield et al. published a paper that 11 infants aged 13–48 months of age whose ABRs were normal at their graduate from NICU. But

Table 6.2 Example of clinical summary of 13 NICU patients with delayed/later hearing impairment

Pt	Sex	GA	BW	APGAR		Diagnosis 1	Diagnosis 2
				1 min	5 min		
1	F	38	2500	9	9	PPHN	Pneumonia
2	M	40	3290	7	8	PPHN	
3	F	40	3220	3	3	PPHN	MAS
4	M	41	3100	6	8	PPHN	MAS
5	F	37	3100	6	9	PPHN	Pneumonia
6	F	42	3280	4	8	PPHN	MAS
7	M	42	3370	6	–	PPHN	MAS
8	M	42	3800	8	–	PPHN	MAS
9	M	40	2920	2	–	MAS	Pneumothorax
10	M	36	2000	8	9	PDA	Atresia ani
11	M	33	2830	3	6	PPHN	Hydrops
12	M	36	3600	1	–	ICH	Hydronephrosis
13	M	38	3300	8	9	DIC	Hemangioma

PPHN persistent pulmonary hypertension, *MAS* massive aspiration syndrome, *PDA* patent ductus arteriosus, *ICH* intracranial hemorrhage, *DIC* disseminated intravascular coagulation

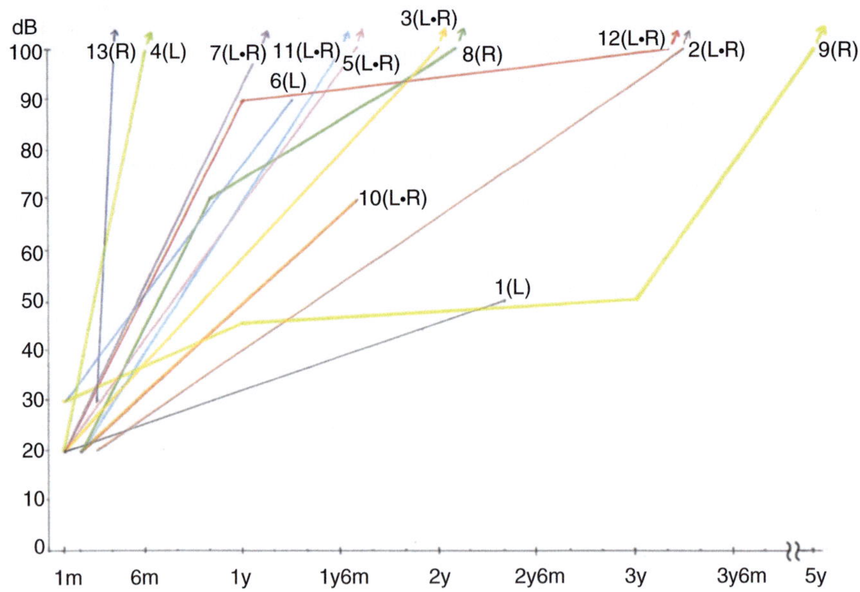

Fig. 6.36 The figure shows confirmed age and speed of hearing decline in 13 patients listed in Table 6.2

later they were diagnosed as hearing impairment. Neild's patients needed long-term mechanical ventilation and 7 among 11 patients had PPHN. They showed severe acidosis and hypoxemia in NICU. This finding means that these patients had the severest cardiopulmonary symptoms and survived their neonatal period. They often had profound and sustained cardiorespiratory symptoms along with severe infections requiring medications such as aminoglycosides, diuretics, and others in NICU. Moreover, they had chronic respiratory disorders due to broncho-pulmonary dysplasia after discharge from NICU [42]. In 1986, Naulty et al. described that 3 among 12 PPHN patients had progressive nature of hearing impairment [43]. Then, Hendricks-Muños et al. reported that 19 among 51 NICU patients (37%) showed hearing impairment [44] and Walton and Hendricks-Munoz [45] found 20 among 40 NICU patients (50%) had hearing impairment, respectively.

Zenri followed sequential ABR and hearing acuity changes in 25 infants diagnosed with PPHN [46]. Seven of these infants had been treated with extracorporeal membrane oxygenation (ECMO). ABRs and hearing evaluations were recorded upon their discharge from the NICU, and their mean age was 1 month. They were then followed-up at an outpatient clinic. During follow-up, 9 of these infants (42.8%) were found to have significant sensorineural hearing loss despite normal ABR at discharge from NICU. Eight of these nine infants with hearing impairment and speech delay were otherwise normal in terms of their physical development. Serial ABR recordings or age/developmnet appropriate audiometry should be routinely included throughout the clinical follow-up of PPHN infants, at least until they are 2 years old. Of course, hearing acuity should be reexamined whenever hearing impairment is suspected in patients. The same applies to infants who have had or currently have severe cardiopulmonary symptoms and impaired hearing acuity is suspected. Their ultimate language ability depends on hearing and intellectual ability. Also, these infants with severe hearing impairment could be candidates for a cochlear implantation. It is extremely important to find hearing impairment to assure their language function doubting hearing impairment in NICU graduates at the age of cochlear implantation. In PPHN, underground diseases such as pneumonia, ascites, massive aspiration, fetal hydrops and diaphragmatic hernia increase pulmonary parenchymal resistance, pulmonary arterial hypertension, and then cardiac right-left shunt through patent arterial duct or foramen ovale occur. In such conditions, profound cardiopulmonary dysfunction and severe anoxia could happen and could induce profound dysfunction in cochlear damage. Besides ECMO (extracorporeal membranous oxygenation) treatment in NICU is done through canulation into internal carotid artery and sacrifice a little bit to intracranial blood volume.

Case Presentation of Patients With or Without PPHN and Delayed Hearing Impairment

Patient 1—male, PPHN (Fig. 6.37).

He was born at 40w of GA with a birth weight of 3300 g. APGAR score was 7 and 8 at 1 and 5 min, respectively. He suffered from PPHN with pneumonia. He needed high-frequency oscillation (HFO) and extracorporeal membrane

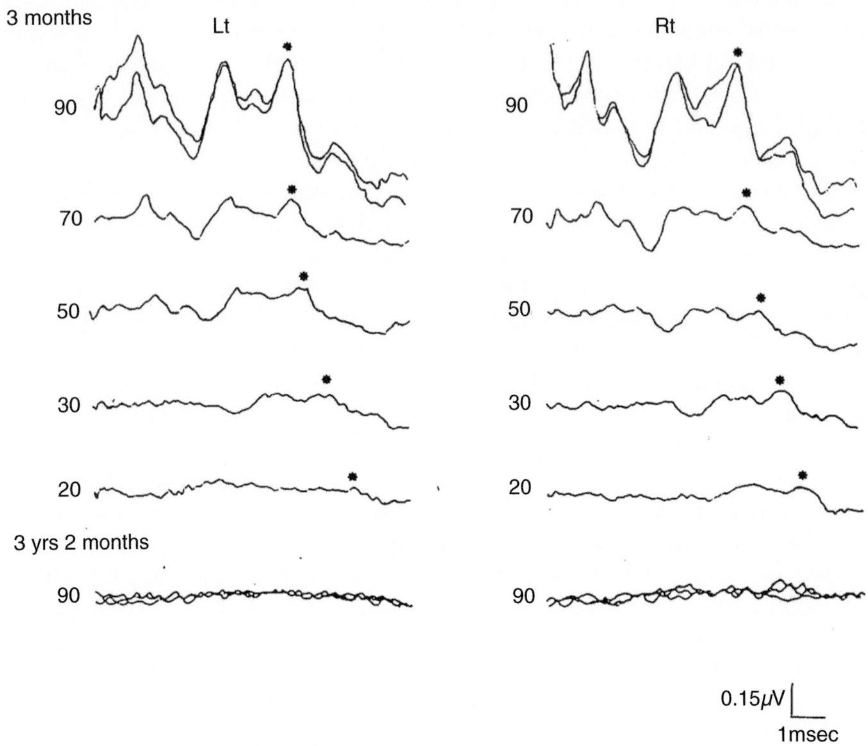

Fig. 6.37 Serial ABR of a male patient with PPHN, recorded at 3 months and 3 and 2/12 years of his age. No response to 90 dB stimuli was confirmed at the later record despite of completely normal ABR at 3 months of his age

oxygenation (ECMO) treatment which revealed his respiratory status was extremely severe. He depended on mechanical ventilation for 58 days in NICU. His ABR at graduate from NICU was normal. Head control was attained at 6 months and he could walk by himself at 17 months of age. He was pointed to delayed speech at 2 years of age and hearing loss was confirmed at 3 years of age. He was trained thereafter with hearing aids because of no response to conditioed orientation response (COR) and no detectable ABR to high sound pressure. His DQ was 68 which suggested mild intellectual disabilities at 3 years of his age.

Patient 2—female, PPHN (Fig. 6.38).

She was born at 37 weeks of gestation with 3100 g of birth weight. Her APGAR score was 6 and 9 for 1 and 5 min. Her ABR was normal on day 21. After she was discharged from NICU, her family gradually noticed her delayed speech with poor response to sounds and voices after her first birthday. When she was 1 year and 7 months of age, ABR showed no response to 90 dB click stimuli. She was confirmed as having a profound hearing impairment. Her mental and motor development were almost within normal range except for her hearing.

Patient 3—male, PPHN (Figs. 6.39, 6.40, and 6.41).

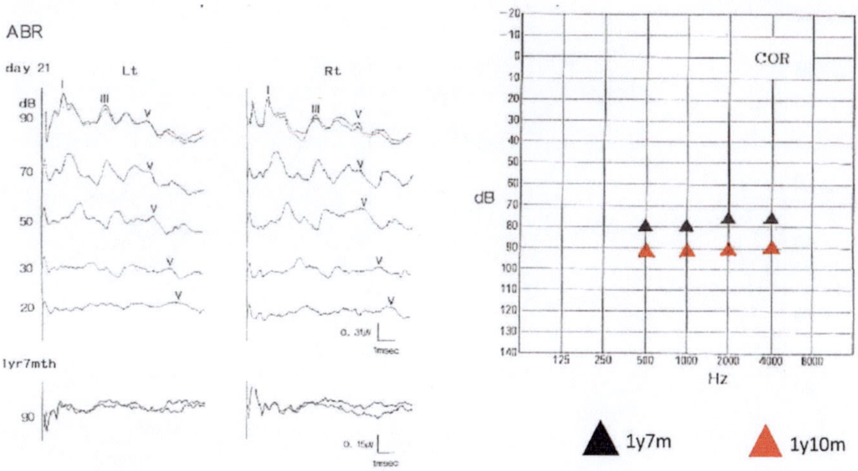

Fig. 6.38 The left half of the figure shows serial ABRs of patient #2. Female. ABR at 1 year and 7 months shows almost no response which suggests profound hearing loss at high-frequency sounds. The right half of the figure is her hearing results using conditioned orientation response (COR) at 1 year 10 months and 1 year 7 months

Fig. 6.39 CT scan at day 39 of patient #3, male, PPHN

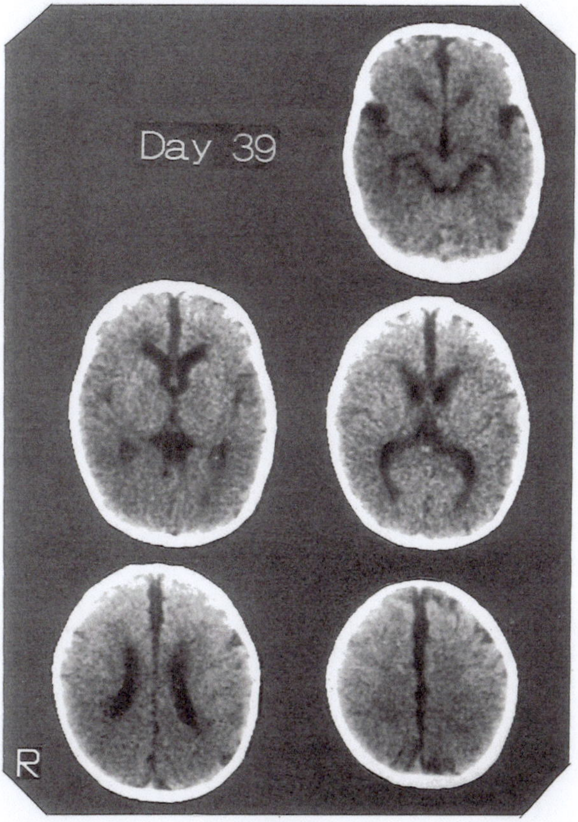

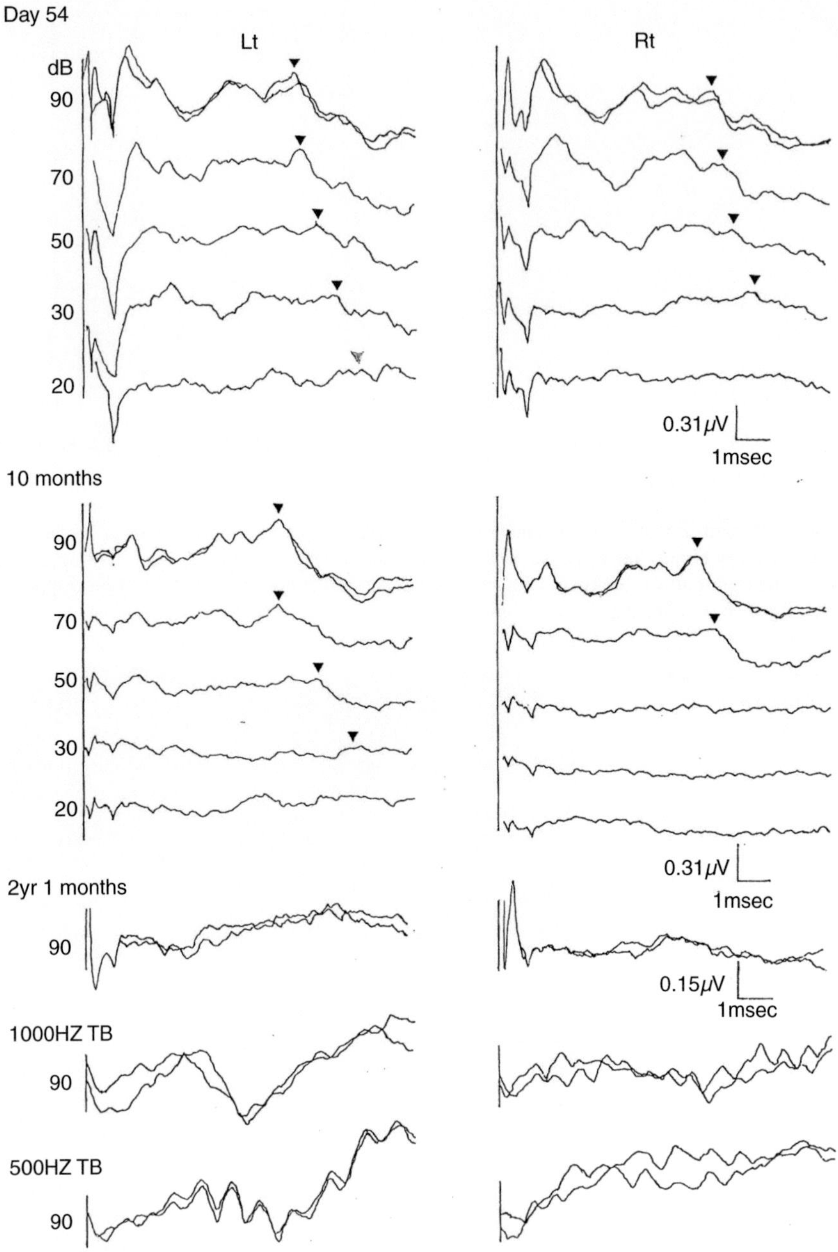

Fig. 6.40 Serial ABRs of patient #3 at day 54, 10 months and 2 years 1 months. ABR was normal at 54 days but the following tests revealed elevation of wave V threshold from right side to both sides

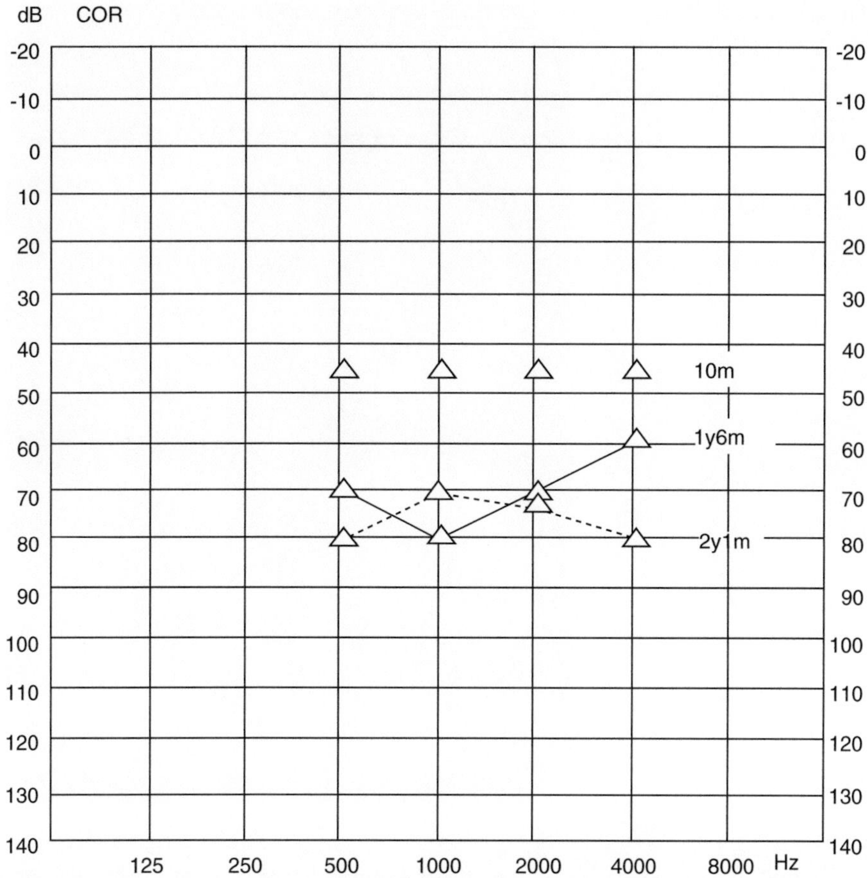

Fig. 6.41 Serial change of hearing revealed by COR in patient #3. Deterioration of his hearing from 45 dB at 10 months to 75 dB at 2 years and 1 month was revealed by COR

He was born at a birth weight of 3800 g at 42 weeks gestation. His APGAR score for 1 min was 8 which means he had no birth asphyxia. He had PPHN during his course in NICU but was well controlled. His ABR was normal at 54 days of his life but at 10 months of age, bilateral wave V threshold, especially on the right side elevated. At 2 years and 1 month, bilateral definitive wave V threshold elevation was apparent. His DQ revealed by Kinder Infant Development Scale (KIDS) was 116 which means better than average. Cranial CT scan on day 39 showed no definitive major lesions.

Patient 4—male, PPHN (Figs. 6.42, 6.43, and 6.44).

He was born at 41 weeks of gestation. His delivery was via Cesarean section because of cephalo-pelvic disproportion. He did not show asphyxia at birth. His birth weight was 3800 g and his amniotic fluid was clouded. One hour after his birth he went into respiratory failure, was intubated, and then placed on mechanical

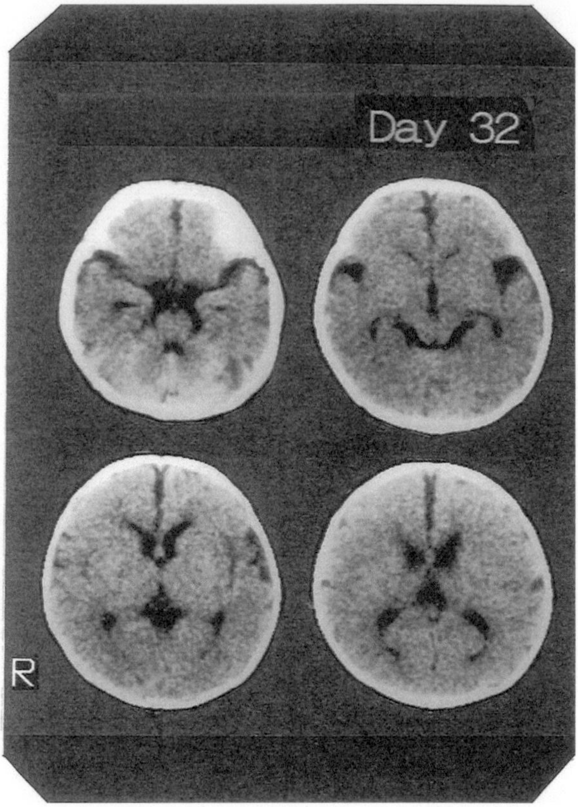

Fig. 6.42 Cranial CT scan at day 32 of patient #4

ventilation for 23 days. PPHN was diagnosed and ECMO therapy was administered for 6 days. He was discharged from the NICU when he was 70 days old. When he was 3 years old, his mental and motor development was normal but his hearing was impaired. His ABR at 25 days after birth was normal. His left ABR apparently deteriorated at 2 years and 5 months (Fig. 6.43). His average hearing threshold revealed by COR was 66 dB at 1 year and 6 months (Fig. 6.44).

Patient 5—female, PPHN (Fig. 6.45).

She was born 2500 g at 38 weeks gestation. APGAR score was 9 and 9. She had Massive Aspiration Syndrome (MAS), PPHN, and needed ECMO treatment. She had moderate hearing impairment as a sequela but her intellectual ability was spared.

Her ABR at 43 days was normal but elevated the threshold of wave V at 2 years and 4 months.

Patient 6—female, PPHN (Fig. 6.46).

Her birth weight was 3300 g of weight at 42 weeks gestation, Her APGAR score was 4 and 8 at 1 and 5 min, respectively. She had MAS, persistent fetal circulation (PFC), and PPHN. She needed ECMO treatment during her stay at NICU.

Hearing loss was diagnosed during her follow-up. Her overall development other than hearing was almost normal.

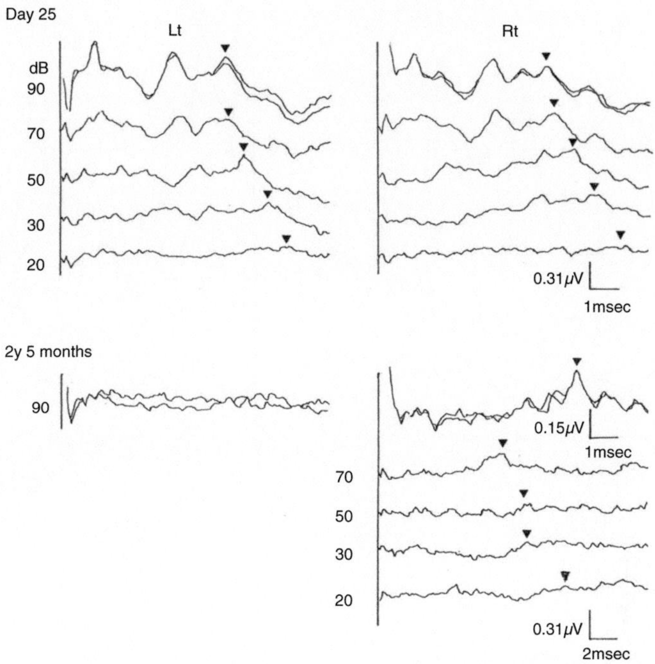

Fig. 6.43 Serial ABRs of patient #4. ABR at day 25 was normal. Unilateral severe hearing loss was suggested at 2 years and 5 months of his age

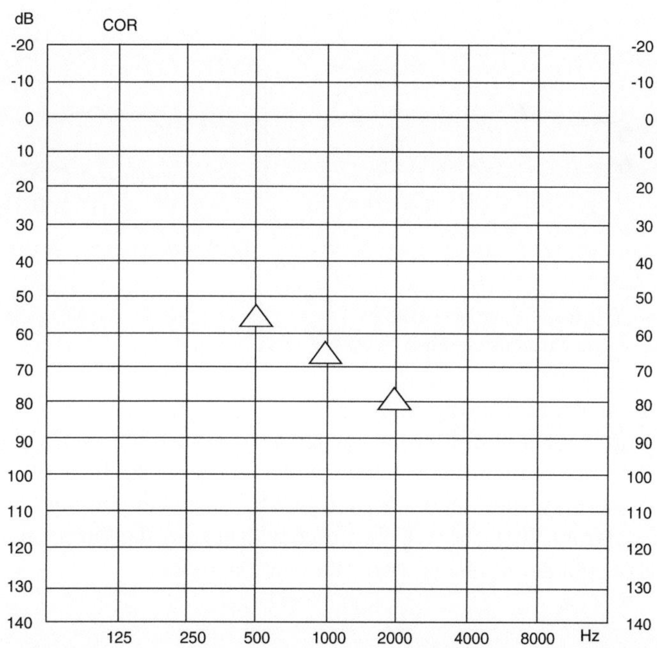

Fig. 6.44 Audiogram of PPHN patient #4 at 1 year and 6 months

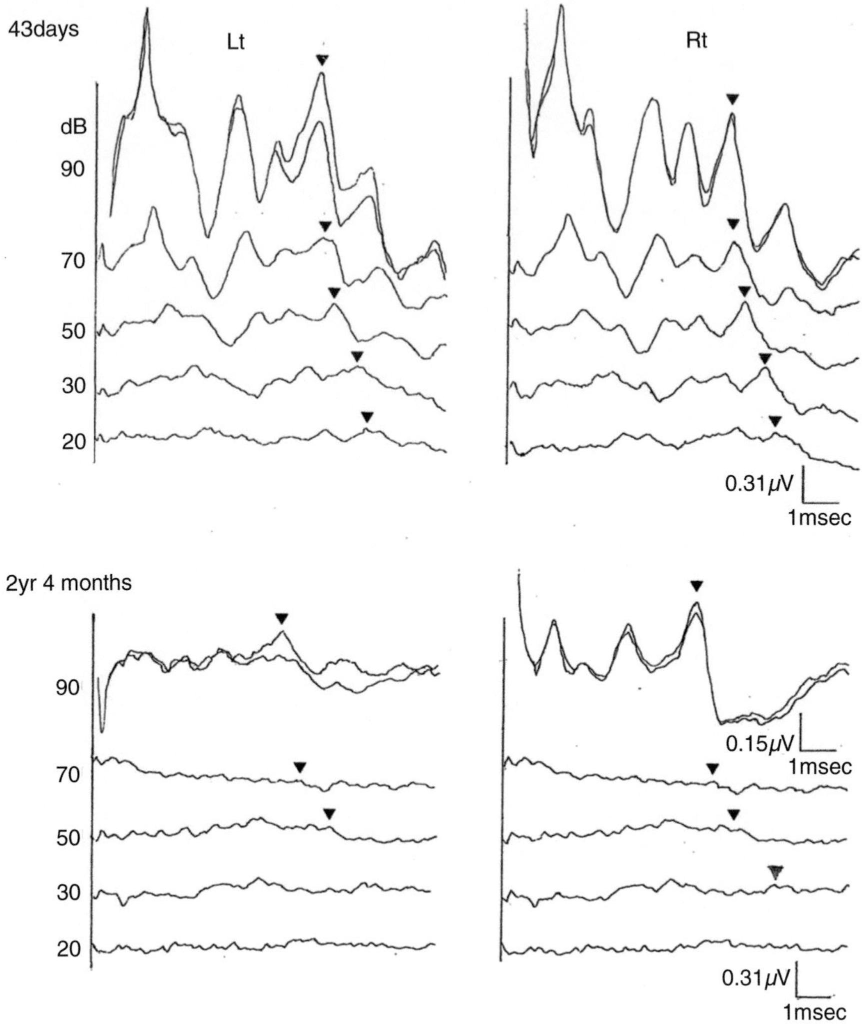

Fig. 6.45 Serial ABRs of patient #5. ABR at 43 days of life was normal. But when she was 2 years and 4 months of age, moderate elevation of wave V was evident

Patient 7—male, PPHN (Fig. 6.47).

He was born 3400 g of birth weight at 42 weeks gestation. His APGAR was 6 at 1 min. He had severe neonatal asphyxia, MAS, and PPHN. His cardiorespiratory dysfunction was so severe that he needed ECMO treatment. During his follow-up after discharge from NICU, he was diagnosed with hearing deterioration. Other than hearing, his overall development was within normal range.

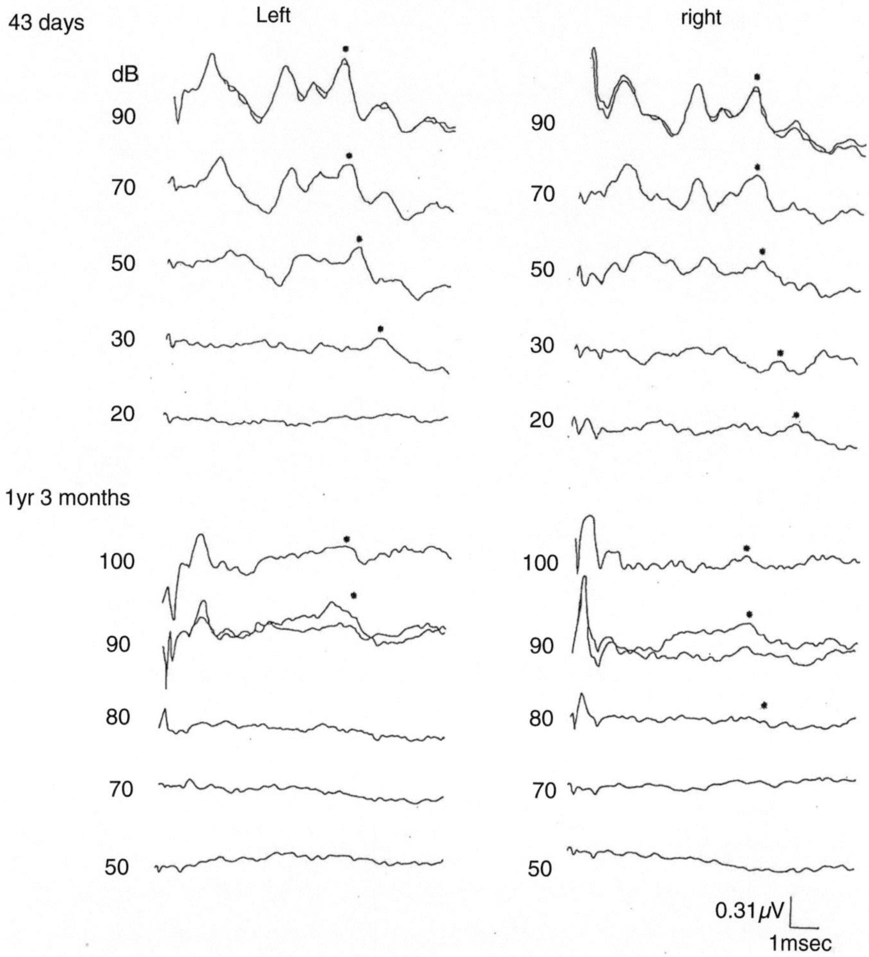

Fig. 6.46 Serial ABRs of patient #6. Her ABR on day 43 was normal to high frequent clicks. ABR at 1 year and 3 months, definitive bilateral threshold elevation was present

Patient 8—female, PPHN (Fig. 6.48).

She was born at full term with 3200 g of her birth weight. Her APGAR score was 1 and 5 for 1 and 5 min. She had MAS and PPHN. Serial ABR recordings revealed a normal record at day 32 but no response at 12 months. Later follow-up at 3 years, she had cerebral palsy, intellectual disabilities along with profound hearing loss.

Patient 9—male, PPHN (Figs. 6.49 and 6.50).

He was born with 2900 g of birth weight at 40 weeks gestation. Massive aspiration syndrome was noted. His APGAR was 2 at 1 min then intubated immediately and was on mechanical ventilation for 3 days. He had pneumothorax and pneumomediastinum. Respiratory failure was severe but could be survived. At 6 years of age, he had cerebral palsy and was intellectually retarded.

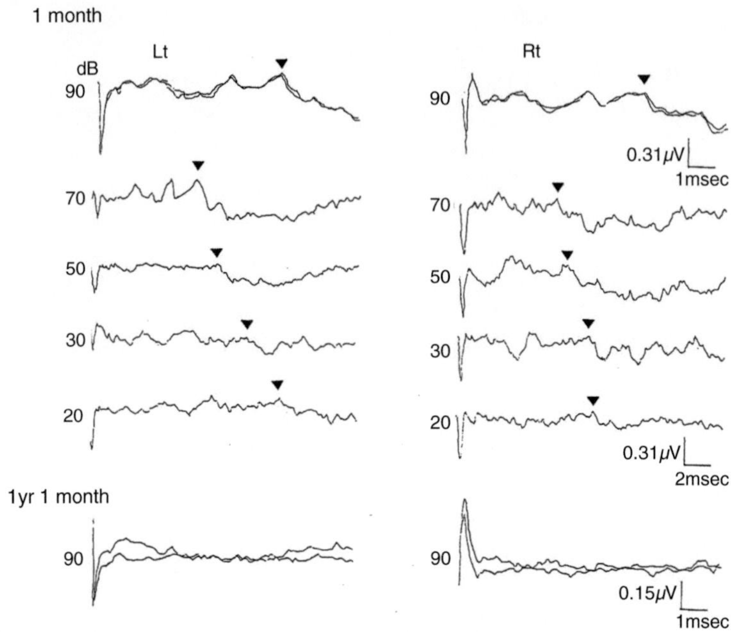

Fig. 6.47 Serial ABR of patient #7. His ABR was completely normal at 1 month of his age but no response 1 year later

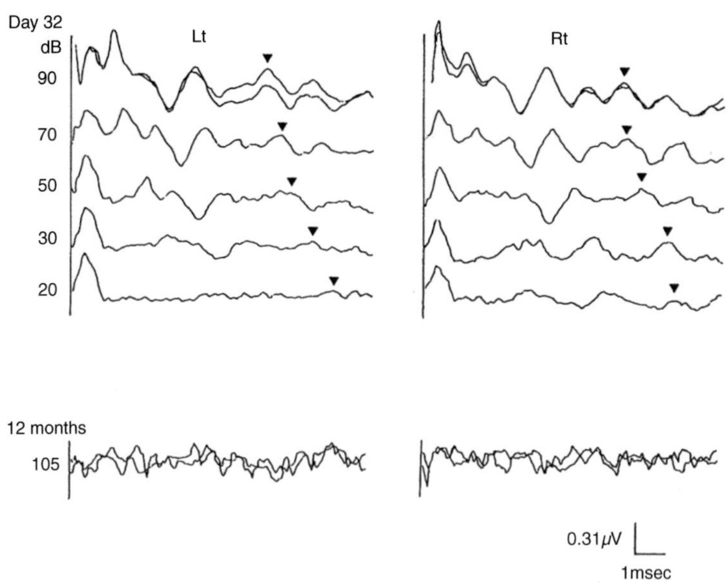

Fig. 6.48 Serial ABR recordings of patient #8. ABRs revealed normal record on day 32 but no response at 12 months

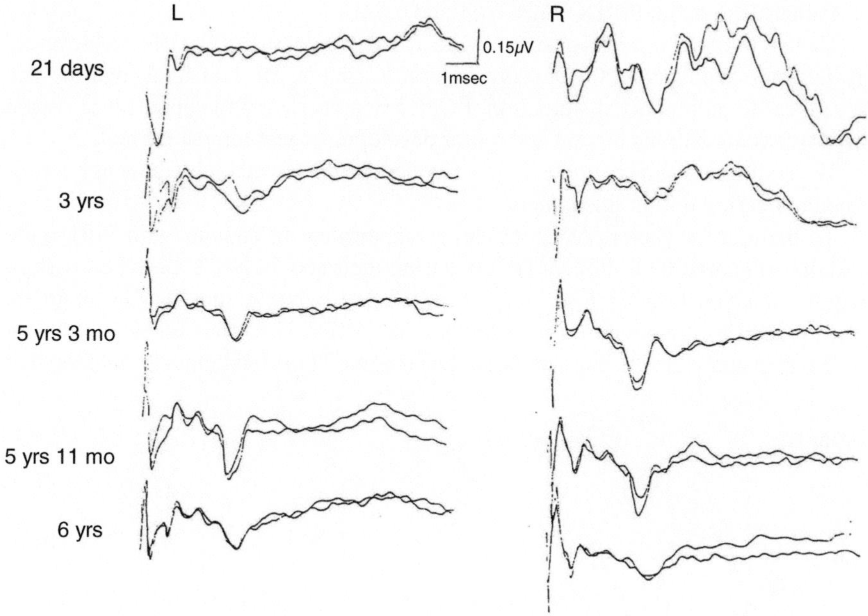

Fig. 6.49 Serial ABRs from 21 days to 6 years in patient #9. From day 21, his left ABR showed abnormal response with marked threshold elevation. On the right side, ABR showed normal configuration at high-intensity click stimuli but gradual deterioration is evident from 5 years and 3 months of his age

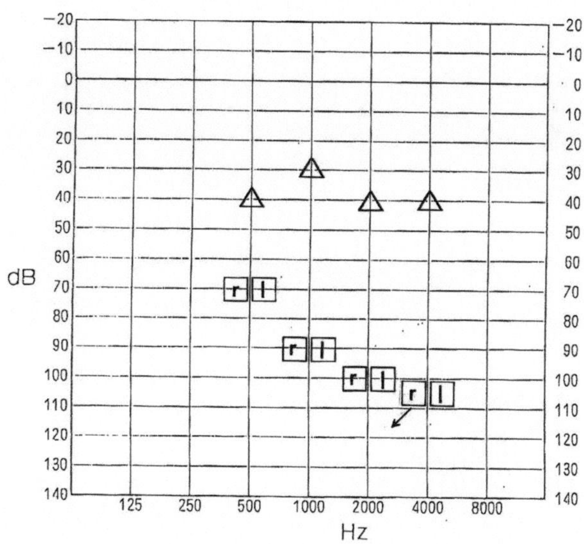

Fig. 6.50 Audiogram by behavior observation audiometry (BOA) at 4 years and 3 months (triangle) and electrically evoked response audiometry (ABR) at 4 years and 9 months (square) of patient #9. ABR threshold was worse than that of BOA at 3 months

Patient 10—male, PPHN (Figs. 6.51 and 6.52).

He was born at 36 weeks gestation with a birth weight of 3600 g. He was severely asphyxiated with his APGAR score of 1 at a minute. He had fetal hydrops and severe cardiopulmonary dysfunction. ECMO was necessary to support him. When he was 3 years old, his mental and motor development was almost normal.

His audiogram shows moderate low frequency and severe high-frequency sensorineural hearing loss in this patient.

To find out the factors of later hearing impairment in patients with PPHN, the authors compared their clinical factors during their stay in NICU based on with or without delayed hearing loss (Table 6.3). Severe hypoxia and ECMO treatment were related to the condition in patients with PPHN. However, ECMO treatment means extremely severe hypoxemia in the patients. Thus, the author concluded that

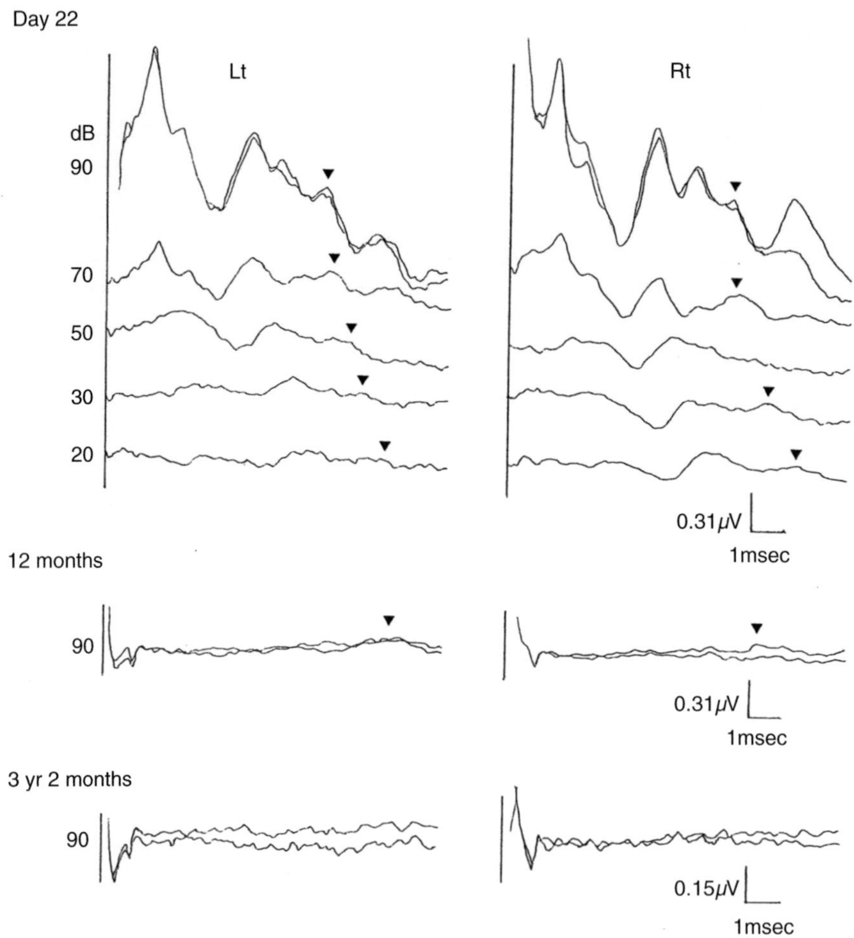

Fig. 6.51 Serial ABRs of patient #10, male, PPHN. On day 22, ABR configuration was normal with normal wave V threshold. At 12 months of age, extreme threshold elevation to 90 dBHL was presented. Follow-up ABR at 12 months showed severe threshold elevation but no response at 3 years and 2 months old

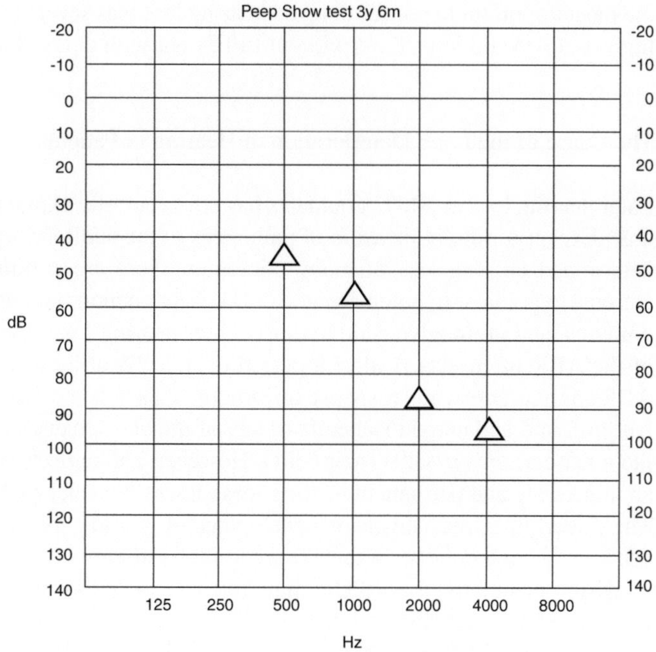

Fig. 6.52 Audiogram revealed by BOA in patient #10. His audiogram shows moderate low frequency and severe high-frequency sensorineural hearing loss in this patient. Behavior Observation Audiometry at 4 years and 4 months

Table 6.3 Perinatal factors and hearing in PPHN. Among 23 patients with PPHN, with or without hearing loss, neonatal risk factors are compared. Usage of ECMO treatment was the most effective component ($p < 0.01$), which means they had the severest respiratory condition in NICU

Hearing	Impaired	Normal	
N	8	15	23
GA (weeks)	40.3 ± 1.9	36.4 ± 6.1	n.s.
BW (g)	3.207 ± 360.0	2563.7 ± 940.0	$p < 0.05$
Apgar (1 min)	6.1 ± 2.0	5.3 ± 2.6	n.s.
Admission (days)	69.5 ± 44.2	68.7 ± 55.9	n.s.
MV (days)	30.9 ± 17.7	20.9 ± 24.4	$p < 0.05$
HFO	37.5%	20%	n.s.
ECMO	75%	0%	$p < 0.01$
pH < 7.25	75%	20%	$p < 0.05$
SpO_2 < 80% 1 h	75%	26.7%	$p < 0.05$
BP < 40 mmHg	50%	20%	n.s.
$PaCO_2$ > 90 mmHg	37.5%	13.3%	n.s.
$PaCO_2$ < 25 mmHg	62.5%	53.3%	n.s.
Gentamicin	100%	93.3%	n.s.
Amikacin	50%	6.7%	$p < 0.05$
Furosemide	100%	73.7%	n.s.
Muscle relaxant	100%	60%	$p < 0.05$
Dopamine	100%	100%	n.s.

Wilcoxon test or χ^2 test

the most important factor for delayed hearing loss was severe hypoxemia. This finding was also valid in patients without PPHN but with delayed hearing loss.

The Cause of the Later Deterioration of Hearing in Patients

Later hearing loss in NICU graduates has not been fully explained and may be variable. Except for direct invasion of pathogens to the auditory organs and genetically determined hearing loss of many etiologies, there are common pathologies like extreme hypoxia or hypotension and concordant phenomena such as acidosis, use of diuretics, and aminoglycoside toxicity. Later hearing loss along with deterioration of the ABR often occurs after a period of intact hearing as confirmed by normal ABR configurations and response thresholds. This delayed hearing loss is enigmatic but profound and anoxia/ischemia or any of the above causes may directly damage the inner ear sensory cells (hair cells). However, anoxia/ischemia usually results in an immediate and permanent hearing loss rather than a delayed and permanent one. The underlying mechanism of developmental hearing loss in PPHN infants and anoxia/ischemia does seem to have a common etiology.

Kirino postulated that PPHN may give rise to "delayed neuronal death" in the hippocampus and confirmed this possibility by means of an excellent experimental technique [47]. This delayed neuronal death has not been confirmed to occur in neural tissue other than the hippocampus. However, Koga et al. suggested the possibility of a similar phenomenon of delayed hearing impairment in the inner ear of gerbils [48]. Their experimental animals lacked the posterior communicating artery which connects to the Circle of Willis. They temporally blocked the blood flow of the bilateral vertebral artery for 5 min and then re-canalized blood flow. Serial recordings of electrocochleogram (ECoG) thresholds revealed immediate elevations of thresholds and loss of action potentials (AP) upon restricting the vertebral artery. Three days after their experiment, the threshold and amplitude of ECoG gradually recovered in all animals. However, on the fifth day post-blockage, the ECoG thresholds of some of these experimental animals again elevated which suggests inner hair cell damage followed by damage to the outer hair cells.

This experiment implies that "delayed neuronal death" in PPHN is primarily localized to the inner ear, but to resolve the difficult clinical questions in such children, more definitive research is necessary.

Other examples of delayed hearing loss in infants, other than non-PPHN NICU graduates, are due to congenital CMV infection, congenital toxoplasmosis, and infants who have survived other difficult episodes in the NICU.

6.3.2 Deterioration of ABR in Degenerative Diseases

The classification of metabolic degenerative diseases is rapidly changing because of the recent developments in molecular biology and genetic analytical techniques. On the other hand, the classical clinical determination of neuropathological findings has become somewhat disvalued. Many of these diseases are often progressive, resulting in severe to profound disability and even death. ABRs are and continue to be useful not only to delineate organic or functional lesions but as a follow-up technique during recovery to assess the effectiveness of gene therapy, enzyme replacement therapy (ERT), and hematopoietic stem cell transplantation (HSCT).

At first, degenerative disease related to infection and immunological factors is shown. Then, the diseases which have been classically characterized by a degenerative loss of white matter (leukodystrophy) and the gray matter are discussed. Many of the diseases are based on metabolic disorders and genetic degenerative pathologies. Genetic aberrations affecting the cerebrum, the cerebellum, and the spinal cord sometimes with the involvement of visceral organs are also discussed with an additional discussion of diseases that mainly affect the peripheral nervous system.

6.3.2.1 Slow Virus Infection

Creutzfeldt-Jakob Disease (CJD) due to abnormal prion, progressive multifocal leukoencephalopathy due to PAPOVA virus, subacute sclerosing panencephalitis (SSPE) due to measles virus are well-known slow virus infections. They have clinical characteristics of a long time incubation period from the onset of infection to the onset of disease, are slowly progressive and result in devastating prognosis. In this section, serial ABRs in three patients with SSPE are shown.

6.3.2.2 Subacute Sclerosing Panencephalitis

The cause is measles infection usually in the early period of life. Subacute Sclerosing Panencephalitis (SSPE) occurs after a few years of latent period of measles infection. During that period measles virus progressively invade into central nervous system and made deterioration of mental and nervous system functions such as intellectual deterioration, motor regression, seizures, character change, and physical functions. It is a devastating disease and causes patients to death. For a long time, there was no way to treat SSPE. But injection of Interferon through spinal fluid or cerebral ventricular space has some effect to improve the symptoms. Oral Isoprinosine Pranobex and Rivabilin have some effecsts to treat SSPE. Introduction of measles vaccine to infants and children dramatically reduces the incidence of measles itself and as a result SSPE. It is going to be a past disease but not yet to be eliminated. Evoked potentials in SSPE have been reported in the literature [49, 50]. Inagaki et al. reported that ABR deterioration in a patient with fulminant type was extremely fast compared with ordinary type of SSPE.

Serial ABRs in three patients with SSPE are shown in Figs. 6.53, 6.54, and 6.55.

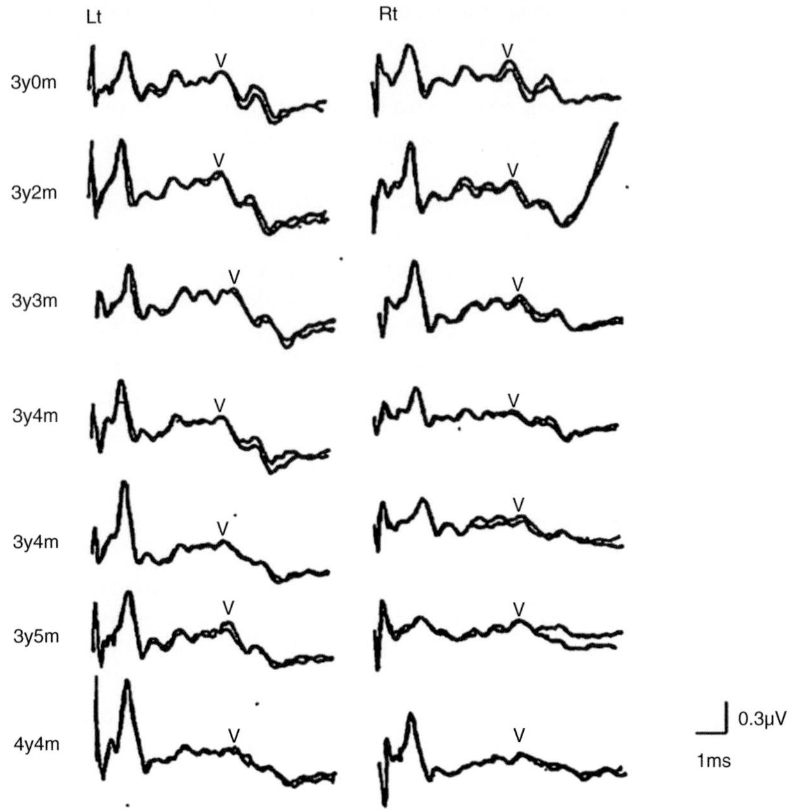

Fig. 6.53 Serial ABRs of SSPE Patient #1, male, 3 years old. Relatively early-onset type. He suffered from measles at 1 year of age, SSPE was diagnosed at 3 years old. Progressive deterioration of ABR is observed [50]

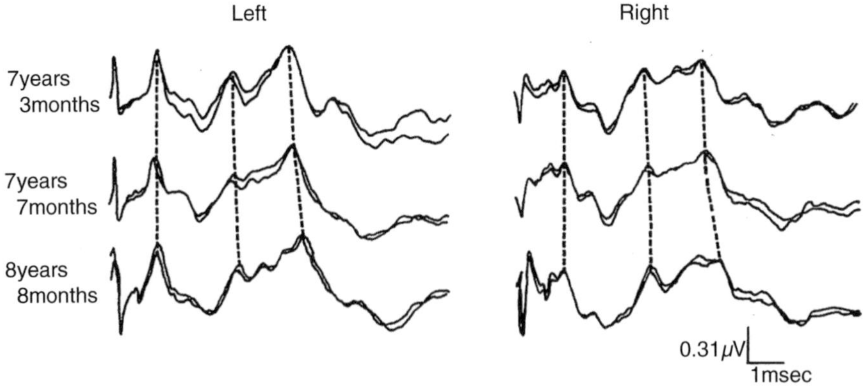

Fig. 6.54 Serial ABRs of SSPE patient #2, female, 7 years old. She suffused from measles at 1 year of age. SSPE was diagnosed at 7 years of age. Physical and mental deterioration progressed slowly and steadily. During one and a half year, waves I and V interpeak latency prolonged

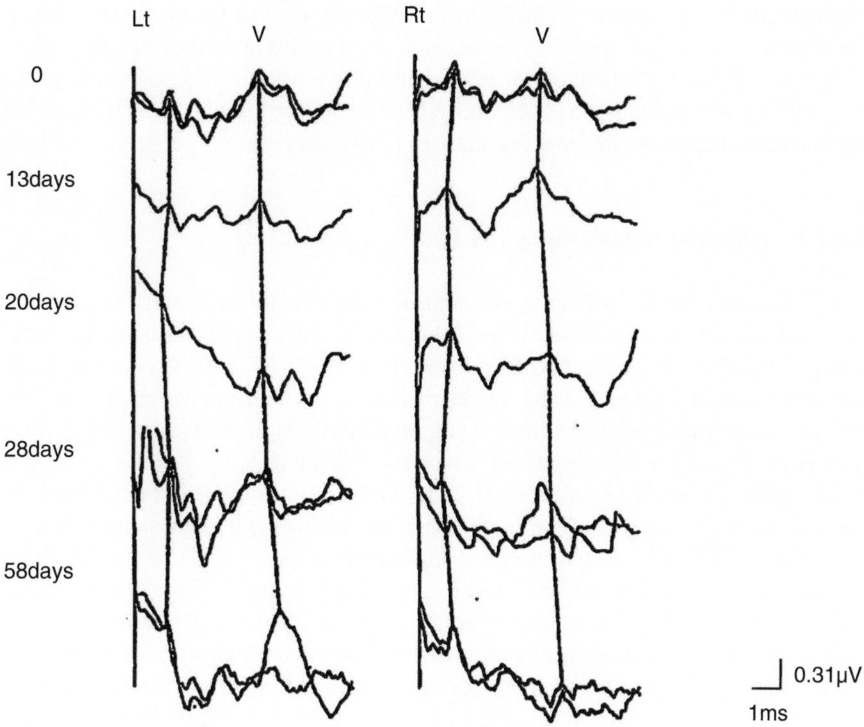

Fig. 6.55 Serial ABRs of SSPE patient #3. Eleven years old female with fulminant type of SSPE. She had measles at 1 year and a half. She developed and diagnosed SSPE at 11 years old. Both her clinical symptoms and ABR deteriorate so rapidly. Serial ABRs are recorded from the first day of admission and followed thereafter [50]

6.3.3 Leukodystrophies

Leukodystrophy is the neuropathology-orientated classification of the diseases which means main brain lesions are white matter instead of gray matter of the brain. The etiology of this neuropathology is variable and the biological/genetic molecular etiology has been studied over many decades. The serial ABR recordings of various leukodystrophy patients are presented below:

1. Adrenoleukodystrophy (ALD)
2. Globoid cell leukodystrophy (GLD)
3. Metachromatic leukodystrophy (MLD)
4. Alexander disease (AXD)
5. Pelizaeus-Merbacher disease (PMD)
6. Others

In this regard, however, Pelizaeus-Merzbacher disease (PMD) at present is not classified as leukodystrophy but a disease of poor myelination as a simplified explanation. White matter of the brain in PMD shows insufficient myelin sheath development instead of destructive process of myelin. But in this section, the author includes PMD into the category of leukodystrophies. Moreover, responsible genes of most leukodystrophies, have become to be already clarified and underlying metabolic mechanisms have become evident.

6.3.3.1 Adrenoleukodystrophy (ALD)

Adrenoleukodystrophy (ALD) is an X-linked recessive and degenerative metabolic disease caused by the mutation of *ABCD1* gene. ALD is classified into eight clinical subtypes: childhood cerebral ALD, adolescent cerebral ALD, adult cerebral ALD, adrenomyeloneuropathy (AMN), Addison's disease, brainstem-cerebellum ALG, female symptomatic type, and male asymptomatic types. In one particular family, a variety of these ALD types were expressed at different ages.

Gene therapy of ALD was introduced to clinical trial study [51] but at this poit, it has been just a pilot study. Thus early diagnosis and hematopoietic stem cell transplantatin (HSCT) are the only rearistic combination of treatment of patients with cerebral type of ALD. ALD has a devastating nature to cause patients to bedridden and to death usually within a few years as a natural course, especially in cerebral types. Childhood cerebral type is most devastating and begins as gait disturbance, decrement of academic achievement, central visual/auditory impairment, character change, and others at 5–10 years of age. It needed early HSCT therapy as best as we can. Recent treatment introduction to adult cerebral type is plausible but it is not a widely used procedure at this point [52].

The AMN (adrenomyeloneuropathy) type usually begins in adults during their thirties or forties, the symptoms of which include gait disturbances as a result of spinal cord pathology and sensory abnormalities of the affected spinal cord segments, often with genitourinary symptoms. In about half of these AMN patients' their symptoms progress to the adult cerebral type.

Soon after the ABR was discovered and became clinically available, ABR recordings have been used to evaluate and monitor the progression of ALD, and the lesions of nervous system of this disease. Ochs et al. [53] recorded serial ABRs of his leukodystrophy patients and demonstrated the sequential changes of the ABR over time [53]. In 2006, Inagaki reported the successive ABR, VEP, and SEP recording in patients with ALD [54].

Examples of serial change of ABR and VEP are shown in Figs. 6.56 and 6.57.

6.3.3.2 Krabbe Disease, Globoid Cell Leukodystrophy (GLD)

Krabbe disease (Globoid cell leukodystrophy, GLD) is a rare autosomal-recessive disease due to the mutation of gene-related to β-galactosyl ceramidase. Deficient production of this enzyme results in demyelination of the central (oligodendroglia) and peripheral (Schwann cell) nervous systems [55]. The clinical manifestations of

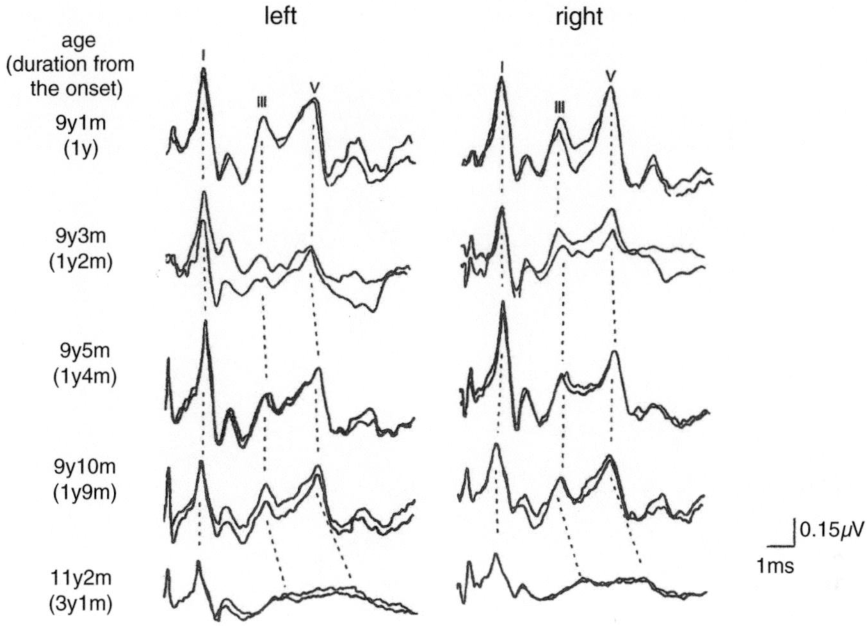

Fig. 6.56 Serial change of ABR in a patient with ALD from 9 to 11 years of age. Progressive prolongation of later components of ABR with elongation of interwave latencies are evident by 1 year and 9 months from the onset of the disease. Wave V, component of ABR gradually delays and seems to disappear [54]

GLD are age related: infantile (3–6 months of onset), late infantile (7 months to 3 years), childhood (4–8 years), and adult (9 years or older). The most typical and most serious is the infantile type. It manifests as poor feeding ability, irritability, and loss of head control. The disease progresses rapidly and infants are usually bedridden before their first birthday and die at 2–3 years of age. Modern medical techniques and skilled caretaking have extended the lifespan of some of these patients to more than 30 years. Nevertheless, Krabbe disease (GLD) is still a devastating genetic disorder.

In 1993 Yamanouchi et al. reported serial auditory evoked response in three patients with GLD [56]. These ABRs showed prolonged latencies of all the waves, increased interpeak latencies, and decreased amplitudes of the later waves which ultimately were not evoked, except wave I which persisted (Fig. 6.58). A characteristic change in these patients was the apparent latency delay of wave I which persisted. A characteristic change in these patients was apparent latency delay of wave I which was parallel to the delayed nerve conduction velocity. This finding is typical for peripheral neuropathy. Serial auditory evoked responses were investigated in three children with GLD. ABR revealed prolongation of each wave component and interpeak latency with decreased amplitudes in later components which finally disappeared except for wave I. Long-latency auditory responses (LLRs) persisted in the advanced stage when all wave components of middle-latency auditory responses

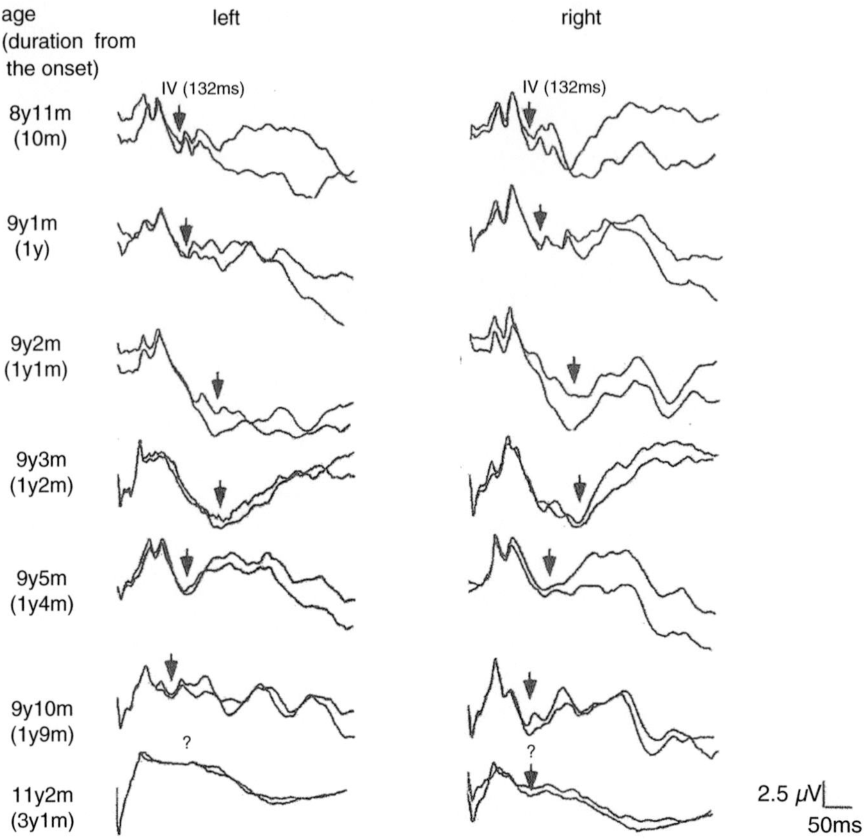

Fig. 6.57 Serial change of VEP in a patient with ALD. Wave shape of VEP gradually comes down during 3 years from the onset of the disease [54]

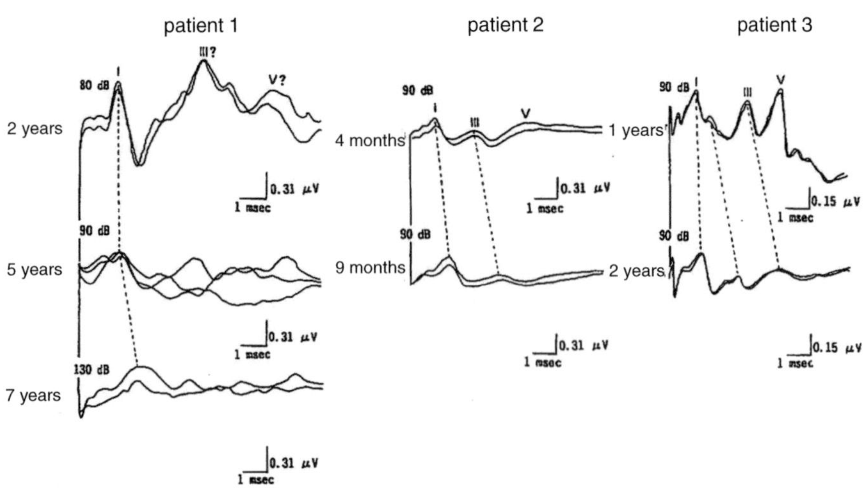

Fig. 6.58 Serial ABR change in three patients with GLD [56]

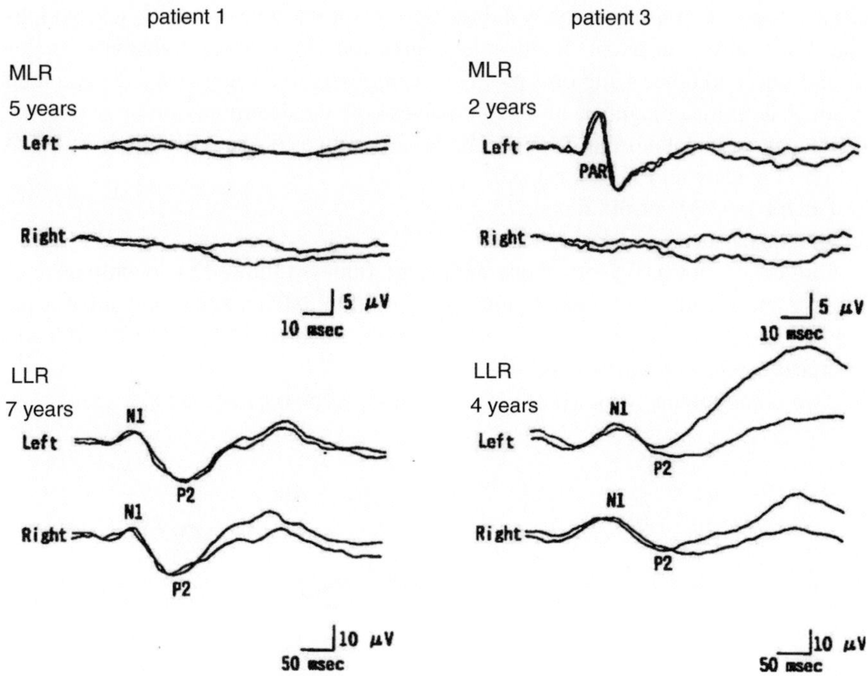

Fig. 6.59 Middle- and long-latency response in two patients with GLD [56]

(MLRs) had disappeared (Fig. 6.59). The results of auditory brainstem responses and MLRs are compatible with magnetic resonance imaging findings and a review of pathologic findings in Krabbe disease, including extensive involvement of brainstem and subcortical structures. It is suggested that the source of LLR waves is different from that of MLR because of the persistent retension of LLR waves. It is speculated that the cerebral cortex and/or subcortical U fibers which are spared in Krabbe disease, have an important role in generating LLR wave components.

Aldosari in 2004 indicated, in his pre-clinical patients, that ABR abnormalities were more diagnostic than visually evoked potentials (VEPs) to ascertain the earliest sign of central nervous system involvement [57].

6.3.3.3 Metachromatic Leukodystrophy (MLD)

Metachromatic Leukodystrophy (MLD) is an autosomal-recessive metabolic disease due to deficiency of arylsulfatase, which is a lysosomal enzyme. As a result, sulfatide is stored in central/peripheral nervous system and visceral organs. Demyelination occurs throughout the entire nervous system. The clinical types are late infantile (onset at 2–4 years old), juvenile (4–6 years old), and adult type (16 year or older). Patients with MLD eventually develop psychomotor deterioration. Death commonly results from pneumonia within 3–10–20 years based on the clinical types. Clumsiness, toe walking, slurred speech, hypertonicity, and peripheral neuropathy can occur. Intellectual regression, dysarthria, clumsiness, motor disabilities, and other symptoms progress relentlessly to a vegetative state and then death. A definitive diagnosis of MLD involves both the determination of an enzyme deficiency and an abnormal *ARSA* gene. Serial changes of the ABRs in three MLD patients are shown in Figs. 6.60, 6.61, and 6.62.

Patient 1—17-year-old female (Fig. 6.60).

Diagnosis; Juvenile type of MLD.

Clinical onset was 6 years of age with forgetfulness followed by incontinence of bladder and rectum, and mental/motor deterioration. ABR shows conductive hearing loss and pontine lesions because of the prolonged latency of bilateral wave I and interpeak latency of waves I and III.

Two other patients with MLD are presented in Figs. 6.61 and 6.62.

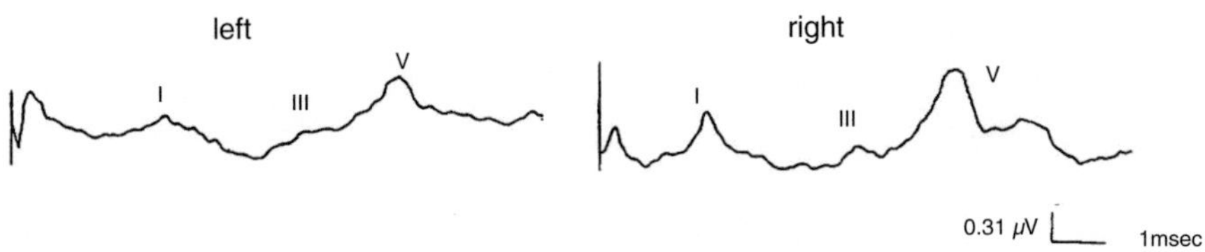

Fig. 6.60 ABR of patient #1 with MLD. Juvenile type. Prolonged latency of both sides of wave I and I–III, I–V interwave latency on the right side. These findings suggest conductive hearing loss in both sides and brainstem dysfunction [58]

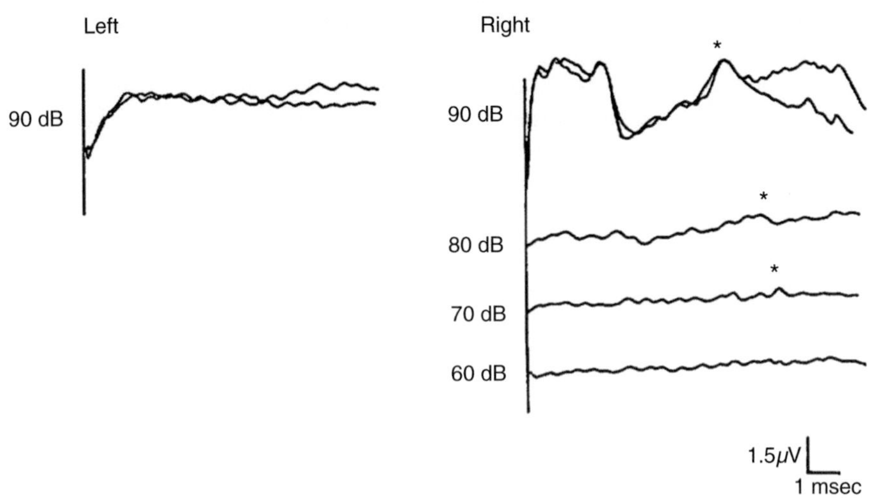

Fig. 6.61 ABR of patient #2 with MLD, 11 months old, male. Infantile type. Prolonged latency of wave I, non-detectable wave III in the right lead and elevated bilateral intensity threshold. Bilateral hearing impairment and apparent brainstem dysfunction are present [59]

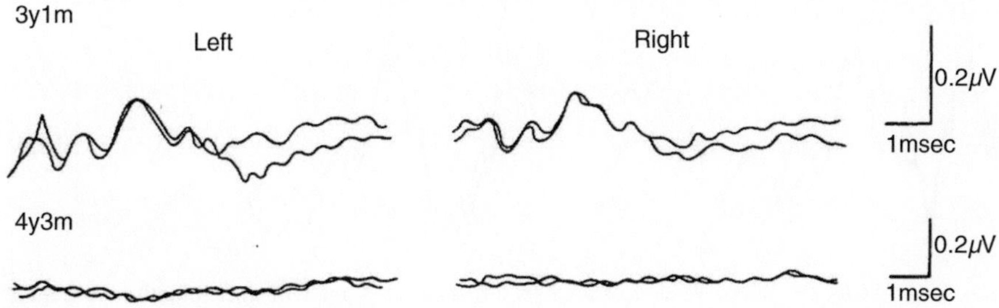

Fig. 6.62 ABR of patient #3 with MLD. Male. His ABR was already abnormal at 3 years 1 month of age but disappeared at 4 years and 3 months of his age. Progressive nature of MLD is evident [23, 24]

6.3.3.4 Alexander Disease (AXD)

A mutation of *giant fibrillary acidic protein gene* (*GFAP gene*) located on chromosome 17q21 is the underlying cause of AXD and determining this mutation is the key to diagnosis. AXD is an autosomal-recessive degenerative disease that results in megalencephaly. A hallmark clinical indicator of this disease is the deterioration of psychomotor ability. Post-mortem neuropathological studies have revealed demyelination of the cerebral white matter, fibral gliosis, and the conspicuous appearance of numerous Rosenthal fibers. AXD is classified as being infantile, juvenile, and adult types and 80% of these cases are of the infantile type with onset between 3 and 24 months. Clinically, it manifests as poor psychomotor ability, enlargement of the cranium, spastic palsy, and epilepsy. MRI scans have revealed symmetrical demyelination, predominantly in the frontal lobes, lesions of the basal ganglia, thalamus, and the brainstem.

ABR recordings of patients with the infantile type of AXD in two patients and one patient with the juvenile type are shown in the figures. Patient 1 had extremely delayed ABR waves at his age of 3 years (Fig. 6.63). Serial changes of ABR in patient 2 show relatively slow change of central conduction during 2 years and 7 months (Fig. 6.64). In patient 3 with juvenile type, the prolonged central conduction seems slow which was in parallel with the relatively stable her clinical condition (Fig. 6.65).

6.3.3.5 Pelizaeus-Merzbacher Disease (PMD)

Pelizaeus-Merzbacher disease (PMD) is an X-linked recessive inherited disease. Mutation or duplication of *proteolipid protein* gene (*PLP1 gene*) located on chromosome Xq22 is the cause of this disease. Abnormal PLP protein induces apoptosis of oligodendrocytes and abnormal PLP synthesis results in generalized dysmyelination sparing the axons. The clinical classification of PMD is threefold: the classical type, the conatal type, and PLP-null syndrome with spastic paraplegia type 2. The involvement

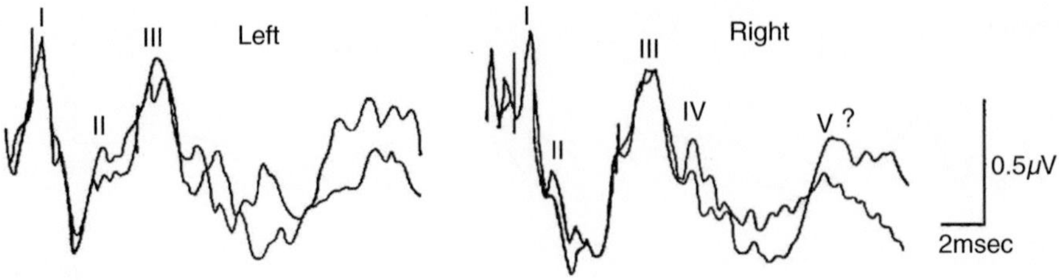

Fig. 6.63 ABRs of patient #1 with Alexander's disease at 3 years of age. Infantile type, male [23, 24]

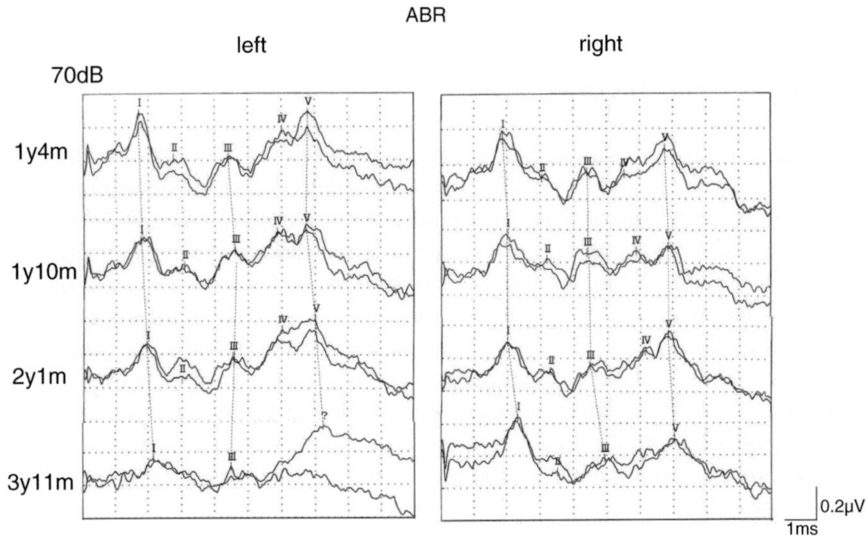

Fig. 6.64 Serial ABRs of patient #2 with infantile type of Alexander disease, female. Slowly progressive prolongation of ABR waves and distortion of wave shape during 2 years and 7 months

of each type is ambiguous, and a transitional type is often diagnosed. The classical type is the severest one and appears shortly after birth. In this form, marked hypotonia and nystagmus are the conspicuous findings followed by head tremor, spastic paralysis, ataxia, and other involuntary movements. Delayed and deteriorating psychomotor disabilities progresses and death occurs between the patient's teens to twenties. Their MRIs reveal overall dysgenesis of their white matter. ABRs from PMD patients are known to include wave I or waves I and II [60]. In spite of this, OAEs are usually normal. This may remind us a type of auditory neuropathy. Auditory discrimination usually remains normal or near normal [61]. Historically, PMD has been thought of as a degenerative disease affecting the myelination of the cortical white matter, however, post-mortem neuropathological findings have shown that PMD is not a demyelinating disease but rather hypoplasia or dysplasia of the white matter. This could explain why

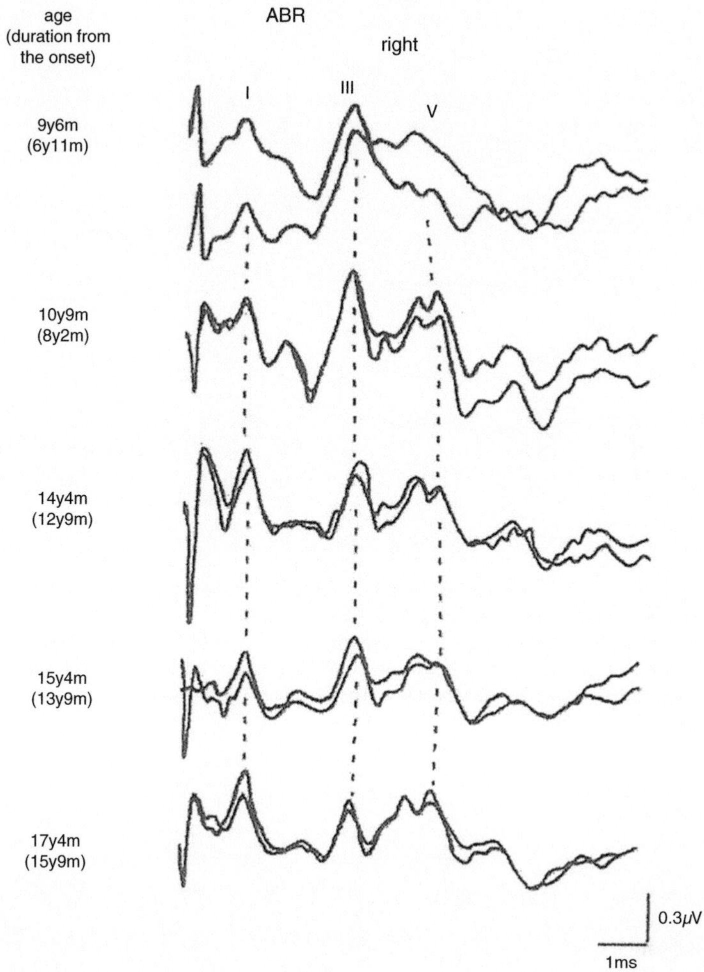

Fig. 6.65 Serial ABRs of patient #3 with Alexander disease. Juvenile type, female. ABR deterioration was not evident for 8 years and 10 months of her disease

serial ABRs show a limited improvement over time such as an evoked wave II or the shortened latency of wave I. ABRs in three patients are presented in Figs. 6.66, 6.67, and 6.68.

Thus, serial ABR shows a limited improvement of ABR such as apparent wave II along with wave I or shortened latency of wave I.

Patient 3 is 55 years old male. From his present history, he has been suffering infantile type of PMD as far. But it is a good fortune that he has enjoyed his life even now despite of slowly progressive nature of the disease.

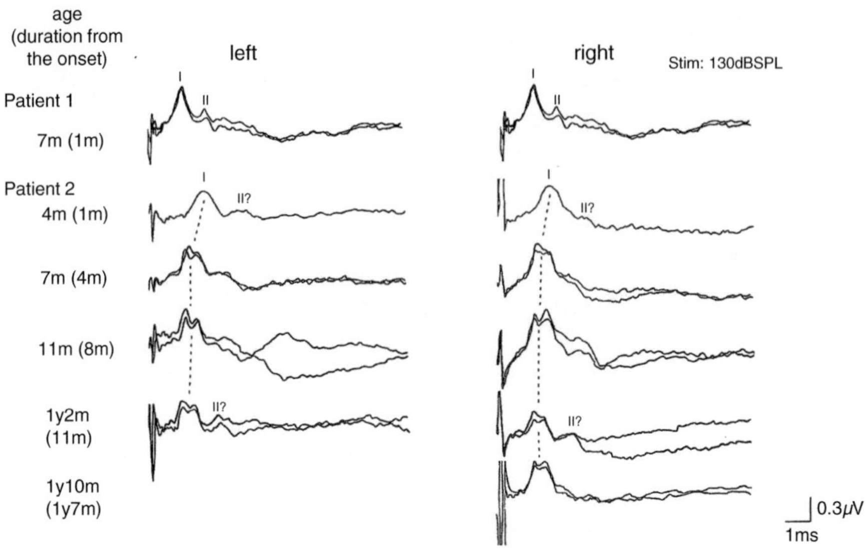

Fig. 6.66 Single ABR at 7 months of Patient #1 with PMD and serial ABRs of patient #2 with PMD. Patient #1 shows only waves I and II bilaterally at 7 months of age. Patient #2 shows serial shortening of wave I latency. It seems wave II sometimes can be apparent. His ABR does not seem to deteriorate during 1 year and 6 months follow-up. But latency of P100 of VEP was apparently prolonged during the same period. Moreover, when he was 3 years and 7 months, VEP could not be recorded

Fig. 6.67 Serial change of flash evoked VEPs of patient #2 with PMD. Contrary to ABRs, VEP seems to show progressive worsening (wave prolongation of a wave of wave IV) during rather a short period. Prolongation of P100 might reflect congenital nystagmus, progress of optic atrophy, and poor vision

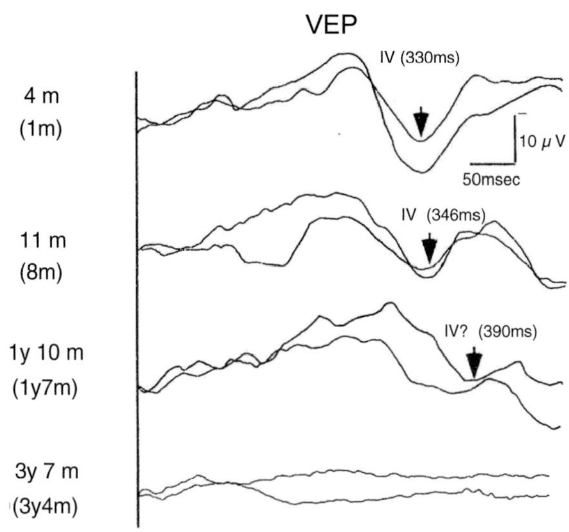

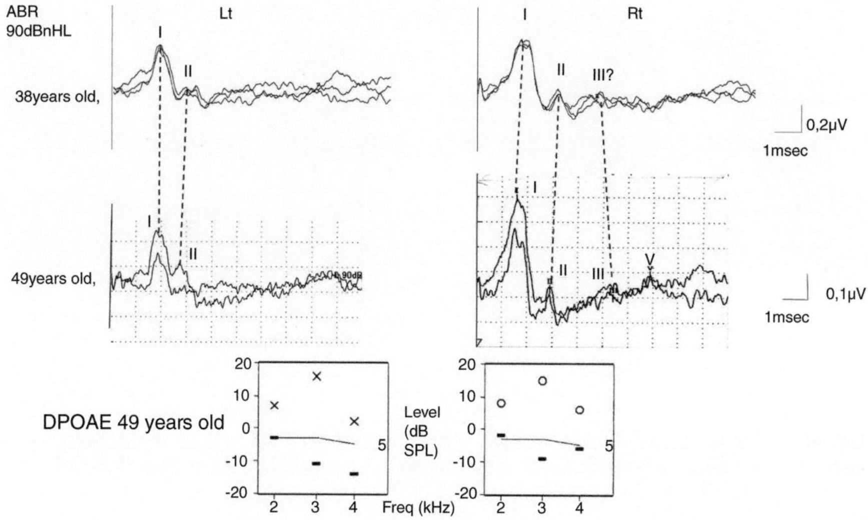

Fig. 6.68 Serial ABR in patient #3 with PMD. Fifty-five years old, male. Infantile type of PMD with longevity as a natural course. Shortening of wave II on both sides and seemingly the appearance or later waves in right side recording. OAE at 49 years of age was completely normal

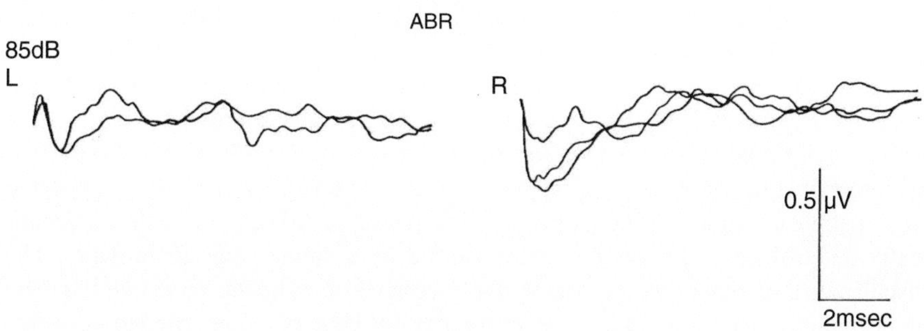

Fig. 6.69 ABR of a patient with leukodystrophy of which lesions were located mainly in the cerebellum and the brainstem. Two years and 7 months old [3]

6.3.3.6 Leukodystrophy of Unknown Origin

Other rare types of leukodystrophy have been found and explored which is not fully understood nor classified appropriately. A patient with such a leukodystrophy was described prior to the advent of molecular biology [62]. This patient's ABR was recorded only once at the age of 4 years just before several months of her death. The post-mortem pathological changes were the severest in her cerebellum and brainstem. These ABR (Fig. 6.69) and pathological findings (Fig. 6.70) are illustrated in the figures.

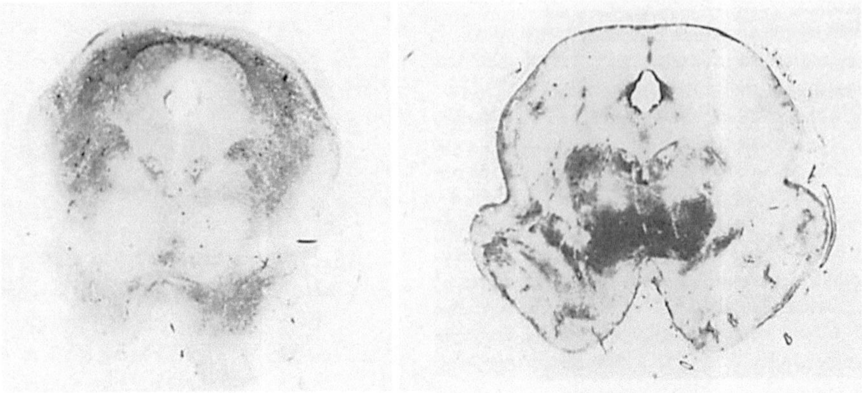

Fig. 6.70 Brainstem pathology of autopsy 4 months after her ABR was recorded. Sections of midbrain and medulla oblongata. Extensive demyelination is present (Kluber-Barrella stain) [62]

6.3.4 Lysosomal Diseases

Lysosomal diseases are inherited metabolic diseases because of genetic deficiency of the enzyme proteins in lysosome. As a result, dicreaced activity of relevant enzymes makes the concerned disease develop. The collective term for such diseases is a lysosomal disease, and more than 60 variants are already known. The Ministry of Health, Labor and Welfare of Japan has designated 30 of them (Table 6.4) as intractable diseases, seeks to inform caretakers and to provide welfare support to such patients/families and encourage clinical research. All these variants are genetically determined progressive diseases caused by a single gene abnormality. The usual mode of inheritance is autosomal-recessive or X-linked recessive. Genetic abnormalities and their defective enzyme proteins have been identified in most diseases. The list of the main lysosomal diseases is shown in Table 6.4.

These metabolic disorders are wide ranging and involve abnormalities in the production of lipids, mucopolysaccharides, ceroid lipofuscin, glycogen, and cholesterol transport.

6.3.4.1 Lipidosis

Tay-Sachs Disease

Tay-Sachs disease is an inherited autosomal-recessive disorder caused by impaired activity of beta-*N*-acetyl hexosaminidase A. Then GM2 ganglioside accumulate in the lysosome and cause damage to the central nervous system. The onset of this disease occurs within 3–5 months after birth. Mental and motor deterioration progresses

Table 6.4 A list of intractable lysosomal diseases compiled by the Ministry of Health, Labor and Welfare in Japan (April, 2022)

Gaucher's disease	
Nieman-Pick disease	Type A
	Type C
GM1 gangliosidosis	
GM2 gangliosidosis	Tay-Sachs disease
	Sandhoff disease A type, B type
Krabbe disease	(Globoid cell leukodystrophy, GLD)
Metachromatic leukodystrophy	(MLD)
Multiple sulfatase deficiency	
Farber disease	
Mucopolysaccharidosis	Type I (Hurler/Scheie syndrome)
	Type II (Hunter syndrome)
	Type III (Sanfilippo syndrome)
	Type IV (Morquio syndrome)
	Type VI (Maroteaux-Lamy syndrome)
	Type VII (Sly disease)
	Type IX (Hyaluronidase deficiency)
Sialidosis	
Galactosialidosis	
Mucolipidoseis	Type II
	Type III
α-Mannnocidosis	
β-Mannnocidosisfucosidosis	
Fucosidosis	
Aspartylglucosaminuria	
Schindler disease/Kanzaki disease	
Pompe disease	
Acid lipase deficiency	
Danon disease	
Free sialic acid storage disease	
Ceroid lipofuscinosis	
Fabry disease	
Cystinosis	

rapidly and relentlessly with fatality between the age of 2 and 4 years. Blindness is one of the early signs. At the relatively early stage, the patients seem to be hypersensitive to sounds but the threshold to sound intensity is usually elevated. This phenomenon is actually a kind of startle response and not real hypersensitivity [63].

The progress of this disease is rapid with a relentless deterioration of psychomotor ability and rigo-spasticity. Deterioration of psychomotor development, and rigo-spastic posture relentlessly progress. An obvious cherry-red spot on the retinal macula is a distinct sign. The ABRs of two patients are shown in Figs. 6.71 and 6.72.

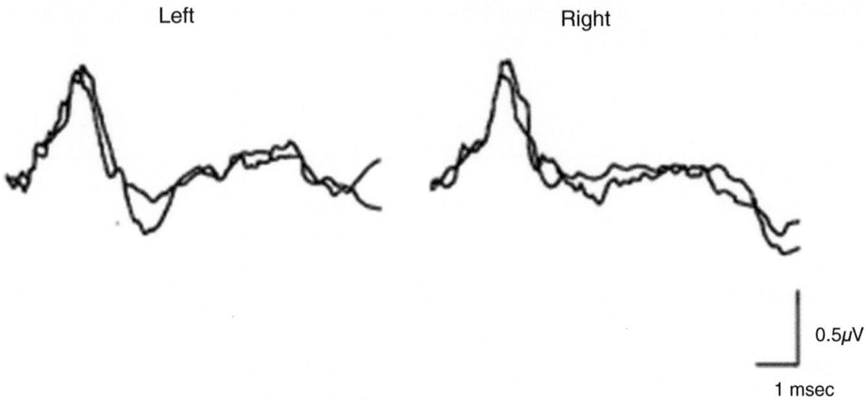

Fig. 6.71 ABR of patient #1 with Tay-Sachs disease. Two years and 4 months, male. Poor vision, hypersensitive sounds, and delayed motor and mental development were his first signs. At 12 months of his age, Tay-Sachs disease was suspected because of cherry red spots in his macula and confirmed as such 3 months later. ABR to 100 dB clicks induce enormous wave I and poor or no formation of later components. Only delayed wave I and amorphous wave V can be seen [63]

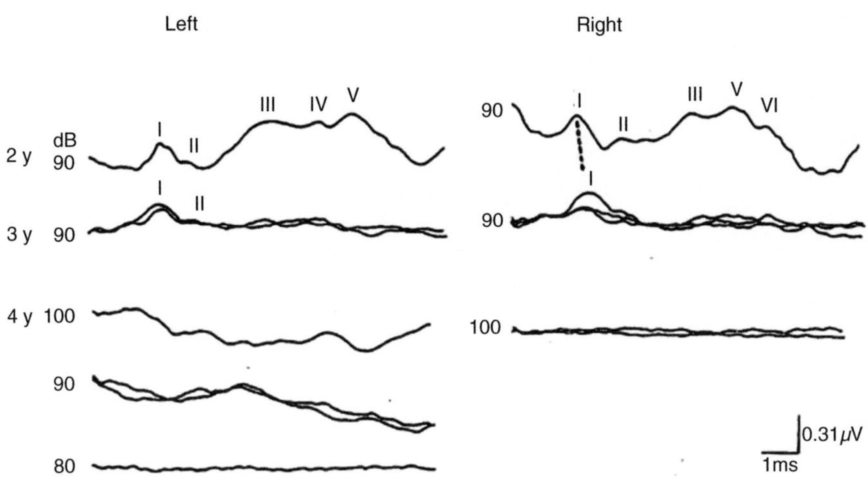

Fig. 6.72 Serial ABRs of patient #2 with Tay-Sachs disease to high-intensity click stimuli. At 2 years of age, his ABR show a relatively normal wave shape. However, progressive deterioration and threshold elevation of his ABR was noted in this patient [64]

Metachromatic Leukodystrophy (MLD)

Refer to the previous section of MLD in leukodystrophy.

Globoid Cell Leukodystrophy (GLD), Krabbe Disease

Refer to the previous section of GLD in leukodystrophy.

Mucopolysaccaridosis (MPS)

Mucopolysaccharidosis is a rare genetic metabolic disease that causes lysosomal enzyme deficiency and leads to the accumulation of glycosaminoglycan in connective tissue and bone. The clinical features of MPS are different for each type with often seen symptoms of coarse face, joint contractures, bone anomalies, hepatosplenomegaly, cardiac valvular disease, progressive hearing loss, and a thick tongue. Intellectual deterioration is a common finding other than Morquio disease.

The classification of MPS is subdivided into more than 13 types and named after the physicians who described each type, for instance, the Hurler, Hunter, Scheie, Sanfillippo, Morquio, and many other types. The involved mutated genes and the deficient enzymes have been identified and form the basis of an objective diagnosis. Treatment attempts have been bone marrow transplants (BMTs) and enzyme replacement therapy (ERT). It has recently been noted that if ERT is initiated during the neonatal period or, if possible, intrauterine, it can delay or even stop the progress of symptoms other than those of the central nervous system. ERT seems to be the best treatment of choice at this point but intrauterine gene therapy ideally may be most appropriate if it is possible. Hearing impairment of MPS can be sensorineural, mixed, and conductive. ABRs of three patients with Sanfilippo disease are shown in Figs. 6.73, 6.74, and 6.75. All patients showed typical clinical history and mixed hearing loss.

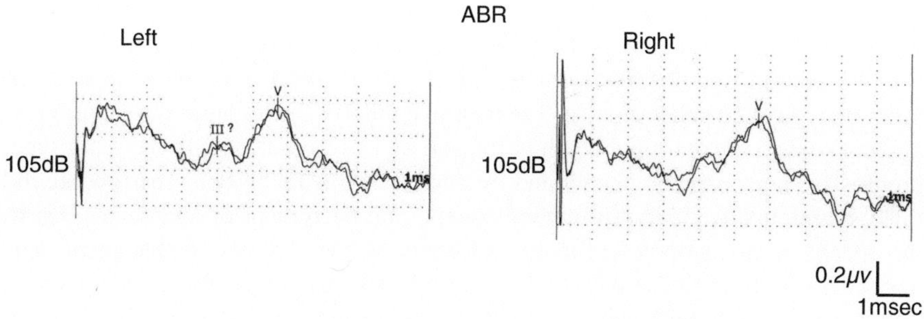

Fig. 6.73 ABR of patient #1 with MPS III. Fourteen years old, female. Bilateral wave I? seems to be present at 2 ms

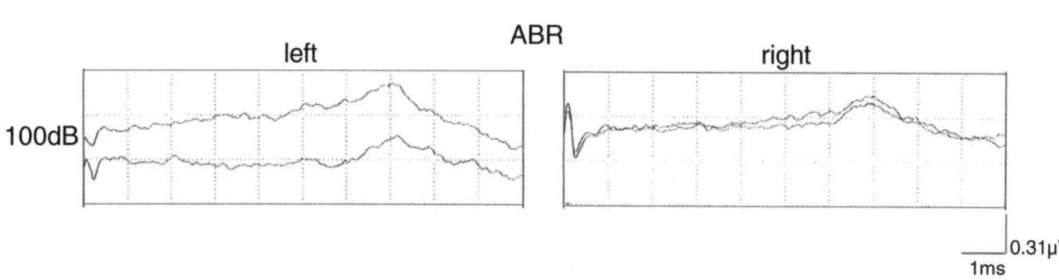

Fig. 6.74 ABR of patient #2 with MPS III. Only wave V is recorded bilaterally by 100 dBHL clicks

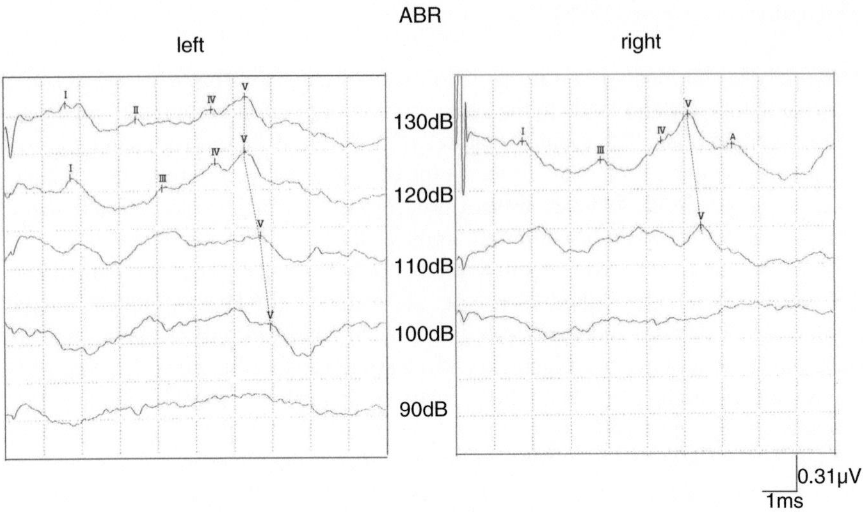

Fig. 6.75 ABR of patient #3 with MPS III. Twenty-three years old, male. Marked threshold elevation of wave V is evident

Gaucher Disease

The cause of Gaucher disease is a deficiency of glucocerebrosidase. In infantile type, central nervous system and reticuloendothelial system are the main targets of the disease. Thus, degradation of intellectual and motor development, hepatosplenomegaly, anemia, and thrombocytopenia are typical clinical signs and symptoms of infantile type of Gaucher disease. The natural course of the infantile type is progressive rigo-spasticity and final death at the age of 1 or 2 years old. In the adult type, progressive hepatosplenomegaly and functional deficiency of bone marrow are the main symptoms. Anemia, thrombocytopenia, and decrement of leukocytes due to the attacks on hematopoietic function of bone marrow. Enzyme replacement therapy (ERT) is effective for symptoms of visceral organs but not for nervous system involvement. Thus, ERT can be effective in adult type but little in infantile type. Thus, gene therapy should be the final goal.

Serial ABRs of patients with infantile and juvenile types are presented in Figs. 6.76 and 6.77.

The former patient passed away at 1 year and 4 months. Autopsy was permitted. A slice of his neuropathological specimen is presented in Fig. 6.78.

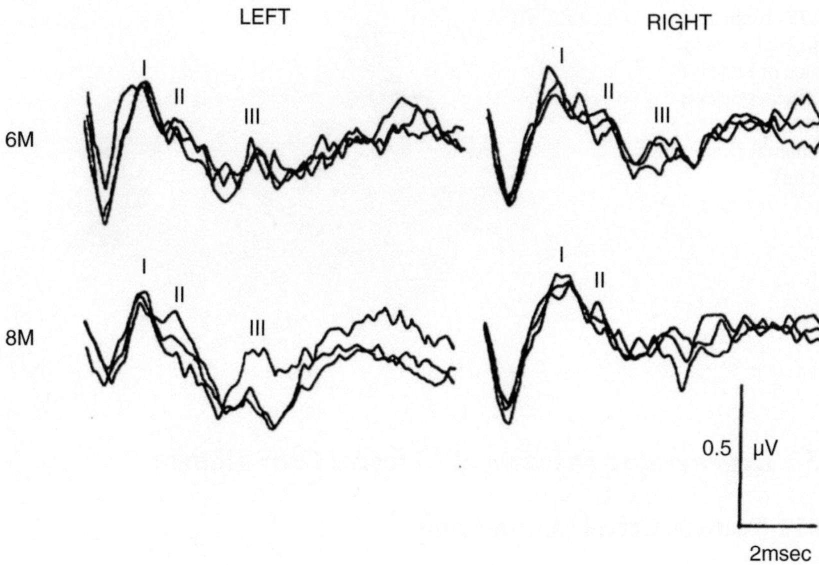

Fig. 6.76 Serial ABRs of patient #1 with Gaucher disease (infantile type). Male. Six and 8 months of age. During 2 months (age 6 months to 8 months), wave III on the right side disappeared. Thus progressive nature of deterioration of ABRs is shown in the figure [65]

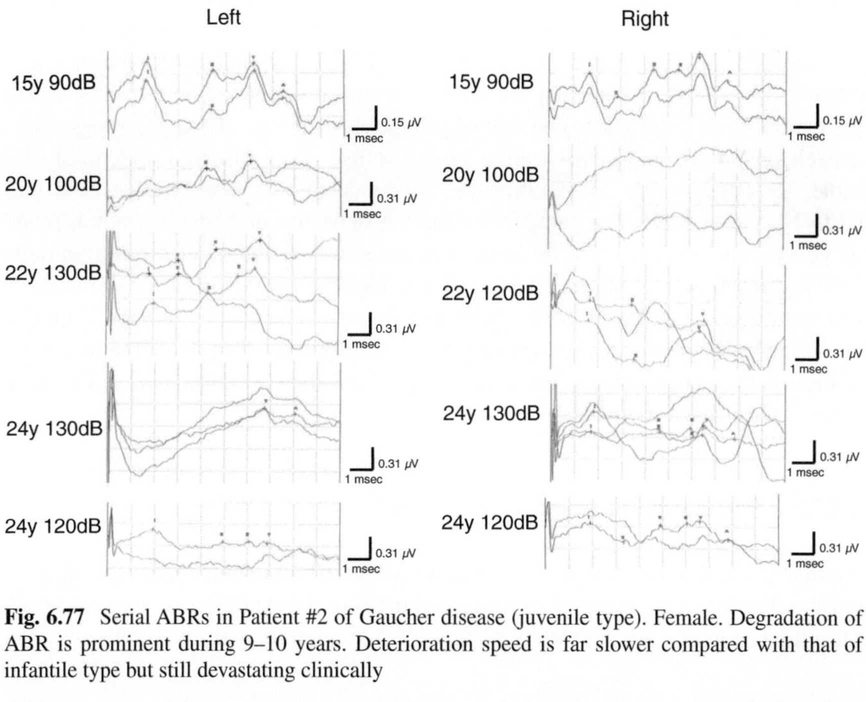

Fig. 6.77 Serial ABRs in Patient #2 of Gaucher disease (juvenile type). Female. Degradation of ABR is prominent during 9–10 years. Deterioration speed is far slower compared with that of infantile type but still devastating clinically

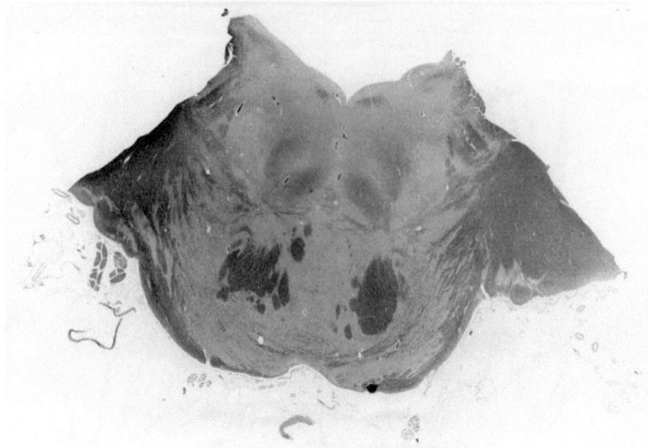

Fig. 6.78 Brainstem pathology of autopsy specimen of Patient #1 with Gaucher disease (infantile type) at 1 year and 4 months (Luxol-Fast blue stain)

6.3.5 Degenerative Diseases of Cerebral Gray Matter

6.3.5.1 Neuronal Ceroid Lipofuscinosis

Neuronal ceroid lipofuscinosis (NCL) is an inherited and rare autosomal-recessive degenerative disease. Recent genetic analysis made clear the responsible genes. Those are named as *CLIN1, CLIN2, CLIN3, and CLIN4.* Chromosomal location of these genes has been identified in the former three genes which were 1p22, 11p15, and 16p12.1. There are four clinical types of NCL classified into age groups: infantile (Santavuori), late infantile (Jansky-Bielshowski), juvenile (Vogt-Spielmeyer), and adult (Kufs). The clinical manifestations of NCL are epilepsy (myoclonic and others), progressive intellectual and motor deterioration, ataxia, and loss of vision ("amaurosis" or blindness). The rate of progression and the clinical findings differ in each age group, but the devastating natural course of this disease is essentially the same. Recent research has verified the existence of two new types, CLN5 and CLIN10, and research is ongoing in this field. A definitive diagnosis of NCL is made by genetic analysis followed by clinical observations including electroretinograms (ERGs), visual evoked potentials (VEPs), and photosensitivity in EEG. Visual signs and symptoms often appear earlier and more conspicuous than in auditory findings.

Serial ABRs of two patients with NCL and serial ERGs of a patient are presented in Figs. 6.79, 6.80, and 6.81. Their VEP (Figs. 6.82 and 6.83) disappear at the early stage of their disease process.

6.3.5.2 Nieman-Pick Disease Type C (NPC)

Nieman-Pick disease type C (NPC) is an inherited autosomal-recessive degenerative disease of the central nervous system and visceral organs. The responsible mutated genes are *NPC1* or *NPC2*. Hepatosplenomegaly becomes obvious

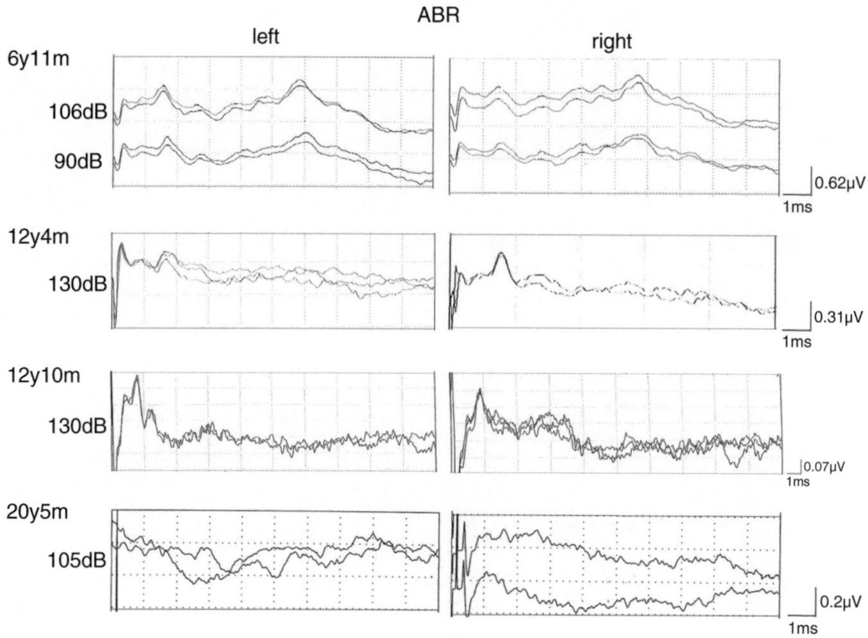

Fig. 6.79 Serial ABRs in patient #1 with NCL, female. Four times recordings from 6 years to 20 years old. Deterioration begins from the later components of ABR

and neurological symptoms such as cataplexy, ataxia, abnormal vertical ocular movement, dysarthria, dystonia, epilepsy, and intellectual deterioration are also prominent clinical findings. Visceral symptoms appear early and neurological symptoms are severe and critical in children but are mild in adults. Clinical types are again classified into age groups: less than 2 months of age; infantile (2 months to 2 years of age), late infantile (2–6 years of age); juvenile (6–15 years of age); adolescent and adult type (6–15 years old). The clinical signs are variable depending on the age at onset. Auditory dysfunction occurs within cochlea and neural auditory pathway [66]. They tried to analyze the auditory function of 50 patients with NPC1 of any type. They could record ABRs of 26 patients with an average interval of 18 months. They described that the most common finding was a loss of wave I and/or wave III occurred in five and three patients. Fillipine staining of form cells in bone marrow or cultured fibroblasts from biopsy specimens has been used to make a definitive diagnosis. Genetic analysis of the mutations of the *NPC1 gene* and *NPC2 genes* determines the diagnosis. Miglustat, an oral inhibitor of glucosylceramide synthase, has been approved for the treatment of NPC.

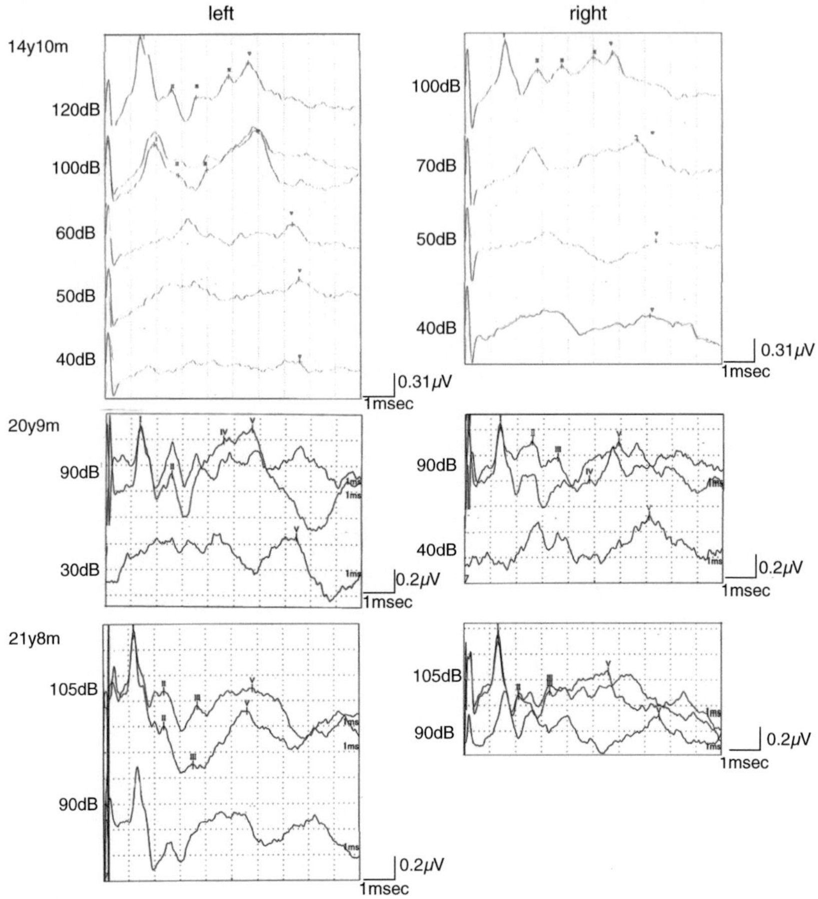

Fig. 6.80 Serial VEPs in patient #1 with NCL. VEP disappeared between her 6 and 11 years of age

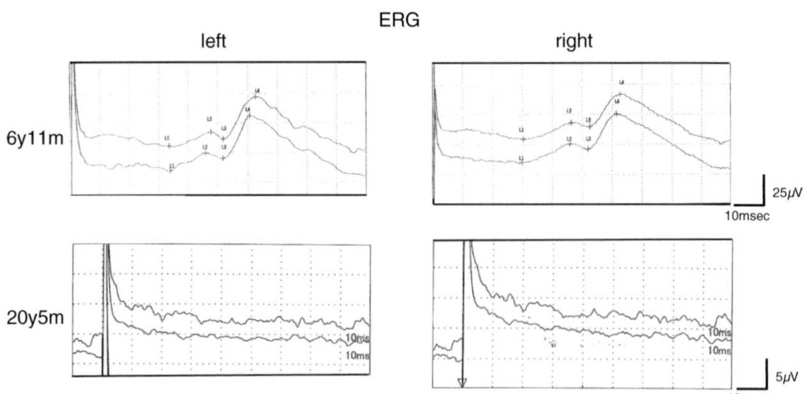

Fig. 6.81 Serial ERGs in patient #1 with NCL. At 6 years and 11 months, oscillation potentials are present but disappeared at 20 years of age

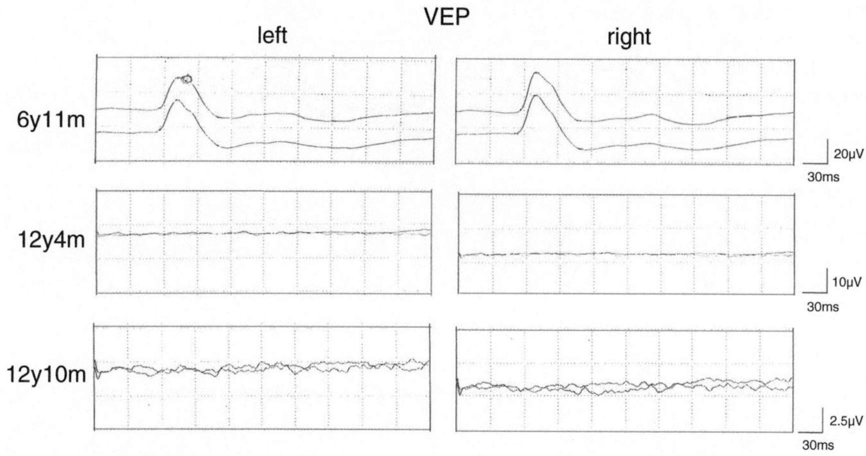

Fig. 6.82 Serial ABRs in patient #2 with NCL. Female. Later components of ABR seem degraded

6.3.5.3 Mitochondrial Diseases

The most important role of mitochondria is the production of energy. It is a subcellular organelle and contains mitochondrial DNA which has genetic codes which are handed down only from maternal code. Abnormalities in the mitochondria cause various levels of dysfunction in cells, tissues, and organs. Many clinical types of mitochondrial diseases are known and the underlying genetic abnormalities have been discerned.

These types include chronic progressive external ophthalmoplegia syndrome, Leigh's encephalopathy, mitochondrial encephalomyopathy with lactic acidosis (MELAS), mitochondrial encephalopathy with ragged red fiber (MERRF), and others.

Each type has a variety of clinical features and gene mutations of mitochondrial DNA. Progressive hearing impairment which includes auditory neuropathy, abnormalities of glucose metabolism, respiratory abnormalities, visual impairment, and psychomotor deterioration could occur in this category of diseases. The severest type of mitochondrial disease is thought to appear as a type of Leigh's encephalopathy. The independency of the genetic mutations and the extent of pathology has been vigorously explored but the relationship between them has yet to be determined.

ABRs of five patients with MELAS (Figs. 6.84, 6.85, 6.86, 6.87, and 6.88), F-VEPs and ERGs of a patient with MELAS (Fig. 6.89) and five patients with Leigh's encephalopathy are shown in Figs. 6.90, 6.91 and 6.92.

Fig. 6.83 VEP of patient #2 with NCL when she was 20 years old. No response could be elicited

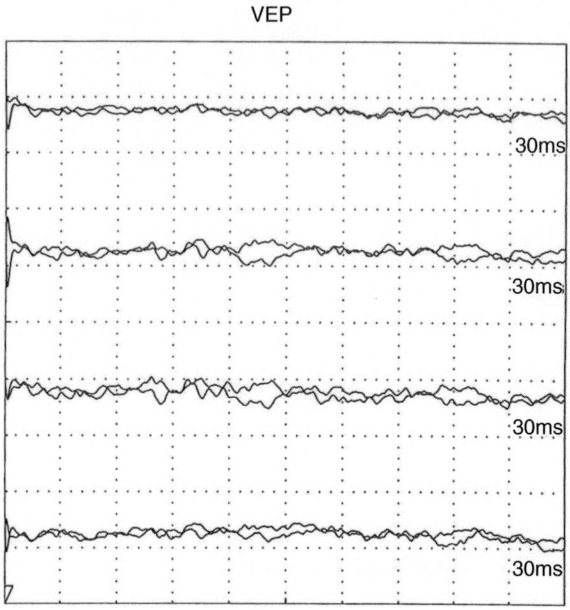

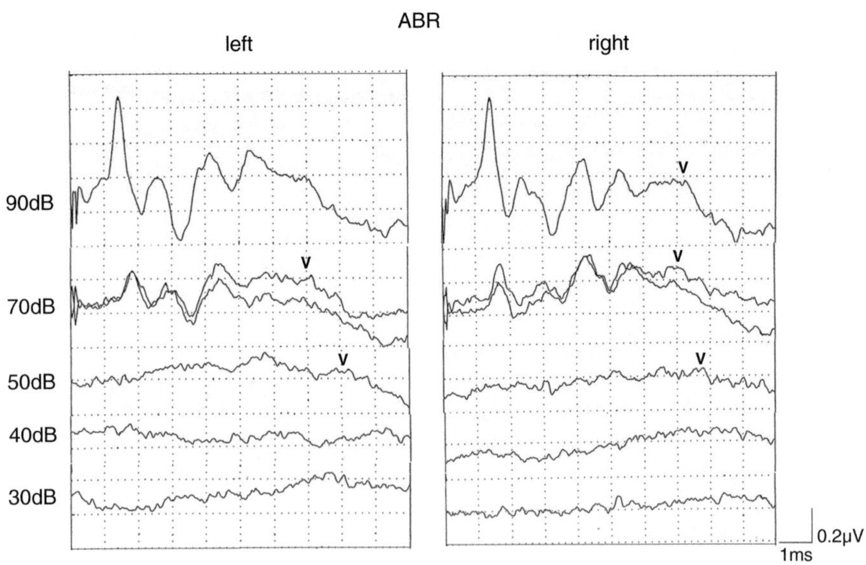

Fig. 6.84 ABRs in patient #1 with MELAS. Male, 2 years and 11 months. Elevated threshold of bilateral wave V is already present suggesting moderate hearing loss at least high-frequency level

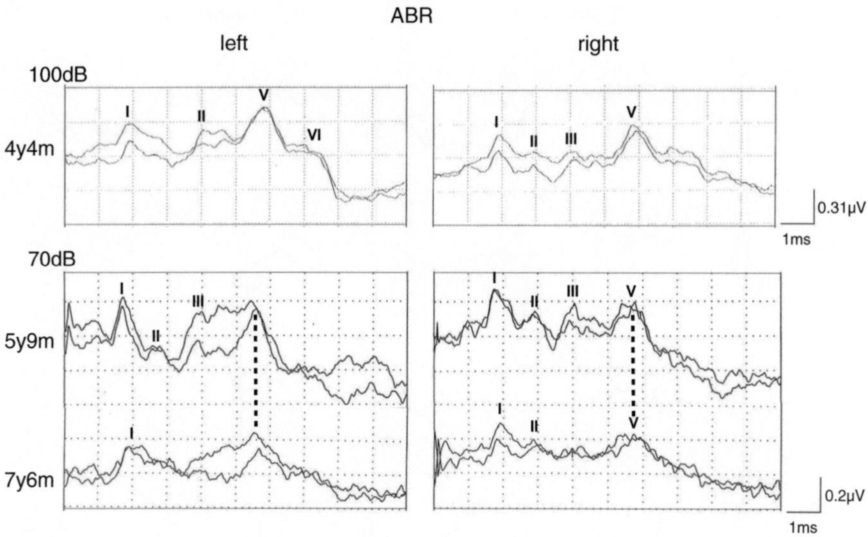

Fig. 6.85 Serial ABRs in patient #2 with MELAS at 4, 5, and 7 years of age. Wave configuration became amorphous as time passed. Deterioration of ABR is certain

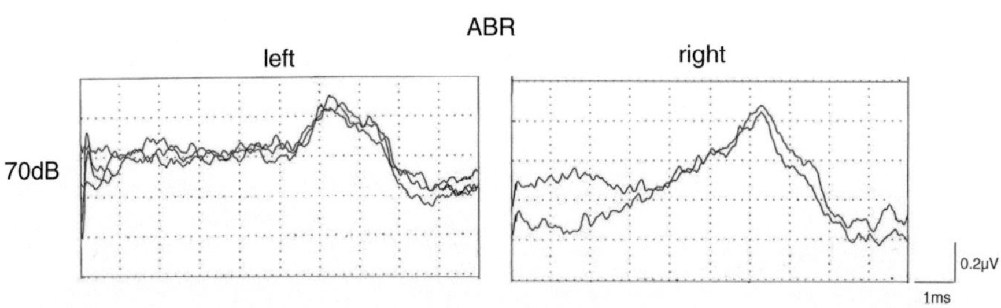

Fig. 6.86 ABR in patient #3 with MELAS at 8 years and 7 months of age. Early components are deficient with only remaining wave V

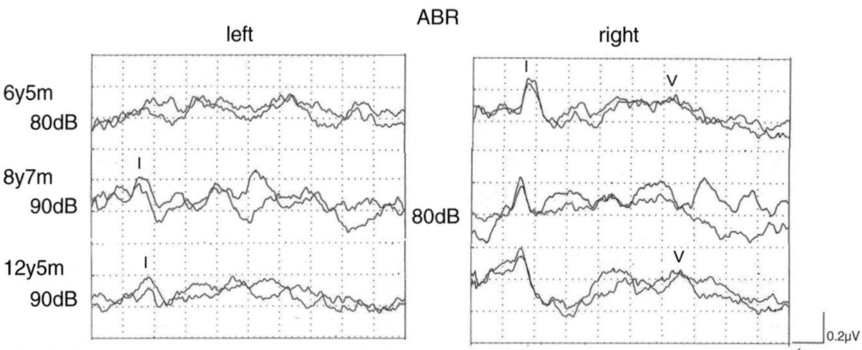

Fig. 6.87 Serial ABRs in patient #4 with MELAS. Bilateral threshold elevation is present. Progress of bilateral hearing loss was present during his clinical course

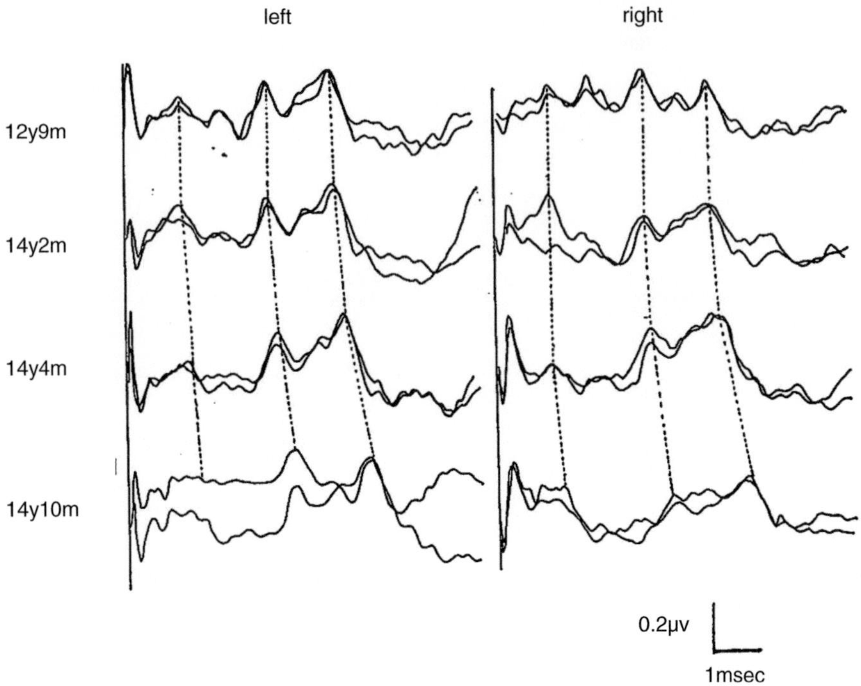

Fig. 6.88 Serial ABRs in patient #5 with MELAS. Progressive prolongation of all waves especially of later components are clear during only 2 years' interval

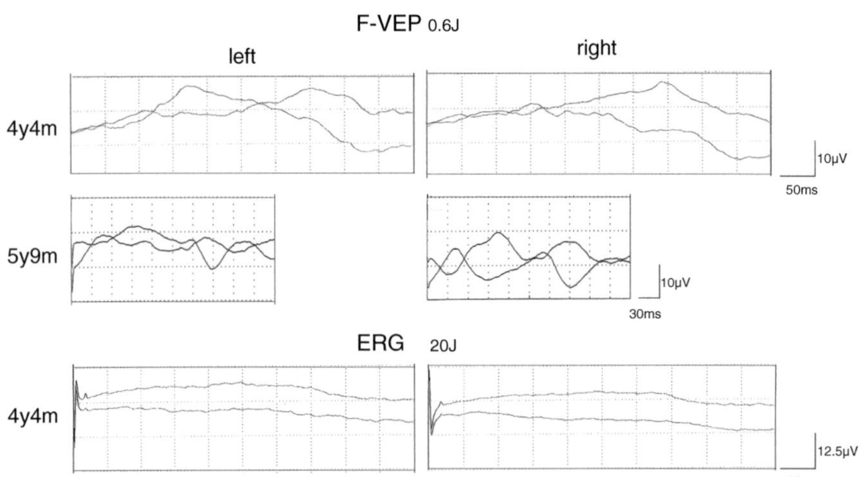

Fig. 6.89 Serial VEP and single ERG in male patient #2 with MELAS. VEP and ERG are not recorded appropriately

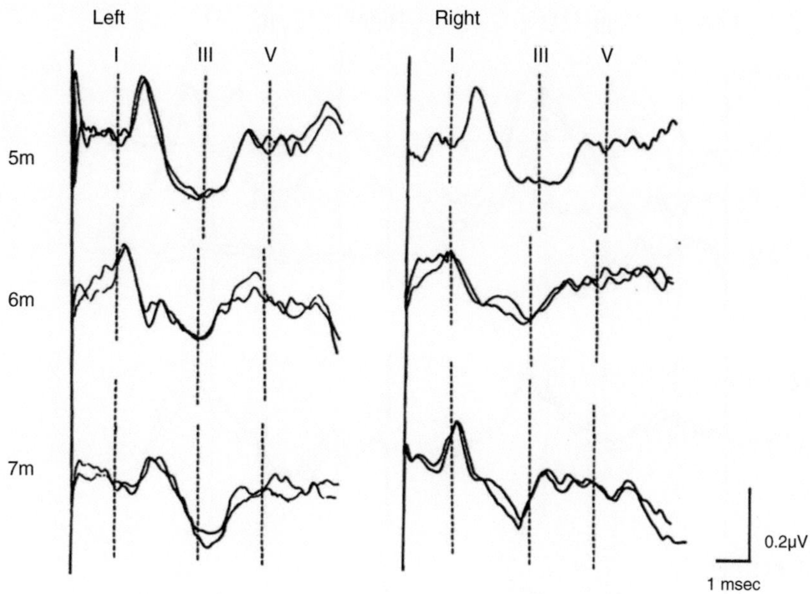

Fig. 6.90 Serial ABRs in patient #1 with Leigh's encephalopathy. Male. From 5 to 7 months of age. During this short period, ABR configuration seemed to worsen. His Abnormal respiration was conspicuous from the onset of the disease [67]

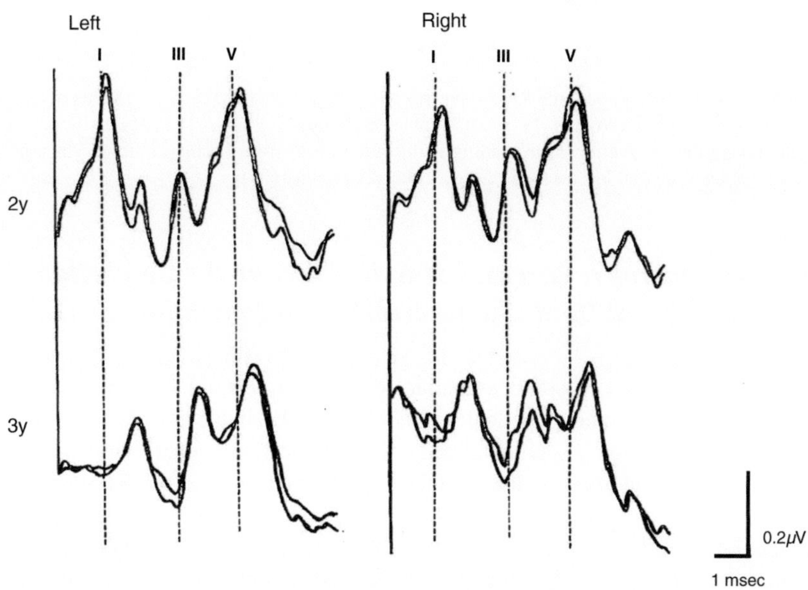

Fig. 6.91 Serial ABRs in patient #2 with Leigh's encephalopathy. Male. From 2 to 3 years of age. Prolonged latency of waves from 2 to 3 years of age suggests pathological or functional deterioration [67]

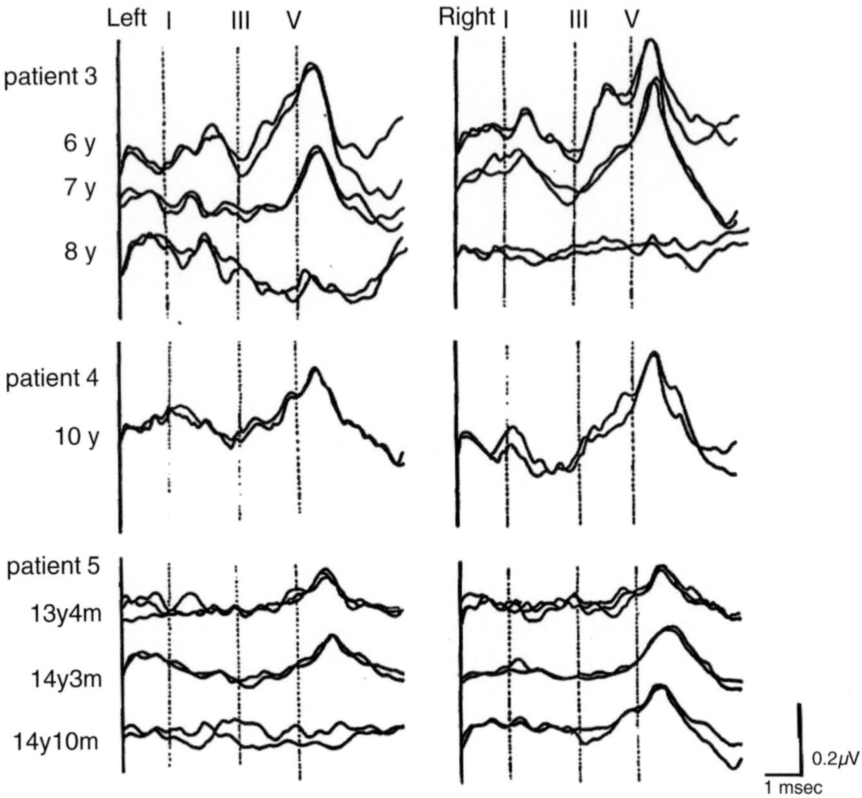

Fig. 6.92 Serial ABRs in patients #3, #4, and #5 with Leigh's encephalopathy. Shapes of waves I and V are apparent but waves II–IV seemed rather ambiguous which may suggest severe pathological change or dysfunction of ascending auditory pathway from cochlear nuclei, via superior olivary nucleus to medial lemniscus in Leigh's encephalopathy [65]

6.3.6 Degenerative Diseases Mainly Effecting the Cerebellum and Spinal Cord (Spinocerebellar Degeneration, SCD)

There are many types of spinocerebellar degeneration (SCD) with two modes of inheritance, sporadic and genetically determined. The latter autosomal-dominant type has been thoroughly segmentalized and the underlying genetic mutation often includes CAG repeat abnormalities. SCD among Japanese, Dentate-Rubro-Pallido-Luysian Atrophy (DRPLA) is the most frequent and one of the devastating degenerative diseases.

Degenerative/hypoplastic cerebellar diseases of infants and children are ataxia telangiectasia, Marinesco-Sjogren syndrome, Arima syndrome [68, 69], and Joubert syndrome [70]. In this section, DRPLA and Joubert syndrome will be briefly explained with serial ABRs in patients with these two diseases.

6.3.6.1 Dentate-Rubro-Pallido-Luysian Atrophy

Dentate-Rubro-Pallido-Luysian Atrophy (DRPLA) is an inherited, progressive, and degenerative disease. The primary central lesions are located in the deep gray matter which includes the dentate nucleus, the red nucleus, the pallidum, and Luy body. DRPLA is explained as triplet repeat disease which is the longer CAG repeat is the indicator of the severity of the disease and diagnostic key of the disease. An increase in the number of CAG repeats of the *DRPLA* gene is responsible for the inherited abnormalities and is the objective basis of the diagnosis.

Clinical features are progressive myoclonus, intractable epilepsy (progressive myoclonus epilepsy, PME), and involuntary movement (myoclonus, chorea, athetosis, and dystonia). In a family, the onset of the disease appears earlier than the onset of the previous generation which derives to the longer repeat of CAG in the younger generation. In such a family, the children and even infants could be affected by the disease. MRIs of these patients show cerebral (mainly frontal lobe), midbrain, cerebellar, and brainstem atrophy. Infants and children also possibly show delayed myelination in those areas. Examples of their ABRs are shown in the figure below. Most patients have abnormal cortically evoked responses such as SEPs and VEPs. The cortical components of the SEP are usually not evoked at an early stage but in some patients with cortical myoclonus occasionally have very large amplitude VEPs or SEPs (giant VEP or giant SEP) possibly because of cortical hypersensitivity.

Examples of serial changes in the ABRs of DRPLA patients are shown in Figs. 6.93, 6.94, 6.95, 6.96, 6.97, 6.98, and 6.99. Serial change of SEP in a DRPLA patient 1 is shown in Fig. 6.100.

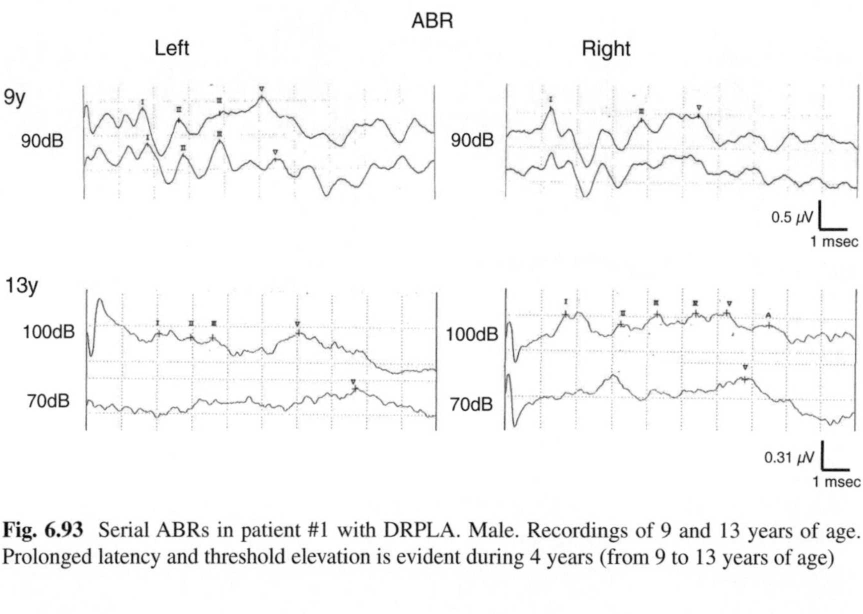

Fig. 6.93 Serial ABRs in patient #1 with DRPLA. Male. Recordings of 9 and 13 years of age. Prolonged latency and threshold elevation is evident during 4 years (from 9 to 13 years of age)

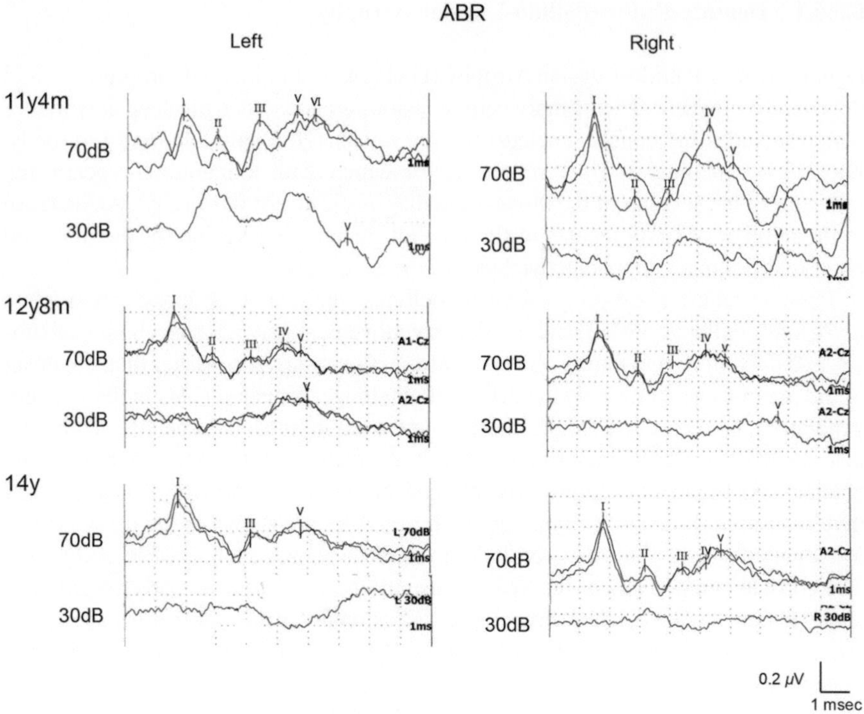

Fig. 6.94 Serial ABRs in patient #2 with DRPLA. Male. Recordings at 11, 12, and 14 years of age. Threshold of wave V elevation is noted during observation period

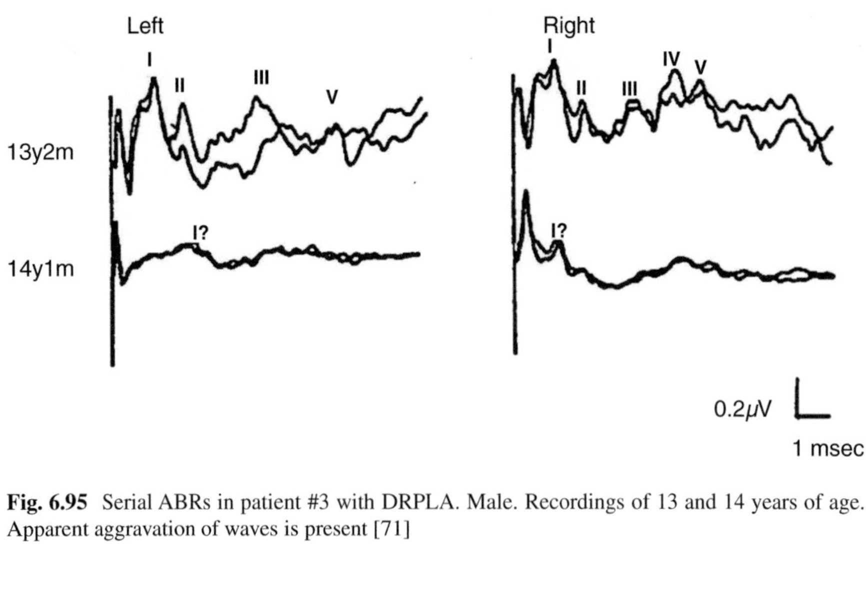

Fig. 6.95 Serial ABRs in patient #3 with DRPLA. Male. Recordings of 13 and 14 years of age. Apparent aggravation of waves is present [71]

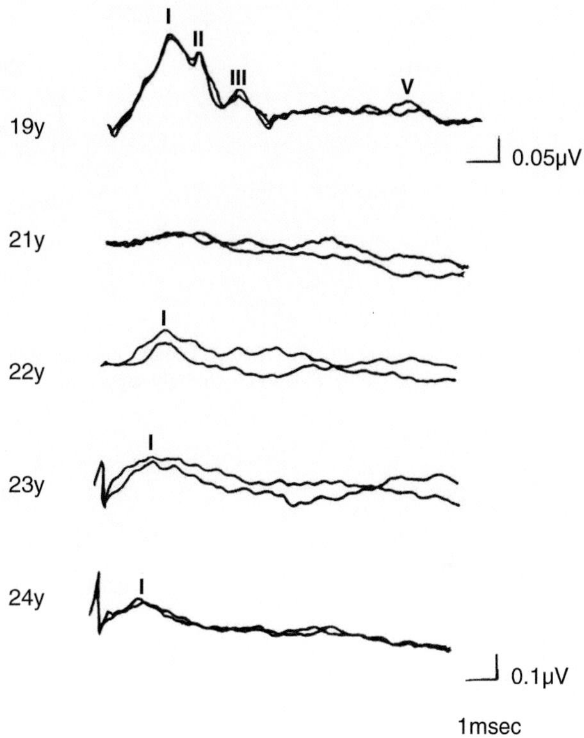

Fig. 6.96 Serial ABRs in patient #4 with DRPLA. Male. Recordings at 19–24 years of age. Progressive worsening of ABRs is present along with intellectual and motor deterioration

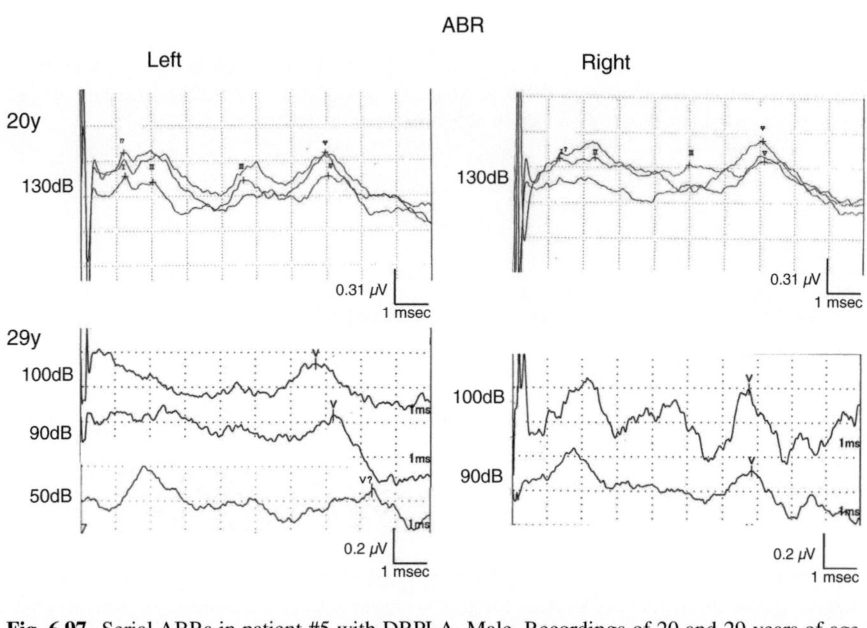

Fig. 6.97 Serial ABRs in patient #5 with DRPLA. Male. Recordings of 20 and 29 years of age. Wave form deterioration and possible threshold elevation is evident

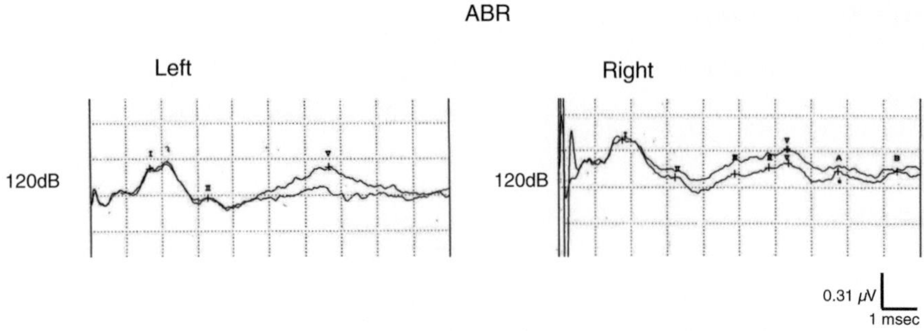

Fig. 6.98 ABR in patient #6 with DRPLA. Female. Recordings at 23 years of age. Marked threshold elevation and pontine dysfunction is strongly suggested

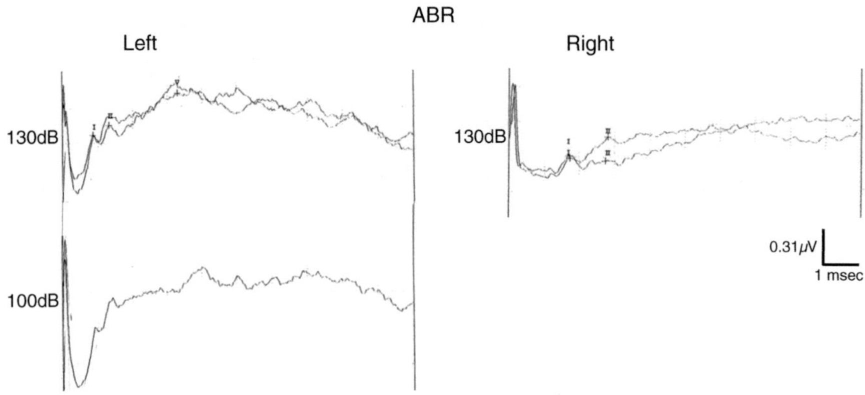

Fig. 6.99 ABR in patient #7 with DRPLA. Male. Recording at 31 years of age. Despite of high sound pressure stimuli, severe dysfunction in pontine auditory pathway is suggested

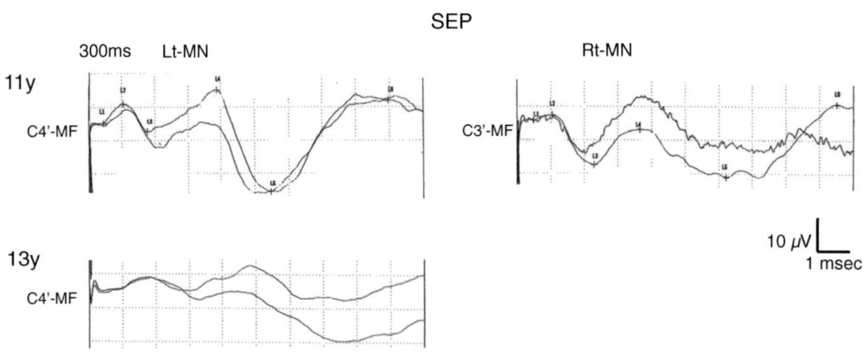

Fig. 6.100 Serial SEP of patient #1 with DRPLA. Giant SEP of more than 25 μV is present at 11 years of age but disappeared at 13 years of age. It seems to reflect the prevalence of cortical hypersensitivity and active myoclonus and myoclonic epilepsy

6.3.6.2 Joubert Syndrome

Joubert described his syndrome in 1969 [70]. The main clinical features are psychomotor retardation, hypotonia, ataxia, abnormal ocular movements, retinal degeneration, renal cysts, hepatic involvement, and abnormal respiration. Cerebral imaging revealed hypoplasia or aplasia of cerebellar vermis and an abnormal brainstem (molar tooth sign). Recently, Joubert's syndrome has been reclassified as "Joubert syndrome and related diseases" in Japan, which includes the Arima syndrome [68, 69]. The underlying gene mutation is variable but cilia abnormalities in the general organ system (including respiratory system) have recently been identified.

In 2002, Kabeya published his findings on serial changes of the ABR and other neurophysiological findings in Joubert's syndrome [72].

Serial ABRs from two patients with Joubert syndrome are shown in Figs. 6.101 and 6.102.

6.3.7 Degenerative Disease of Peripheral Nervous System

These peripheral degenerative diseases are classified as hereditary motor and sensory neuropathies (HSMNs) type I to Type VII, hereditary sensory and autonomic neuropathies (HSAN) type I–V, giant axonal neuropathies, hereditary tomaculous (swelling of the myelin) neuropathy, and hereditary brachial plexus neuropathies.

6.3.7.1 Charcot-Marie-Tooth Disease

Charcot-Marie-tooth disease (CMTD) is a peripheral HSMN which impairs both the spinal and cranial nerves which are peripheral neurons. One of the first reports of auditory neuropathy by Starr included two patients with CMTD [73]. The precise

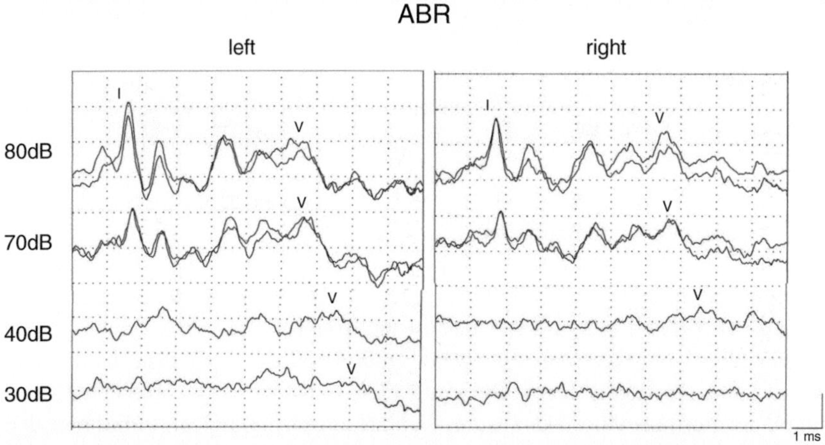

Fig. 6.101 ABR in patient #1 with Joubert syndrome, 7 months old. His ABR shape was almost normal at 7 months of age despite of elevated wave V threshold in the right side

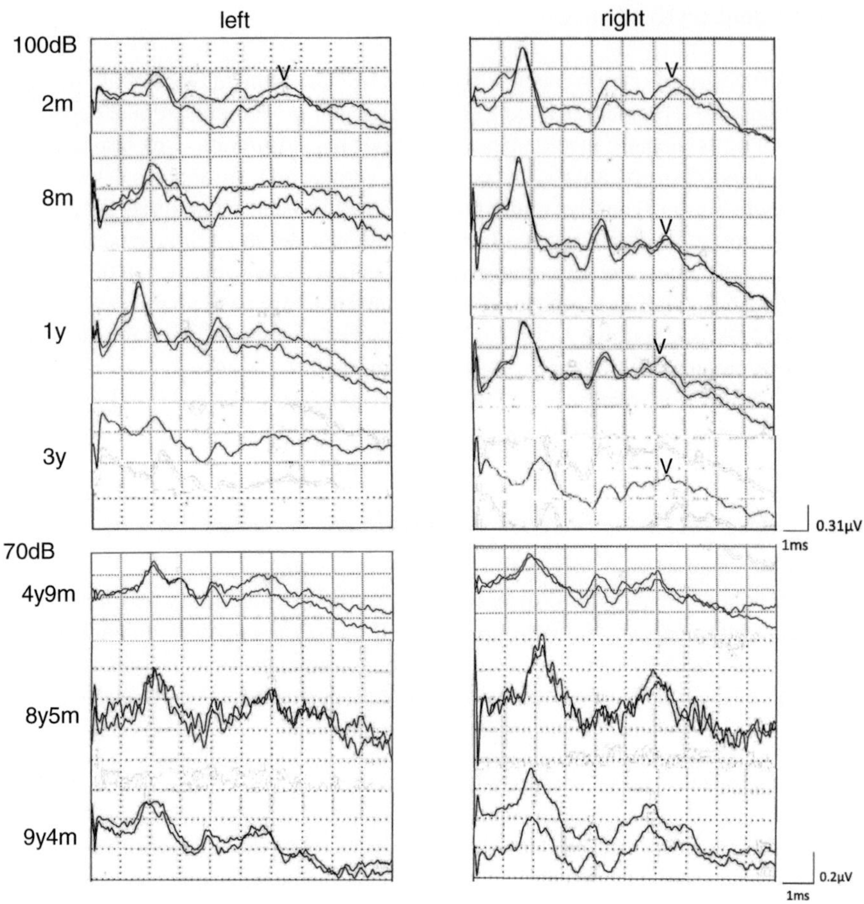

Fig. 6.102 Serial ABR in patient #2 with Joubert syndrome. Female. Seven times recordings from 2 months to 9 years old. Amplitude reversal of waves I and V is present. Pathological meaning is yet to be determined

description of a variety of auditory neuropathies is described in the later section written by Kaga.

6.3.7.2 Giant Axonal Neuropathy

Giant axonal neuropathy is an inherited autosomal-recessive disorder. A mutation of the *gigaxonin (GAN1) gene* is the cause of the disease. The initial symptoms are hypotonia, distal muscle weakness, weak tendon reflexes, gait disturbance, and curly hair. Its onset usually occurs from infancy to toddlers. It is a combined disease of central and peripheral nervous systems [74]. Neurophysiological studies revealed delayed motor and sensory conducting velocity with intact intellectual ability. ABRs of two patients are shown in Figs. 6.103 and 6.104. The interwave latencies of these patients are extremely prolonged.

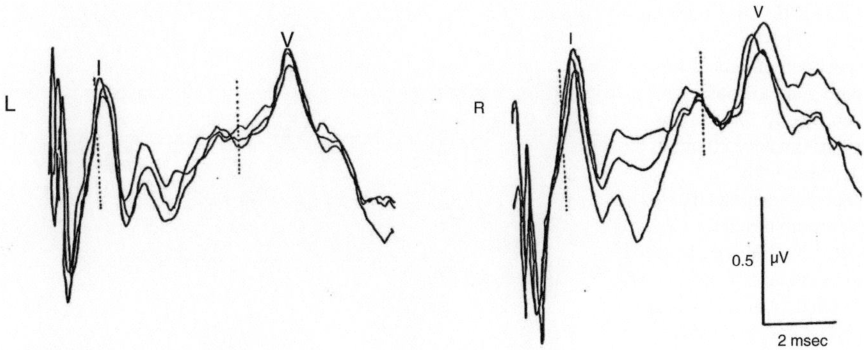

Fig. 6.103 ABR of patient #1 with Giant axonal neuropathy, male. Seven years old. Prolonged latency of wave V is seen. Bilateral dotted lines are average latencies of waves I and V of age matched healthy children [3]

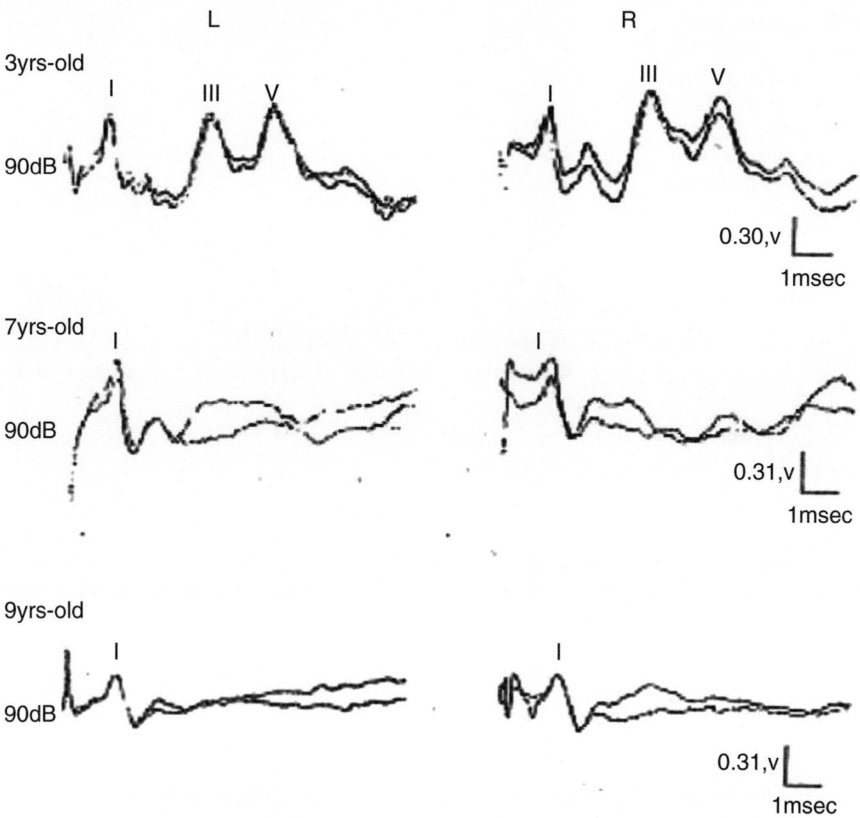

Fig. 6.104 Serial ABRs in a patient #2 with giant axonal neuropathy. Male. Recordings at 3–9 years of age. Definitive worsening of wave shapes beginning from the later components

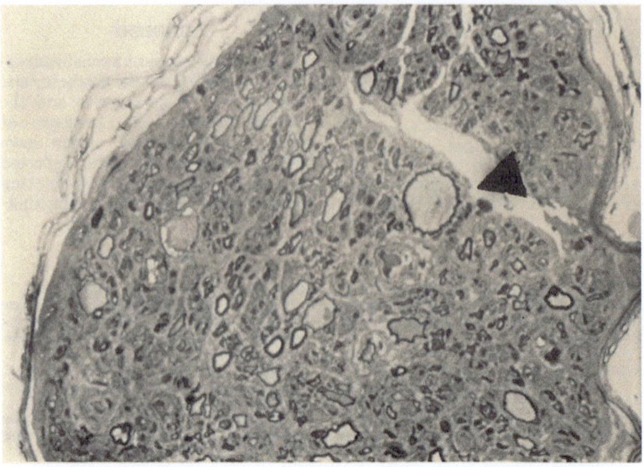

Fig. 6.105 Ultrastructure of sural nerve. Biopsy specimen of patient #1 with giant axonal neuropathy. Giant axon approximately 20 μm in diameter with neurofilamentous masses. Neurotubules and mitochondria are displaced to marginal zone of swelled axon (uranyl acetate and lead citrate, ×7000) [74]

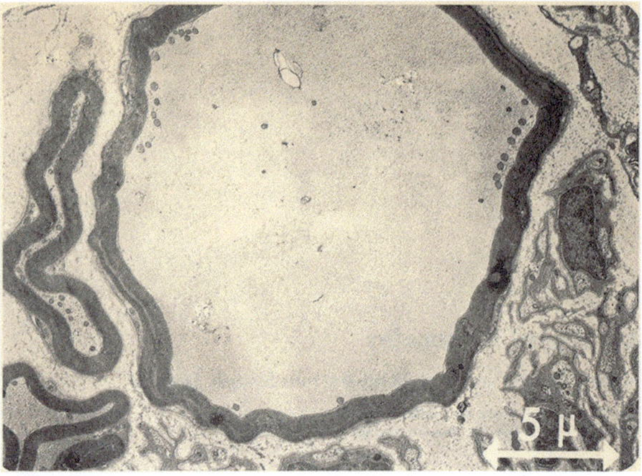

Fig. 6.106 Sural nerve biopsy specimen of patient #1 with giant axonal neuropathy, some large axons with thin myelin sheaths are seen. Largest measured 32 μm in diameter in transverse section (Toluiodin blue staining, ×500) [74]

Sural nerve biopsy specimen of patient 1 has revealed enlarged axonal neuropathy as shown in Figs. 6.105 and 6.106.

Acknowledgments The author deeply appreciates Dominic Hughes, PhD for his sincere and critical reading/English editing and Keiko Okawara, B.A. for her marked contribution to help every aspect of this section. Thousands of infants and children who cooperated in the clinical situation are sincerely acknowledged.

References

1. Jewett D, Romano MN, Williston JS. Human auditory evoked potentials: possible brain stem components detected on the scalp. Science. 1970;167:1517–8.
2. Sohmer H, Feinmesser M. Cochlear and cortical audiometry conveniently recorded in the same subject. Isr J Med Sci. 1970;6:219–23.

3. Kaga M. ABR: application to clinical pediatrics. Jpn J Pediatr Med. 1981;13:1817–24. Japanese.
4. Otawara S, Iyoda K, Kohno C. Sudden infant death syndrome and ABR. Jpn J Pediatr Med. 1983;15:475–82. Japanese.
5. Eggermont JJ, Salamy A. Maturational time course for ABR in preterm and full term infants. Hear Res. 1988;33:35–48.
6. Iwasaki S, Kaga K. Chronological changes of auditory brainstem responses in Cockayne's syndrome. Int J Pediatr Otorhinolaryngol. 1994;30:211–21.
7. Worthington DW, Peters JF. Quantifiable hearing and no ABR: paradox of error? Ear Hear. 1980;1:281–5.
8. Kraus N, Ödzmar Ö, Stein LS, Reed N. Absent auditory brainstem response; peripheral hearing loss of brainstem dysfunction? Laryngoscope. 1984;94:400–6.
9. Eggermont JJ. Development of ABR parameters in a preterm and a term born population. Ear Hear. 1988;9:283–9.
10. Hecox K, Galambos R. Brainstem auditory evoked responses in human infants and adults. Arch Otolaryngol. 1974;99:30–3.
11. Kaga K, Tanaka Y. Auditory brainstem response and behavioral audiometry. Arch Otolaryngol. 1980;106:564–6.
12. Birnholz JC, Benacerraf BR. The development of human fetal hearing. Science. 1983;222:516–8.
13. Ruben RJ. The ontogeny of human hearing. Acta Otolaryngol. 1992;112:192–6.
14. Hepper PG, Shahidullah BS. Development of fetal hearing. Arch Dis Child Fetal Neonatal Ed. 1994;71:F81–7.
15. Woods JR Jr, Plessinger MA, Mack CE. Fetal auditory brainstem evoked response (ABR). Pediatr Res. 1984;18:83–5.
16. Eggermont JJ. Development of auditory evoked potentials. Acta Otolaryngol. 1992;112:197–200.
17. Wennberg RP, Ahlfors CE, Bickers R, McMurtry CA, Shetter JL. Abnormal auditory brainstem response in a newborn infant with hyperbilirubinemia: improvement with exchange transfusion. J Pediatr. 1982;100:624–6.
18. Salamy A, Eldredge L, Tooley WH. Neonatal status and hearing loss in high risk infants. Pediatrics. 1989;114:847–52.
19. Coenraad S, Goedegebure A, Hoeve LJ. An initial overestimation of sensorineural hearing loss in NICU infants after failure on neonatal hearing screening. Int J Pediatr Otorhinolaryngol. 2011;75:159–62.
20. Hof JR, Stokroos RJ, Wix E, Chenault M, Gelders E, Brokx J. Auditory maturation in premature infants: a potential pitfall for early cochlear implantation. Laryngoscope. 2013;123:2013–8.
21. Psarommatis I, Florou V, Fragkos M, Douniadakis E, Kontrogiannis A. Reversible auditory brainstem responses screening failure in high risk neonates. Eur Arch Otorhinolaryngol. 2011;268:189–96.
22. Psarommatis I, Voudouris C, Kapetanakis I, Athanasiadi F, Douros K. Recovery of abnormal ABR in neonates and infants at risk of hearing loss. Int J Otolaryngol. 2017;2017:7912127.
23. Kaga M. ABR in pediatrics. JOHNS. 1989a;5:364–72. Japanese.
24. Kaga M. ABR: application to neonates and infants. Perinat Med. 1989b;19:245–51. Japanese.
25. Weston PF, Manson JI, Abbott KJ. Auditory brainstem-evoked response in childhood brainstem glioma. Childs Nerv Syst. 1986;2:301–5.
26. Yagi T, Kaga K, Baba S. A study of cases with partial disappearance of the waves in the auditory brain stem response. Arch Otorhinolaryngol. 1980;226:251–8.
27. Kaga M, Nihei K. Appearance of wave III of auditory brainstem response after removal of a cerebellar tumor. Brain Dev. 1993;15:305–7.
28. Kimura J, Mitsudome A, Yamada T, Dickins QS. Stationary peaks from a moving source in far-field recording. Electroencephalogr Clin Neurophysiol. 1984;58:351–61.

29. Desmedt JE, Huy NT, Carmeliet J. Unexpected latency shifts of stationary P9 somatosensory evoked potential far-field with changes in shoulder position. Electroencephalogr Clin Neurophysiol. 1983;56:628–34.
30. Özmar Ö, Kraus N, Stein L. Auditory brainstem response in infants recovering from bacterial meningitis: audiologis evaluation. Arch Otolaryngol. 1983;109:13–8.
31. Spankovich C, Lustig LR. Restoration of brain stem auditory-evoked potential in maple syrup urine disease. Otol Neurotol. 2007;28:566–9.
32. Kaga M, Ohuchi M, Kaga K, Tanaka Y. Normalization of poor auditory brainstem response in infants and children. Brain Dev. 1984b;6:458–66.
33. Friede RL. Developmental neuropathology. 2nd and expanded ed. Berlin: Springer-Verlag; 1989.
34. Carducci F, Onorati P, Condoluci C, Di Gennaro G, Quarato PP, Pierallini A, Sarà M, Miano S, Cornia R, Albertini G. Whole-brain voxel-based morphometry study of children and adolescents with Down syndrome. Funct Neurol. 2013;28:19–28.
35. Shiohama T, Jacob Levman J, Nicole Baumer N, Takahashi E. Structural magnetic resonance imaging-based brain morphology study in infants and toddlers with down syndrome: the effect of comorbidities. Pediatr Neurol. 2019;100:67–73.
36. Tintore M, Rovira A, Arrambide G, Mitjana R, Río J, Auger C, Nos C, Edo MC, Castilló J, Horga A, Perez-Miralles F, Huerga E, Comabella M, Sastre-Garriga J, Montalban X. Brainstem lesions in clinically isolated syndromes. Neurology. 2010;75:1933–8.
37. Kaga M. Auditory brainstem response in chromosomally abnormal children. J Jpn Pediatr Soc. 1988;92:15–20. Japanese.
38. Smith DW. Recognizable patterns of human malformation. 3rd ed. Philadelphia: Saunders; 1982.
39. Kaga M, Maeda K, Nihei K, Mogi F. Auditory evoked potentials in chromosomal aberration. J Mental Health. 1986;33:195–203. Japanese
40. Sohmer H, Freeman S, Gafni M. The depression of the auditory nerve-brain-stem evoked response in hypoxaemia—mechanism and site of effect. Electroencephalogr Clin Neurophysiol. 1986;64:334–8.
41. Sell EJ, Gaines JA, Gluckman C, Williams E. Persistent fetal circulation. Neurodevelopmental outcome. Am J Dis Child. 1985;139:25–8.
42. Nield TA, Schrier S, Ramos AD, Platzker AC, Warburton D. Unexpected hearing loss in high-risk infants. Pediatrics. 1986;78:417–22.
43. Naulty CM, Weiss IP, Herer GR. Progressive sensorineural hearing loss in survivors of persistent fetal circulation. Ear Hear. 1986;7:74–7.
44. Hendricks-Muñoz KD, Walton JP. Hearing loss in infant with persistent fetal circulation. Pediatrics. 1988;81:650–6.
45. Walton JP, Hendricks-Munoz K. Profile and stability of sensorineural hearing loss in persistent pulmonary hypertension of the newborn. J Speech Hear Res. 1991;34:1362–70.
46. Zenri H, Yao N, Condou M, Nakamura H, Tateishi T, Kawano T, Kaga M. Outcome of hearing acuity in infants with persistent pulmonary hypertension of the newborn. Acta Neonatologica Japonica. 1996;32:278–83.
47. Kirino T. Delayed neuronal death in the gerbil hippocampus following ischemia. Brain Res. 1982;239:57–69.
48. Koga K, Hakuba N, Watanabe F, Shudou M, Nakagawa T, Gyo K. Transient cochlear ischemia causes delayed cell death in the organ of Corti: an experimental study in gerbils. Comp Neurol. 2003;456:105–11.
49. Hecox KE, Cone B. Prognostic importance of brainstem auditory evoked responses after asphyxia. Neurology. 1981;31:1429–34.
50. Inagaki M, Kaga M, Nihei K, Naitoh H, Takayama S, Sugai K. The value of serial auditory brainstem response in patients with subacute sclerosing panencephalitis. J Child Neurol. 1999;14:422–7.
51. Cartier N, Hacein-Bey-Abina S, Bartholomae CC, Veres G, Schmidt M, Kutschera I, Vidaud M, Abel U, Dal-Cortivo L, Caccavelli L, Mahlaoui N, Kiermer V, Mittelstaedt D, Bellesme C, Lahlou N, Lefrère F, Blanche S, Audit M, Payen E, Leboulch P, l'Homme B, Bougnères P, Von

Kalle C, Fischer A, Cavazzana-Calvo M, Aubourg P. Hematopoietic stem cell gene therapy with a lentiviral vector in X-linked adrenoleukodystrophy. Science. 2009;326:818–23.
52. Matsukawa T, Yamamoto T, Honda A, Toya T, Ishiura H, Mitsui J, Tanaka M, Hao A, Shinohara A, Ogura M, Kataoka K, Seo S, Kumano K, Hosoi M, Narukawa K, Yasunaga M, Maki H, Ichikawa M, Nannya Y, Imai Y, Takahashi T, Takahashi Y, Nagasako Y, Yasaka K, Koshi Mano K, Kawabe Matsukawa M, Miyagawa T, Hamada M, Sakuishi K, Hayashi T, Iwata A, Terao Y, Shimizu J, Goto J, Mori H, Kunimatsu A, Aoki S, Hayashi S, Nakamura F, Arai S, Momma K, Ogata K, Yoshida T, Abe O, Inazawa J, Toda T, Kurokawa M, Tsuji S. Clinical efficacy of haematopoietic stem cell transplantation for adult adrenoleukodystrophy. Brain Commun. 2020;2:fcz048.
53. Ochs R, Markand ON, DeMyer WE. Brainstem auditory evoked responses in leukodystrophies. Neurology. 1979;29:1089–93.
54. Inagaki M, Kaga Y, Kaga M, Nihei K. Multimodal evoked potentials in patients with pediatric leukodystrophy. Clin Neurophysiol (Suppl). 2006;59:251–63.
55. Suzuki Y, Suzuki K. Krabbe's globoid cell leukodystrophy: deficiency of galactocerebrosidase in serum, leukocytes and fibroblasts. Science. 1970;171:73–5.
56. Yamamouchi H, Kaga M, Sakuragawa N, Arima M. Auditory evoked responses in Krabbe disease. Pediatr Neurol. 1993;9:387–90.
57. Aldosari M, Altuwaijri M, Husain AM. Brain-stem auditory and visual evoked potentials in children with Krabbe disease. Clin Neurophysiol. 2004;115:1653–6.
58. Matsui K, Fukumizu M, Yoshikawa H, Kaga M, Kurokawa T, Takashima S. Electrically elicited blink reflex and auditory brainstem response in leukodystrophy. J Jpn Pediatr Soc. 1991;95:2628–33. Japanese.
59. Kaga M, Tanaka Y, Takamizawa M, Naitoh H, Nihei K. Clinical diagnoses of pediatric patients without detectable auditory brainstem response (ABR). No to Hattatsu. 1989;21:550–6. Japanese.
60. Garg BP, Markand ON, DeMyer WE. Usefulness of BAER studies in the early diagnosis of Pelizaeus-Merzbacher disease. Neurology. 1983;33:955–6.
61. Kaga K, Tamai F, Kodama M, Kodama K. Three young adult patients with Pelizaeus-Merzbacher disease who showed only waves I and II in auditory brainstem responses but had good auditory perception. Acta Otolaryngol. 2005;125:1018–23.
62. Kaga M, Kawasaki M, Mizuno Y, Ohuchi M, Nagashima K, Mohri N. Cerebello-brainstem orthochromatic leukodystrophy with floppiness and bulbar palsy. Clin Neuopathol. 1984a;3:178–84.
63. Yoshikawa H, Kaga M, Sakuragawa N, Kaga K. Neuro-otologic studies of startle reaction to sound in a case with Tay-Sachs disease. No to Hattatsu. 1989;21:583–5. Japanese.
64. Ozawa H, Hashimoto T, Kaga M. Evoked potentials in children with Tay-Sachs disease. Clin Electroencephalogr. 1999;41:128–31. Japanese.
65. Kaga M, Azuma C, Imamura T, Murakami T, Kaga K. Auditory brainstem response (ABR) in infantile Gaucher disease. Neuropediatrics. 1982;13:207–10.
66. King KA, Gordon-Salant S, Yanjanin N, Zalewski C, Houser A, Porter FD, Brewer CC. Auditory phenotype of Niemann-Pick disease, type C1. Ear Hear. 2014;35:110–7.
67. Kaga M, Naitoh H, Nihei K. Auditory brainstem response in Leigh's syndrome. Acta Paediatr Jpn. 1987;29:254–60.
68. Arima M, Ono K, Hisada K, Handa T. A familial syndrome of maldevelopment of the brain, polycystic kidneys, congenital tapetoretinal dysplasia with coloboma and unilateral ptosis. No to Hattatsu. 1971;3:330–2. Japanese.
69. Matsuzaka T, Sakuragawa N, Nakayama H, Sugai K, Kohno Y, Arima M. Cerebro-oculo-hepato-renal syndrome (Arima' syndrome): a distinct clinicopathological entity. J Child Neurol. 1986;1:338–46.
70. Joubert M, Eisenring JJ, Robb JP, Andermann F. Familial agenesis of the cerebellar vermis. A syndrome of episodic hyperpnea, abnormal eye movements, ataxia, and retardation. Neurology. 1969;19:813–25.
71. Kaga M, Murakami T, Naitoh H, Nihei K. Studies on pediatric patients with absent auditory brainstem response (ABR) later components. Brain Dev. 1990;12:380–4.

72. Kabeya M, Satoh H, Fujisaki T, Takahashi S. The auditory brain response (ABR) in an infant with Joubert syndrome. Audiol Japan. 2002;45:680–4.
73. Starr A, Picton TW, Sininger Y, Hood LJ, Berlin CI. Auditory neuropathy. Brain. 1996;119(Pt 3):741–53.
74. Mizuno Y, Otsuka S, Takano Y, Suzuki Y, Hosaka A, Kaga M, Segawa M. Giant axonal neuropathy: combined central and peripheral nervous system disease. Arch Neurol. 1979;36:107–8.

Chapter 7
Hypoxic and Anoxic Brain Damage

Kimitaka Kaga

Abstract The ABRs of 16 infants and children, who had incurred brain damage as a sequela of hypoxic or anoxic incidents following near-suffocation or near-drowning, were obtained. There were eight patients assigned to the near-drowning (hypoxic) group and eight to the near-suffocation (anoxic) group. Clinically, all of these patients variably presented with cerebral palsy, mental retardation and/or epilepsy and had poor responses to VRA. Of the patients in the near-drowning group the ABR responses were abnormal in five of them, i.e., only waves I, II, and III were evoked in three of the cases and the amplitude of waves IV and V was low in two of the cases. Of the near-suffocation group ABRs were generally normal. This difference in the ABRs between the two groups suggests that, in infants and children, anoxic brain damage due to near-drowning might involve not only the cerebral cortex and subcortical white matter but also the upper brain stem and midbrain. To further study these different effects hypoxia and anoxia seen to have on the central nervous system, we recorded ABRs from the cat which were artificially respirated. Respiration was periodically arrested and then restored over various lengths of time. The ABRs were found to change within 7 min of respiratory arrest but they did not change after 3 min.

Keywords ABR · Near-suffocation · Hypoxic brain damage · Near-drowning · Anoxic brain damage · Hypothermia · Respiratory arrest

7.1 Hypoxic and Anoxic Brain Damage in Infants and Children

Following the perinatal period, hypoxic or anoxic brain damage occasionally occurs in infants and children as a result of accidents involving near-suffocation or near-drowning.

K. Kaga (✉)
National Institute of Sensory Organs, National Hospital Organization, Tokyo Medical Center, Audiology Clinic, Kamio Memorial Hospital, Tokyo, Japan
e-mail: kimitaka.kaga@kankakuki.jp; kimikaga-tky@umin.ac.jp

© Springer Japan KK, part of Springer Nature 2022
K. Kaga (ed.), *ABRs and Electrically Evoked ABRs in Children*, Modern Otology and Neurotology, https://doi.org/10.1007/978-4-431-54189-9_7

It has been reported that age underlies ischemic alterations of the brain due to hypoxic or anoxic accidents [1]. Hypoxic brain damage of fetuses and newborn infants accounts for a high proportion of children with cerebral palsy, mental retardation, epilepsy, and sensory/neural hearing loss [2–4]. We studied visual reinforcement audiometry (VRA) and ABRs in infants and children who were involved in sudden near-suffocation (hypoxic) or near-drowning accidents (anoxic).

7.2 Hypoxic Brain Damage in Near-Suffocation (Hypoxic) Group

Accidents of near-suffocation were caused by airway obstruction during nursing, sleeping on a futon (Japanese bedding) or during general anesthesia. Of the eight cases in this study with mental retardation, cortical blindness was noted in five cases, cerebral palsy in four cases, epilepsy in three cases, and cortical deafness in 1.

With the exception of two cases among eight cases, there was no reaction to sound stimuli by VRA. One of these infants reacted only to high intensity stimuli and the other one case showed a reaction to a low intensity level where healthy children normally react. However, ABRs overall were normal except from the left ear of Case 6 in which the neurological problems included left microtia and aural atresia. A typical ABR (Case 7) with no VRA responses is shown in Fig. 7.1. The VRA results and ABRs for the near-suffocation (hypoxic) group are summarized in Table 7.1.

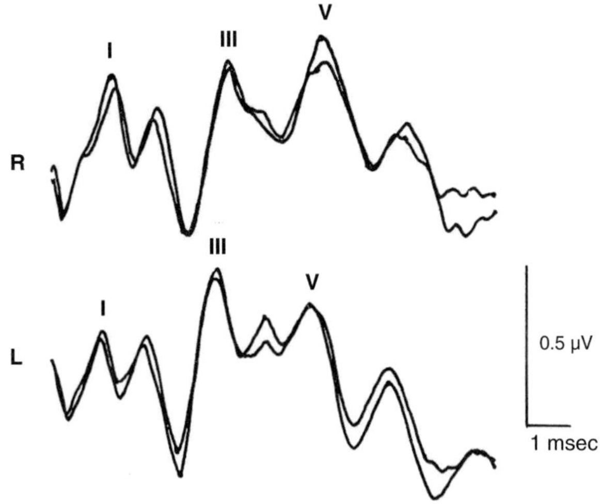

Fig. 7.1 Case 7. 10-month-old boy. A typical ABR from the near-suffocation (hypoxic) group. The VRA showed no response but the ABR was normal. R:right ear stimulus, L:left ear stimulus

Table 7.1 Near-suffocation (hypoxic) group

Case	Age at ABR	Neurological problems	VRA (dBHL)	ABR
1	13 months	Cerebral palsy, cortical blindness	No reaction	Normal
2	3 months	Cerebral palsy	No reaction	Normal
3	2 years	Cerebral palsy	90 dBHL	Normal
4	4 months	Epilepsy, cortical blindness	45 dBHL	Normal
5	8 months	Cortical deafness	No reaction	Normal
6	16 months	Epilepsy, cortical blindness	No reaction	Normal
7	10 months	Epilepsy, cortical blindness	No reaction	Normal
8	9 years	Cerebral palsy, cortical blindness	No reaction	Normal

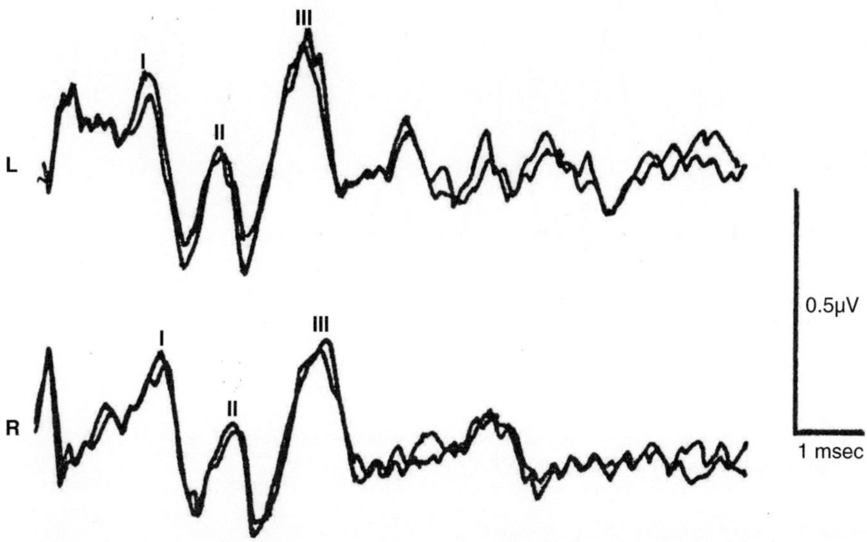

Fig. 7.2 Case 2. 16-month-old boy. An abnormal ABR with waves I, II, and III only of Case 2 of the near-drowning (anoxic) group. VRA showed no response

7.3 Brain Damage in the Near-Drowning (Anoxic) Group

These children incurred an airway obstruction due to near-drowning in a bathtub, in a washing machine, river, pond, or pool. Most of these children suffered from epilepsy and 2 cases were associated with mental retardation.

Of this group, VRA showed no response in six cases but normal responses in two cases. ABRs were abnormal in five cases: waves I, II, and III only were present in three cases and the amplitudes of waves IV and V were diminished in two cases. Figures 7.2 and 7.3 illustrate the abnormal ABRs from Case 2 and Case 5, respectively.

VRA and ABR findings from the near-drowning group (anoxic) are summarized in Table 7.2.

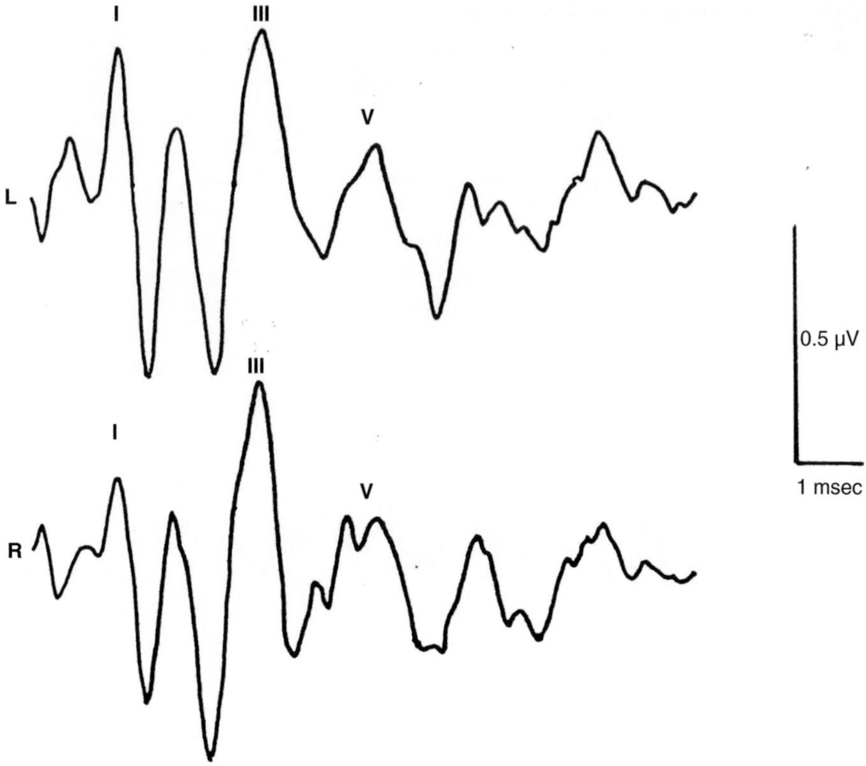

Fig. 7.3 Case 5. 3-year-old girl. An abnormal ABR with low amplitude of wave IV and V in Case 5 of the near-drowning (anoxic) group. VRA showed no response

Table 7.2 Near-drowning (anoxic) group

Case	Age at ABR	Neurological problems	VRA (dBHL)	ABR
1	14 months	Cerebral palsy	No response	Normal
2	16 months	Cerebral palsy	No response	R: Waves I, II, III L: Waves I, II, III
3	2 years	Cerebral palsy	60 dBHL	Normal
4	2 years	Cerebral palsy	No response	R: Waves I, II, III L: Waves I, II, III
5	3 years	Cerebral palsy	No response	R:Low amplitudes of waves IV, V L: Low amplitudes of waves IV, V
6	5 years	Cerebral palsy	No response	R: Waves I, II, III L: Waves I, II, III
7	6 years	Pseudobulbar palsy, epilepsy	Normal	R:Low amplitudes of waves IV, V L: Low amplitudes of waves IV, V
8	7 years	Epilepsy	Normal	Normal

7.4 Pathophysiology of Hypoxic and Anoxic Brain Damage Due to Near-Suffocation and Near-Drowning Accidents

Although this study revealed normal ABRs in the near-suffocation (hypoxic) group, ABRs from the near-drowning (anoxic) group revealed abnormal ABRs consisting of only waves I, II, and III or low amplitudes of waves IV and V. These abnormalities in the anoxic group suggests upper brainstem or midbrain pathophysiology in that the origins of ABR waves IV and V in humans have been demonstrated to be located in the lateral lemniscus and inferior colliculus [5–7]. On the other hand, in all cases in the near-suffocation (hypoxic) group, ABRs were normal. However, there is not much difference in the clinical neurological findings between these two groups. It may be that the differences in the ABR findings between the two groups indicates that near-drowning (anoxia) might cause more severe upper brainstem or midbrain damage than near-suffocation (hypoxia). The duration of hypoxia might have been longer and resuscitation attempts may have been delayed in the near-drowning (anoxic) group relative to the near-suffocation (hypoxia) group [8].

The degree of susceptibility and its location in regions of the brain following hypoxia or anoxia varies. The degree of pathology to hypoxia and anoxia is usually greater in the parietal and occipital lobes and is less obvious towards the temporal and frontal poles [1]. Heavily damaged centers include especially the lenticular nucleus, notably the globus pallidus, athetosis being a noteworthy clinical residual. The hippocampus and dentate nuclei are also susceptible. Regions of the cortex and subcortical white matter show varying degrees of degeneration [2].

On the basis of these ABR recordings of anoxia (near-drowning) children (absent waves IV and V, low amplitude of wave V), it can be deduced that hypoxia results in damage to the inferior colliculus [5–7].

It has been reported that in children who incurred a near-drowning (anoxic) event, their central nervous systems were severely damaged, and their prognoses depended on the age of the event, duration of anoxia, time lapse prior to resuscitation, depth of coma, pH of blood gases, and amount of CT abnormalities [9–11]. Neurological signs varied across these children, possibly because of variation within these cases in terms of their prognoses.

Finally, in neither of these (hypoxic nor anoxic) groups we were able to elicit auditory behavioral responses by VRA. We suggest that the absence of these responses most likely resulted from cortical and subcortical brain damage but not due to peripheral hearing loss.

7.5 Effects of Deep Hypothermia and Circulatory Arrest on the ABR and the EEG Undergoing Cardiac Surgery

At low temperature, changes in nerve function excitability occur, such as decreased resting potentials, decreased amplitude of action potentials, reduced conduction velocities and increased synaptic transmission delays [12]. ABR is a possible monitor of brainstem function at low temperature.

We investigated effects of cooling, circulatory arrest, and rewarming on the ABR and the electroencephalography (EEG) during surgical hypothermia undergoing cardiac surgery for children with congenital heart disease [13]. The latency of the ABR waves was prolonged and the amplitude of the EEG became smaller with decreased body temperature. The latency of the later wave components was prolonged more than that of the earlier wave components. All waves disappeared below 25 degrees and during artificial cardiac arrest. When the body temperature was raised, the later wave component began to reappear and the amplitude of the EEG became bigger above 25 degrees; the latency of all wave components shortened with temperature until normal responses were obtained at 34 degrees (Fig. 7.4).

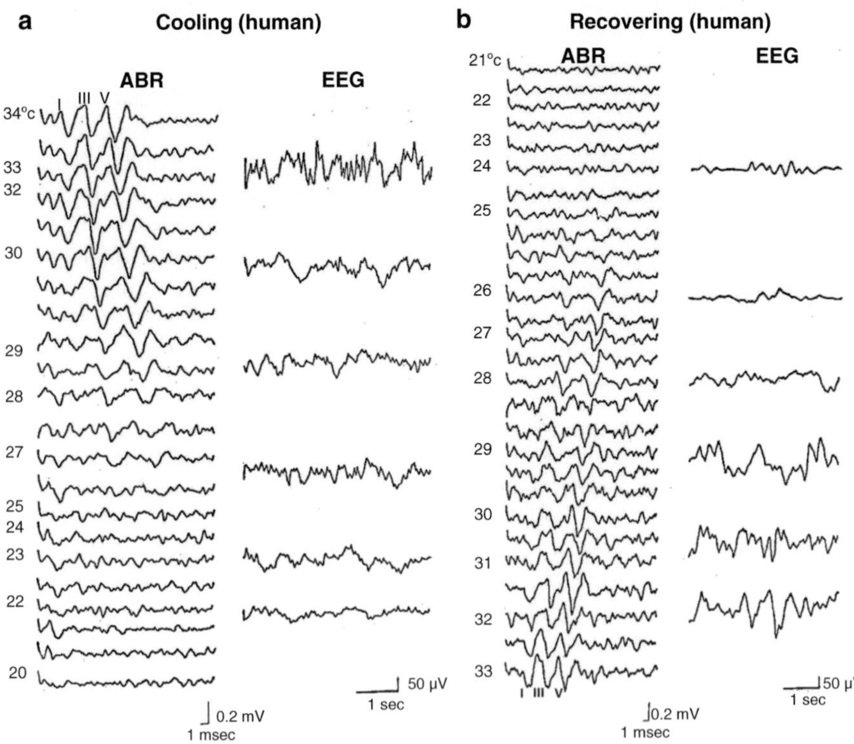

Fig. 7.4 ABR and EEG during hypothermia undergoing cardiac surgery. (**a**) Effects of cooling the patient's body on ABR and EEG, (**b**) Effects of recovering the patient's body temperature on ABR and EEG

These changes of the ABR can be explained by a decrease in the generator potential in the receptor organ and delay in synaptic transmission and in nerve conduction of brainstem at lower temperature. These effects are stronger for waves which depend on polysynaptic neuronal circuit.

The later ABR wave components are generated more rostrally along the auditory pathway and reticular formation in the brainstem. Therefore, the greater prolongation of the later wave is probably a reflection of more susceptibility to cooling for their generators' polysynaptic inputs.

Our study showed that the ABR was a useful monitor for evaluating brainstem function during deep hypothermia as well as the EEG for evaluating cerebral function.

7.6 ABRs from the Cat During Artificial Respiratory Arrest and Restoration

In our cat experiment, under artificial respiration and anesthetized with i.v. nembutal and myoblock, ABR changes were recorded at 3 and 7 min following cessation of respiration. After 3 min of respiratory cessation, the latencies of wave I, III, and IV did not change. However, after 7 min of respiratory cessation, the latency of wave V increased although the latencies of wave II and III did not. In temporal bone histological studies of cases of anoxia, the organ of Corti and the spiral ganglion have shown no appreciable alterations nor is the dorsal cochlea nucleus affected. On the other hand, the inferior colliculi seem to be affected by anoxia [2]. Prolonged latency of wave V may be related to susceptibility to anoxia of the inferior colliculi (Fig.7.5). In young rabbits experiment, severe hypoxia for 2 h produced significant prolongation and decreased amplitude of the long latency components of the ABR [14].

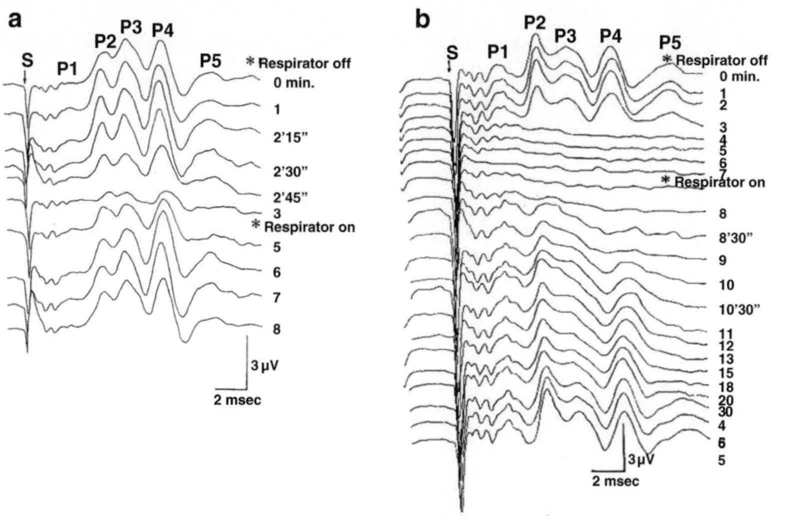

Fig. 7.5 ABRs of the anesthetized cat following termination and restoration of respiration. (**a**) 3 min of respiratory termination and recovery. (**b**) 7 min of respiratory termination and recovery

References

1. Brierley JB, Graham DI. Cerebral hypoxia. In: Adams JH, Corsellis JAN, Duchen LW, editors. Greenfield's neuropathology. London: Edward Arnold Ltd.; 1987. p. 125–207.
2. Dublin WB. Fundamentals of sensorineural auditory pathology. Springfield, IL: Charles C Thomas; 1976. p. 190–5.
3. Hecox K, Cone B. Prognostic importance of auditory evoked responses after asphyxia. Neurology. 1981;31:1429–33.
4. Kaga K, Kitazumi E, Kodama K. Auditory brainstem response of kernicterus infants. Int J Pediatr Otolaryngol. 1979;1:255–64.
5. Hashimoto I, Ishiyama Y, Yoshimoto T. Brainstem auditory-evoked potentials recorded directly from human brainstem and thalamus. Brain. 1981;104:841–59.
6. Jewett DL, Williston LS. Auditory-evoked far field averaged from the scalp of humans. Brain. 1971;94:681–96.
7. Møller R, Jannetta PJ. Neural generators of the auditory brainstem response. In: Jacobson JT, editor. The auditory brainstem responses. San Diego: College Hill; 1987. p. 13–31.
8. Kaga K, Ichimura K, Kitazumi E, Kodama K, Tamai F. Auditory brainstem responses in infants and children with anoxic brain damage due to near-suffocation or near-drowning. Int J Pediatr Otolaryngol. 1996;36:231–9.
9. Murray RR, Kapia A, Blanco E, Kagon-Hallet KS. Cerebral computed tomography in drowning victims. AJNR. 1984;5:177–9.
10. Orlowski JP. Prognostic factors in pediatric cases and the near-drowning. J Am Coll Emerg Physicians. 1979;8:176–9.
11. Taylor SB, Quencer RM, Holzman BH, Naidich TP. Central nervous system anoxic-ischemic insult in children due to near-drowning. Radiology. 1985;156:641–6.
12. Hubbard JI, Jones SF, Landau EM. The effects of temperature change upon transmitter release, facilitation and post-tetanic potentiation. J Physiol. 1971;216:591–609.
13. Kaga K, Takiguchi T, Myokai K, Shinoda A. Effects of deep hypothermia and circulatory arrest on the auditory brain stem responses. Arch Otorhinolaryngol. 1979;225:199–205.
14. Inagaki M. Effect of hypothermia and anoxia on ABR in rabbit. In: Kaga K, editor. ABR Handbook. Tokyo: Kanehara & Co., LTD; 1998. p. 17–9.

Chapter 8
Only Wave I, II of the ABR with Residual Hearing Acuity

Kimitaka Kaga

Abstract In the audiological and neurological diagnosis of infants and children with neurological disease, ABRs play a very important role. There are particular pediatric neurological diseases which show only waves I and II on the ABR, specifically Pelizaeus–Merzbacher disease of dysmyelination, adrenoleukodystrophy or leukodystrophy, i.e., Gaucher's disease, Tay–Sachs disease of metabolismm, and brainstem tumors with mild or moderate sensory/neural hearing loss. This study demonstrates that the loss of ABR waves following Waves I and II does not necessitate the loss of hearing.

Keywords Dysmyelination · Adrenoleukodystrophy · Metabolic disease · Brainstem tumor

8.1 Introduction

There are particular pediatric neurological diseases in which only Waves I and II are evoked on the ABR (absent or reduced Wave V). Nevertheless, most of these patients demonstrate preservation of their hearing. Patients with five of these particular neurological diseases were evaluated clinically and by ABR.

8.2 Pelizaeus–Merzbacher Disease

Pelizaeus, R reported the first case of Pelizaeus–Merzbacher disease (PMD) in 1885. PMD is an inherited X-linked recessive disorder which results in dysmyelination or hypomyelination of the central nervous system and is neuropathologically

K. Kaga (✉)
National Institute of Sensory Organs, National Hospital Organization, Tokyo Medical Center, Audiology Clinic, Kamio Memorial Hospital, Tokyo, Japan
e-mail: kimitaka.kaga@kankakuki.jp; kimikaga-tky@umin.ac.jp

© Springer Japan KK, part of Springer Nature 2022
K. Kaga (ed.), *ABRs and Electrically Evoked ABRs in Children*, Modern Otology and Neurotology, https://doi.org/10.1007/978-4-431-54189-9_8

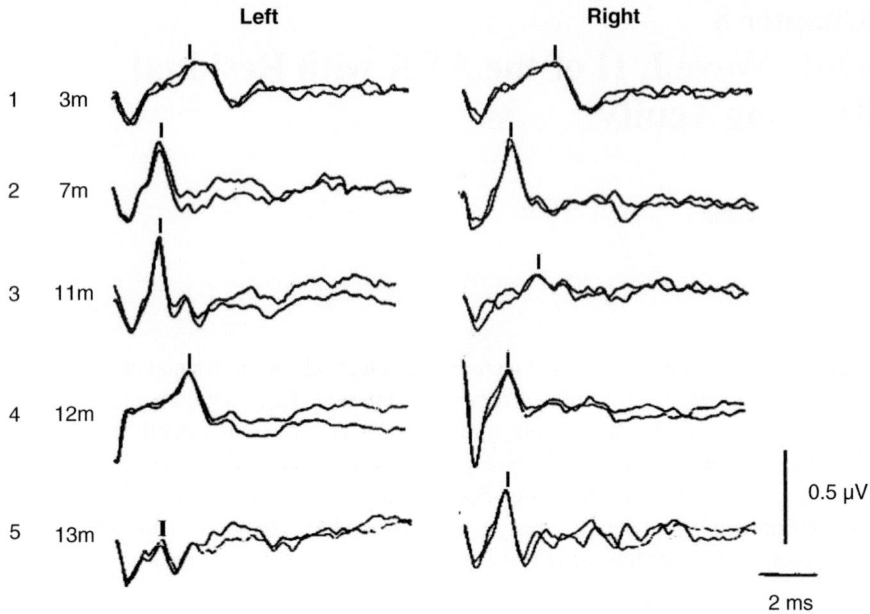

Fig. 8.1 ABRs of five different PMD infants. Only waves I or II are evoked throughout

regarded as a type of leukodystrophy. This disease is manifested during the prenatal period and is caused by a mutation of a gene on the X chromosome responsible for the production of a proteolipid. Clinically, these patients present with horizontal nystagmus and severe rigidity of the extremities. Although the patients showed only waves I and II on their ABRs (Fig. 8.1), they had relatively good behavioral audiometry by VRA as low as 30 dBSNL. The loss of the latter ABR evoked waves can be interpreted as due to the dysmyelination of axons resulting in desynchronization of subsequent neurons responsible for the production of these latter waves. T2-weighted brain MRIs of a PMD infant with only waves I and II on their ABR for both ears revealed high-intensity signals in the subcortical area (Fig. 8.2) [1].

8.3 Adrenoleukodystrophy

In 60 reported cases by Poser [2], adrenoleukodystrophy has been associated with diffuse cerebral sclerosis with skin pigmentation and, in some cases, evidence of adrenal insufficiency. This condition is found almost exclusively in males in a pattern that suggests an X-linked recessive transmission.

Both myelinoclastic and demyelinating diffuse sclerosis have been found in association with adrenal insufficiency. The signs and symptoms of adrenal insufficiency tend to precede the neurologic disorder. Correction of this Addisonian state does not alter the inevitable progression of diffuse sclerosis.

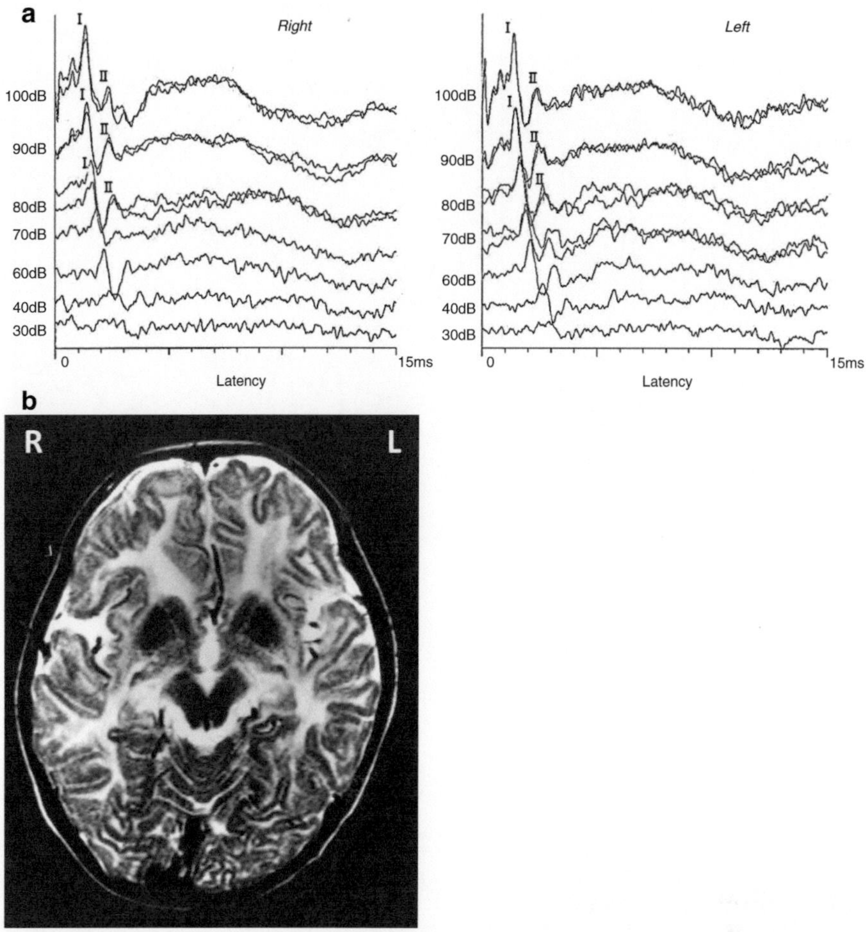

Fig. 8.2 ABRs with waves I and II only (**a**) and T2-weighted MRI of a PMD infant showing a high-intensity signal in the subcortical area (**b**)

In one particular case, postmortem pathologic examination of the brain revealed either myelinoclastic diffuse sclerosis or extensive demyelination. Peripheral neuropathy may dominate the clinical picture, leading to the diagnosis of adrenoneuropathy, as supported by abnormal ABR studies [3].

This particular child was normal until 5 years of age. His illness began with a gait disturbance, dysarthria, and hearing loss. Later, spastic paralysis, serious deafness, and blindness developed. This child's ABR was normal at onset but soon became abnormal. Initially, an increase in the interpeak interval between waves I and V was noted. This was followed by the disappearance of the later ABR waves (waves III and V) as his general condition deteriorated. Just prior to his death at age 7, only a prolonged wave I and II was recorded by ABR (Fig. 8.3). He ultimately died of respiratory failure. Postmortem pathology revealed demyelination of the auditory

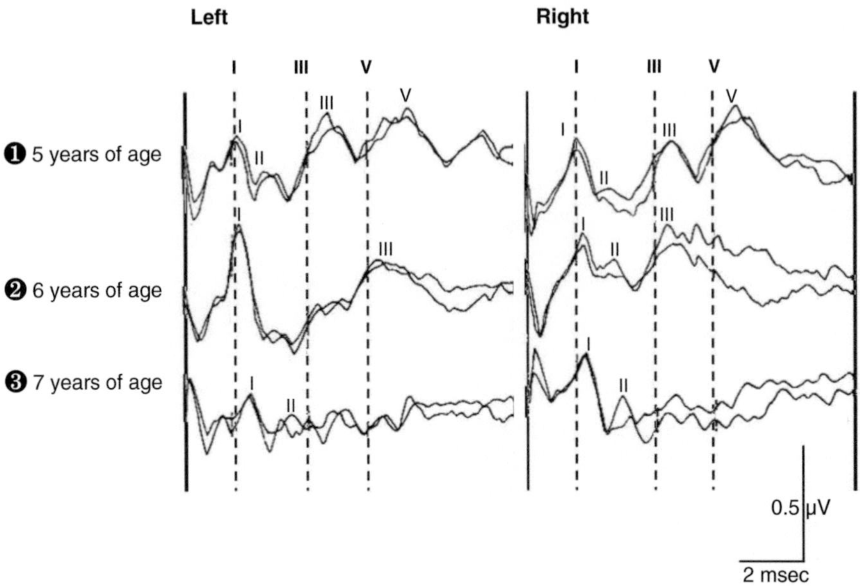

Fig. 8.3 ABR of an adrenoleukodystrophy boy just prior to death

nerves and remarkable neuronal loss in the auditory pathways of the brainstem. In particular, there was complete degeneration of the white matter with concomitant ganglionic cell changes. These findings suggest that, in adrenoleukodystrophy, degeneration of the brainstem progresses rostrally to caudally.

8.4 Metabolic Disease

8.4.1 Gaucher's Disease

Gaucher's disease is classified into three types based on the age of its onset, i.e., whether effecting adults, infants, or juveniles [4]. Infantile Gaucher's disease, type 2, or "acute neuronopathic Gaucher's disease," usually presents within 6 months of birth, the neonatal period often being normal. The first signs of hepatosplenomegaly, failure to thrive, or difficulty feeding can occur singularly or in combination. Motor delay is evident by 6 months and it progresses to cranial nerve and extrapyramidal tract involvement. Seizures are uncommon. Death, usually from pulmonary infection, generally occurs before the second birthday.

Kaga, M et al. [5] were able to record only ABR waves I and II and a small wave III from an infant with infantile Gaucher's disease at 6 months of age and only waves I and II by 8 months of age even though the autopsy showed relative preservation of the nuclei and tracts of the auditory pathways in the brainstem.

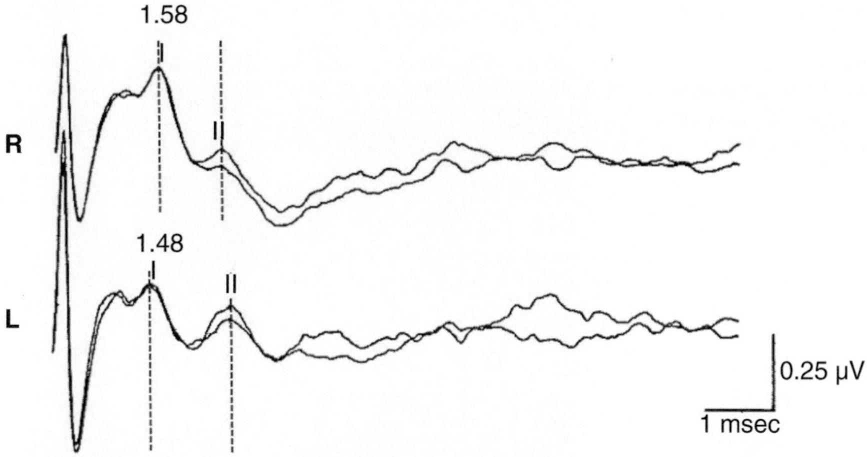

Fig. 8.4 ABR at 4 months of age. Only waves I and II were elicited from each ear. R, right; L, left

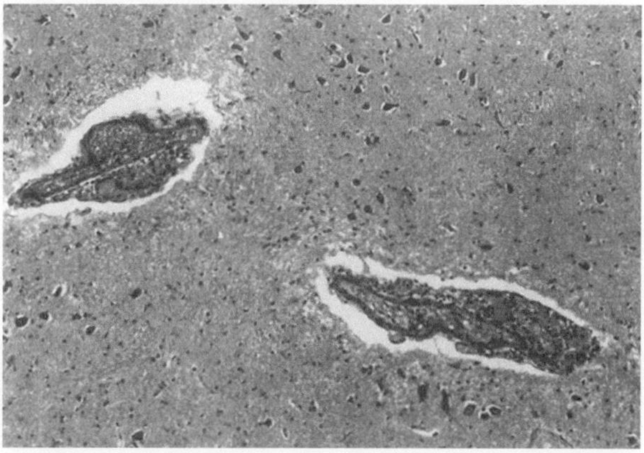

Fig. 8.5 Large Gaucher's cells in the anterior ventral nucleus of the thalamus. (H&E, ×100)

We also followed the ABR and neuropathologic changes in a female infant who died at 6 months of age because of typical (Type 2) infantile Gaucher's disease. This patient was hospitalized for hepatosplenomegaly and failure to thrive. Her ABR showed only waves I and II. (Fig. 8.4).

Postmortem neuropathological examination discerned Gaucher's cells in the perivascular region of the cerebrum and in the anterior ventral nucleus of the thalamus (Fig. 8.5). Gliosis was also noted in the dorsal part of the brainstem but not in its ventral part (Fig. 8.6) [6]. Neuronal cells in the superior olivary nucleus (SON) were also missing and marked gliosis was noted in the cochlear nucleus (Fig. 8.7). The disappearance of wave III and subsequent waves of the ABR can be attributed to these pathological findings [7]. In our study, ABR abnormalities were well correlated with specific brainstem pathologies.

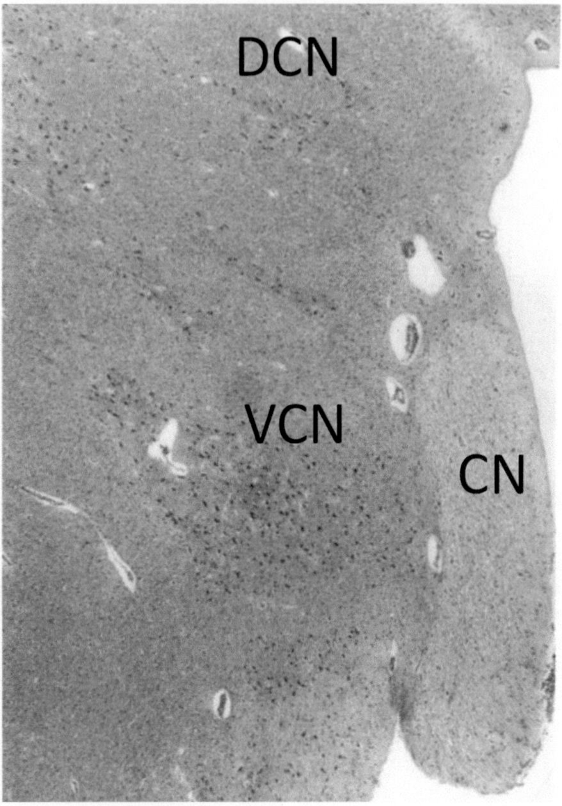

Fig. 8.6 Gliosis in the cochlear nerve (CN) and in the cochlear nucleus. *VCN*. Ventral cochlear nucleus; *DCN* dorsal cochlear nucleus. (H&E, ×40)

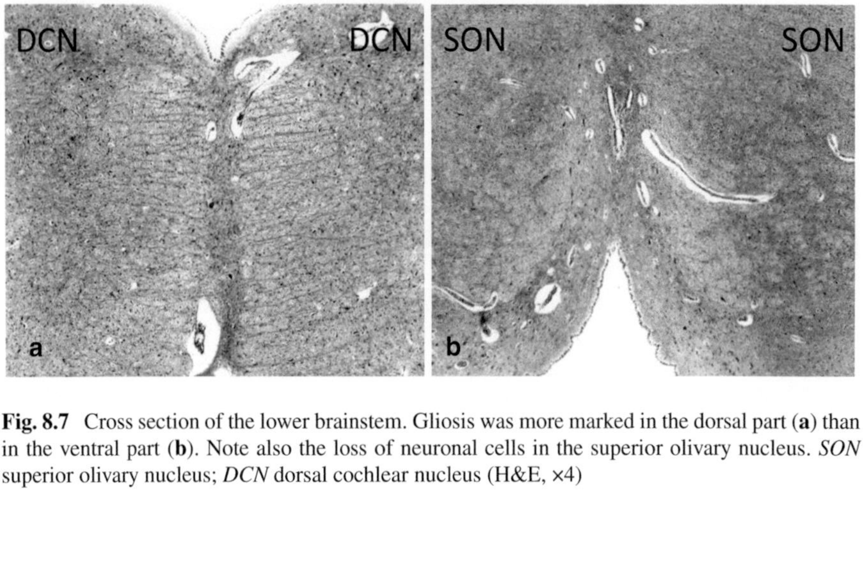

Fig. 8.7 Cross section of the lower brainstem. Gliosis was more marked in the dorsal part (**a**) than in the ventral part (**b**). Note also the loss of neuronal cells in the superior olivary nucleus. *SON* superior olivary nucleus; *DCN* dorsal cochlear nucleus (H&E, ×4)

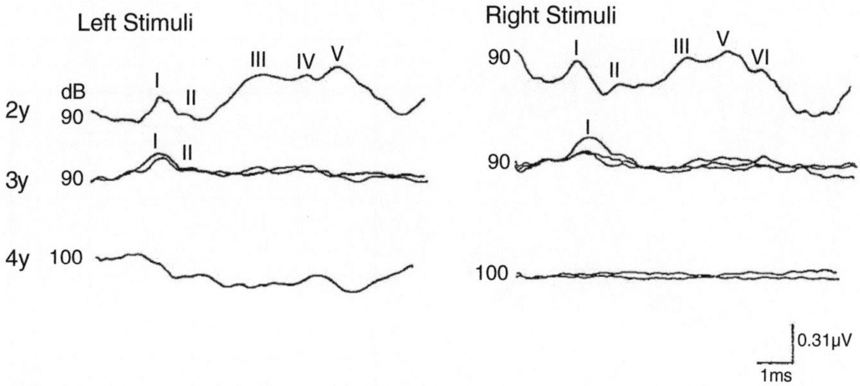

Fig. 8.8 Progressive ABR wave changes of a child with Tay–Sachs disease. At 2 years of age, all waves (I, III, and V) were prolonged. At the age of 3 years, only waves I and II were recorded and at the age of 4 years no ABR waves could be evoked

8.4.2 Tay–Sachs Disease

8.4.2.1 Case Report

This is a case of a 4-year-old boy with Tay–Sachs disease. Up until 3 months after birth his development was normal. Head control was acquired at 6 months. Afterwards, his motor development was seriously delayed with hypotenuse of his extremities. At the age of 12 months, he developed a macular cherry-red spot and an abnormal β hexosaminidase A titer. At the age of 1 year and 3 months, he developed a spastic myoclonus and loss of reaction to visual and auditory stimuli. On this basis, he was diagnosed with Tay–Sachs disease. At the age of 2, his EEG showed irregular slow waves of low amplitude and his ABR showed prolonged wave V latencies and increased waves I to V latency intervals. At the age of 3 years, his ABR showed only waves I and II. Wave II disappeared 1 year later (Fig. 8.8) [8].

Tay–Sachs disease is an infantile encephalopathy caused by a mutation at the α-Locus of the HEXA gene on chromosome 15. Tay–Sachs disease clinically manifests by dementia at about 6 months of age with visual loss, myoclonus seizures, and a macular cherry-red spot on the retina. Progressive vegetative states and death usually occur by the sixth year of age [9].

8.5 Brainstem Tumor

8.5.1 Case Report

Case 1

This case was a 7-year-old girl with a brainstem tumor. She presented with diplopia and right proptosis with left hemiparesis. Upon cerebral angiography she was

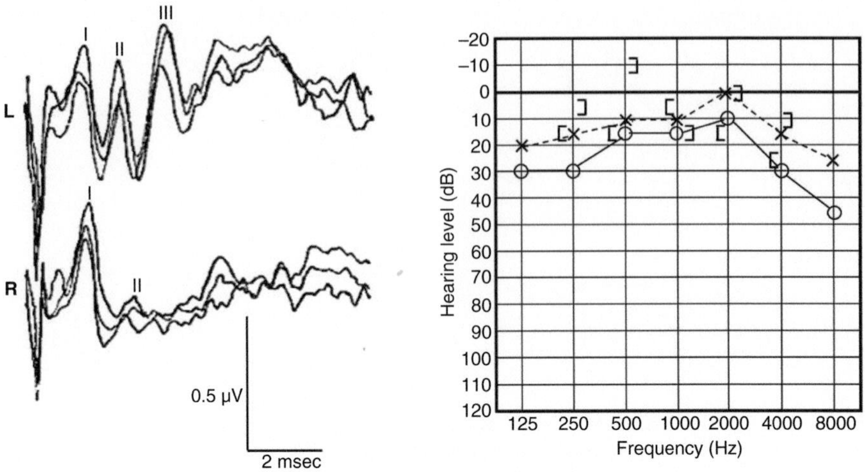

Fig. 8.9 Case 1. Abnormal ABRs of a girl with pontine glioma in the right pons

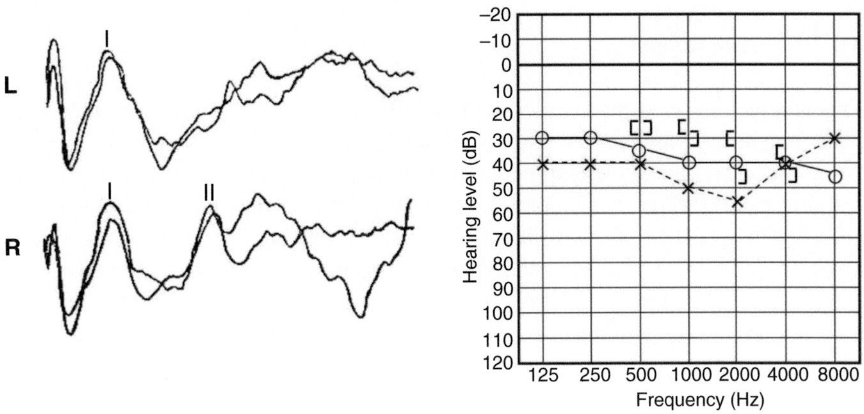

Fig. 8.10 Case 2. Abnormal ABRs of a boy with extensive glioma in the midbrain and pons

diagnosed with a right pontine angle tumor. Her ABR elicited only waves I and II from right ear stimuli and normal waves I, II, and III and a prolonged wave V from left ear stimuli (Fig. 8.9) [10]. Pure tone audiometry sound showed a very mild hearing loss in her right ear.

Case 2

This is a case of a 14-year-old boy with a brainstem tumor. He presented with a left facial nerve paralysis and right hemiparalysis and he complained of headache. Following brain angiography, and ultimately by surgery, he was diagnosed with an extensive tumor of his midbrain and pons. His ABRs elicited only wave I from right ear stimuli and wave I, II and III only from the left (Fig. 8.10) [9]. Pure tone audiometry indicated only a bilateral mild sensory/neural hearing loss.

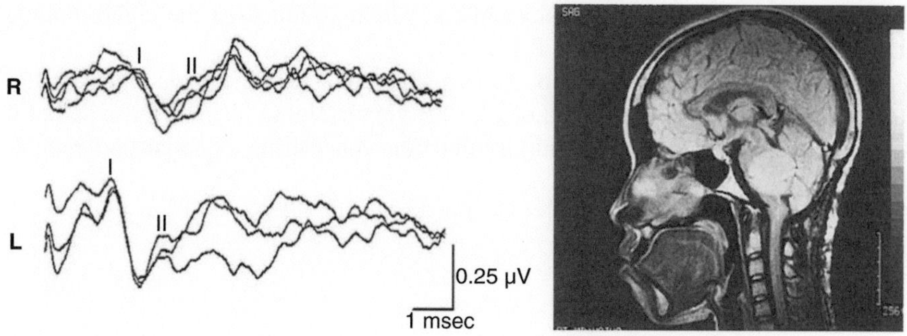

Fig. 8.11 Case 3. Abnormal ABRs of a girl with extensive glioma in the brainstem

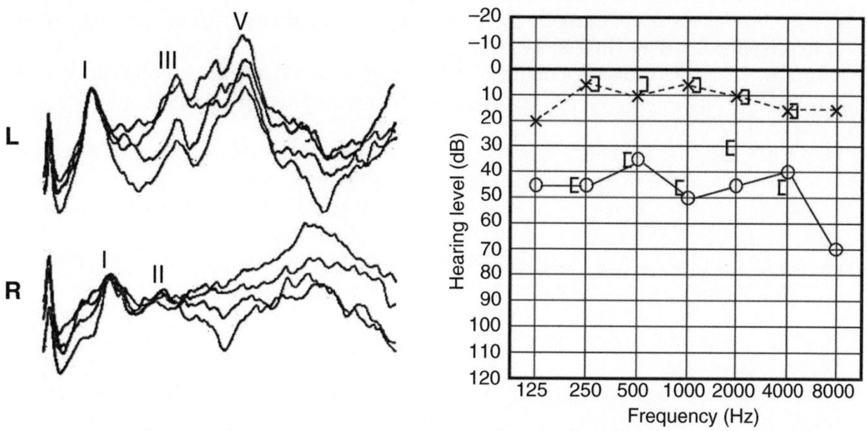

Fig. 8.12 Case 4. ABRs and pure tone audiograms of a boy with the right CP angle tumor

Case 3

This was a 15-year-old girl who complained of diplopia and unsteadiness. A sagittal view of her brain MRI disclosed a large tumor in her brainstem (Fig. 8.11) which was determined to be a glioma. Her ABR responses included only waves I and II provoked bilaterally. Her pure tone audiometric results were normal bilaterally. She subsequently underwent brainstem irradiation to decrease the glioma and was given chemotherapy [10].

Case 4

A case of a 16-year-old girl with a brainstem tumor. At presentation, she complained of a right ear hearing loss and right facial nerve paresis. A CT scan revealed a cerebellopontine angle tumor on her right brainstem. Her ABR responses consisted of only waves I and II to right ear stimuli but normal wave production and latencies from her left ear. Her pure tone audiometric findings indicated a moderate sensory/neural hearing loss in her right and normal hearing in her left ear. She underwent neurosurgery for this cerebellopontine angle tumor, and it was found that her facial nerve on the right side had a schwannoma which compressed the eighth cranial nerve which was extirpated (Fig. 8.12) [11].

In children, brainstem tumors occur frequently in the pontine angle region. ABRs and MRIs of these brainstem pathologies are very useful to localize these pathologies and to grade their extent. Auditory function, considering this brainstem pathology, is generally well preserved.

References

1. Kaga K, Tamai F, Kodama M, Kodama K. Three young adult patients with Perizaeus-Merzbacher disease who showed only wave I and II in auditory brainstem responses but had good auditory perception. Acta Otolaryngol. 2005;125:1018–23.
2. Poser CM. Adrenoleukodystrophy. In: Roland LP, editor. Merits textbook of neurology. 7th ed. Philadelphia: Lea & FEBIGER; 1984. p. 449.
3. Kaga K, Tokoro Y, Tanaka Y, Ushijima H. The progress of adrenoleukodystrophy as revealed by auditory brainstem evoked responses and brainstem histology. Arch Otorhinolaryngol. 1980;228:17–27.
4. Lake BD. Infantile Gaucher's disease. In: Adames JH, Corsellis JAN, Duchen LW, editors. Gaucher disease. 4th ed. London: Edward Arnold; 1984. p. 522–6.
5. Kaga M, Azuma C, Imamura T, Murakami T, Kaga K. Auditory brainstem response (ABR) in infantile Gaucher's disease. Neuropediatrics. 1982;13:207–10.
6. Lacey DJ, Terplan K. Correlating auditory evoked and brainstem histological abnormalities in infantile Gaucher's disease. Neurology. 1984;34:539–41.
7. Kaga K, Ono M, Yakumaru K, Owada M, Mizutani T. Brainstem pathology of infantile Gaucher's disease with only wave I and II of auditory brainstem response. J Laryngol Otol. 1998;112:1069–73.
8. Ozawa H, Hashimoto T, Kaga M. ABRs of two children with Tay-Sachs disease. Clin EEG. 1999;41:128–31.
9. Johnson WG. Lysosomal disease and other storage disease. In: Roland LP, editor. Merits textbook of neurology. 7th ed. Philadelphia: Lea & FEBIGER; 1984. p. 391–7.
10. Kaga K, Takahashi K, Yagi T, Suzuki J-I. Auditory brainstem response. J Med Technol. 1977;21:63–71.
11. Kaga K. Generators of auditory evoked potentials. Adv Neurol Sci. 2002;46(1):110–27.

Chapter 9
Auditory Agnosia and Later Cortical Deafness in a Child over 29 Years Follow-Up

Kimitaka Kaga and Mitsuko Shindo

Abstract There are two types of central auditory disorders due to pathology of the bilateral auditory cortices: *auditory agnosia* with some residual hearing; *cortical deafness* with total hearing loss. In this chapter we present and discuss our long-term experience with a male patient who, at a young age, was diagnosed with auditory agnosia which progressed to cortical deafness as a teenager.

At his age of 1 year and 3 months he incurred herpes simplex encephalitis which caused bilateral temporal lobe and auditory cortex lesions resulting in his auditory agnosia. We followed this patient until he was 29 years old. His subjective hearing decreased over time from normal hearing to profound hearing loss although his peripheral hearing organs and brainstem auditory pathways were preserved until his age of 29. He was not able to speak nor comprehend spoken language and was educated at a school for the deaf from kindergarten to high school by visually based communication techniques such as cued speech, finger spelling, sign language, and written language. Upon graduating from high school, he commutes to a day-care facility where work continues to improve his communication using sign language and written conversation.

Keywords Auditory agnosia · Cortical deafness · Herpes simplex · Auditory cortex · Auditory radiation

K. Kaga (✉)
National Institute of Sensory Organs, National Hospital Organization, Tokyo Medical Center, Audiology Clinic, Kamio Memorial Hospital, Tokyo, Japan
e-mail: kimitaka.kaga@kankakuki.jp

M. Shindo
National Institute of Sensory Organs, National Hospital Organization, Tokyo Medical Center, Tokyo, Japan
e-mail: kimikaga-tky@umin.ac.jp

© Springer Japan KK, part of Springer Nature 2022

K. Kaga (ed.), *ABRs and Electrically Evoked ABRs in Children*, Modern Otology and Neurotology, https://doi.org/10.1007/978-4-431-54189-9_9

9.1 Bilateral Auditory Cortex Lesions and Hearing

Obviously, normal hearing acuity plays a major role in the development of speech and language. The auditory system essentially consists of the peripheral end organs and the central auditory system. The cause of auditory imperception (agnosia) in patients with bilateral auditory cortex lesions remains controversial. Again, bilateral auditory cortex lesions can manifest as auditory agnosia, preservation of some residual hearing, or cortical deafness, a total loss of hearing. In adults, cortical deafness is usually caused by two episodes of cerebral infarction. However, in pediatric cases, auditory agnosia is frequently caused by herpes encephalitis [1]. Adult cases have been extensively studied but long-term follow-up studies of pediatric cases have rarely been reported [2]. The progression of residual hearing changes over time of these pediatric patients is not well documented. It is enlightening and instructive to be able to observe, measure, and record these patients' changing ability to communicate during their development from an educational and rehabilitative point of view.

9.2 Case Report: Long-Term Follow-Up of a Pediatric Patient over 29 Years Who Manifested Auditory Agnosia and Later Cortical Deafness Caused by Herpes Encephalitis

This is a case report of a pediatric patient with auditory agnosia as a sequela of herpes encephalitis, onset at 1 year 3 months. This patient was followed up and evaluated neurologically, neuropsychologically, educationally and by rehabilitative aspects until he was 29 years old.

His brain MRI findings at ages of 2, 4, and 29 years are shown in Fig. 9.1. In the horizontal section at the top of the image, a high signal intensity is evident in the superior temporal gyrus bilaterally at T2 weighting and lesions of the auditory cortex can be seen bilaterally at T1. In the coronal sections, at the bottom of the image, lesions of the auditory cortex are evident bilaterally.

In this patient case, his pure tone audiometric test results remained normal from initial onset until he attained school age and he was able to hear his mother call him from downstairs and respond. Around the time he graduated from high school at the school for the deaf, he had developed a profound hearing loss bilaterally which progressed until his age of 29 when his hearing loss was off-scale and could not be measured, indicative of severe profound hearing loss (Fig. 9.2).

Objective audiometry at age 29, by DPOAE, was normal bilaterally (Fig. 9.3). ABR testing at 5 years old, using click stimuli, displayed normal waveforms with waves I, III, and V evoked at 80 dBSNL and a threshold of wave V at 20 dBSNL. At 29 years of age, both ears displayed normal wave forms with waves I, III, and V evoked at 80 dBSNL. His left ear gave a threshold of wave V at 20 dBSNL and his right ear at 30 dBSNL (Fig. 9.4).

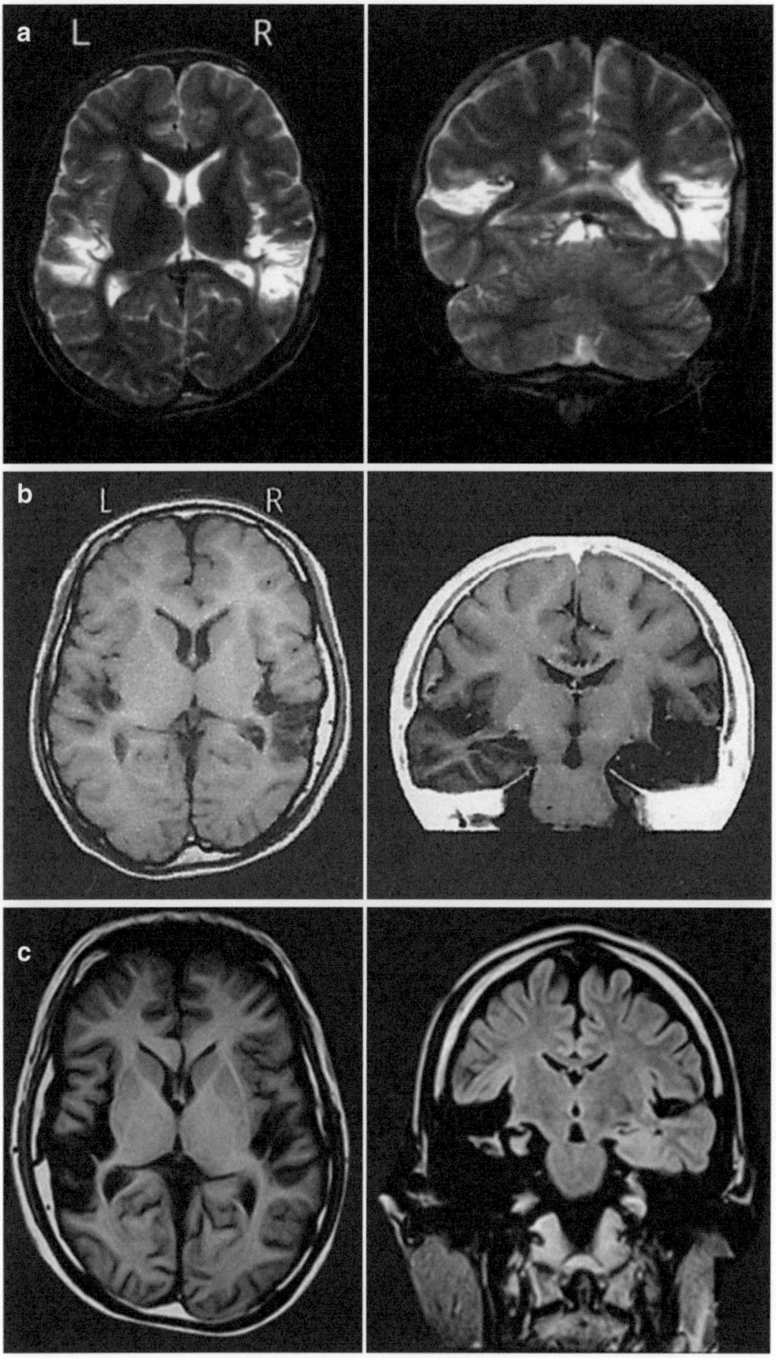

Fig. 9.1 Brain MRIs of a patient with auditory agnosia and later cortical deafness with bilateral lesions of auditory cortex. (**a**) 2 years old, T2, (**b**) 4 years old, T1, (**c**) 29 years old, T1

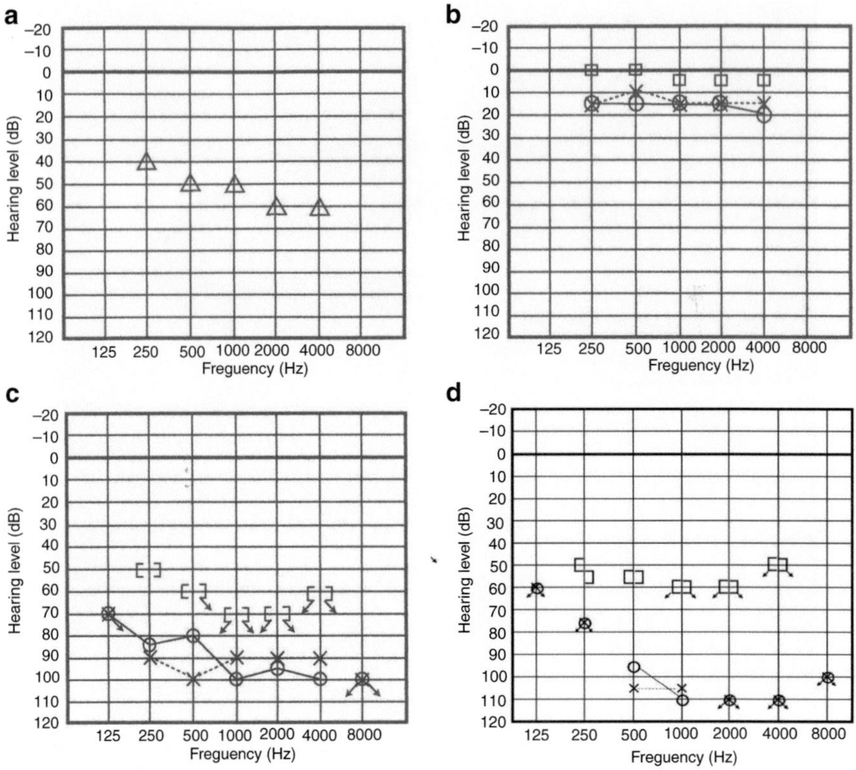

Fig. 9.2 Progressive changes of pure tone audiometry testing over 29 years from a patient with auditory agnosia and later cortical deafness. (**a**) 2 years old, (**b**) 5 years old, (**c**) 18 years old, (**d**) 29 years old

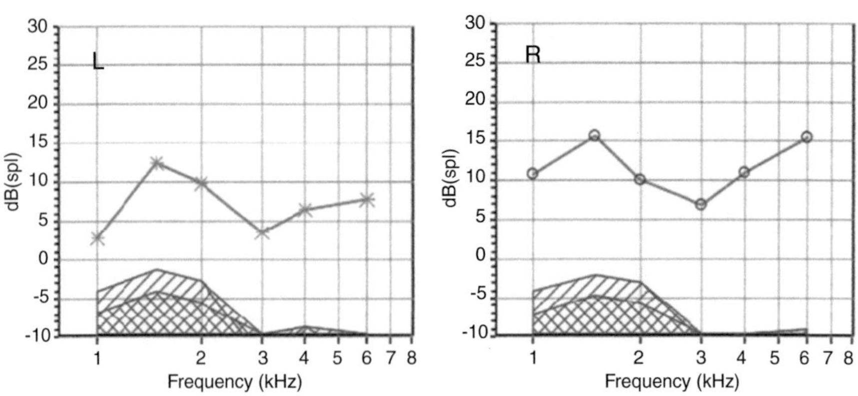

Fig. 9.3 DPOAE testing of a patient with cortical deafness at 29 years old

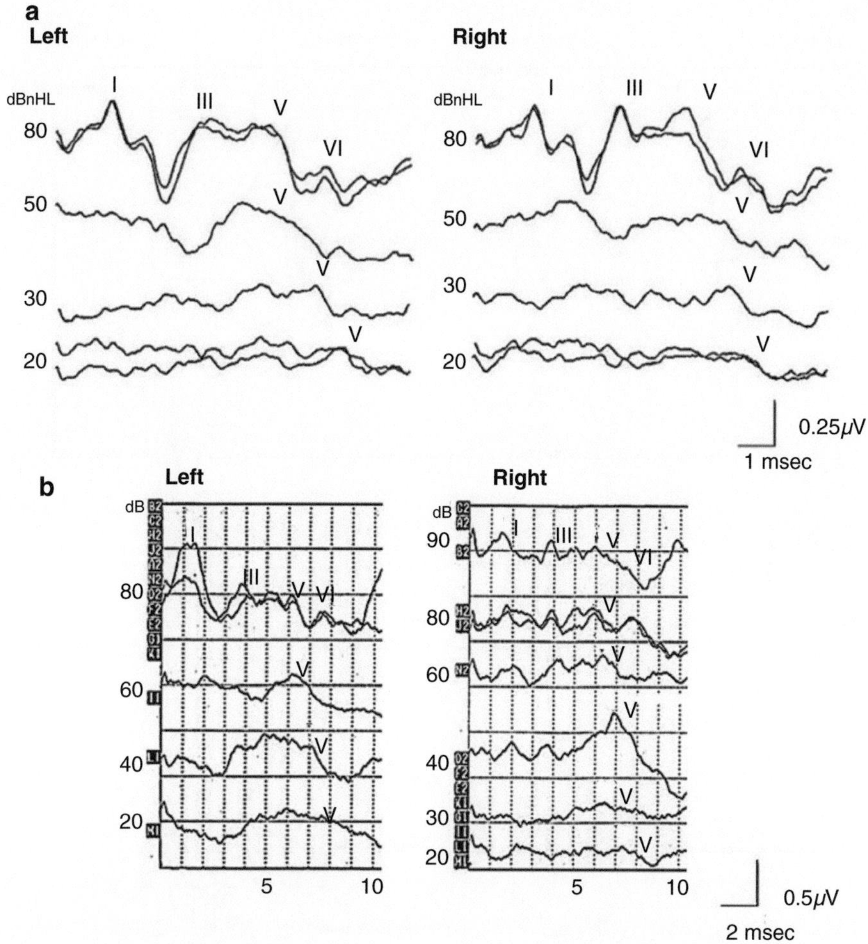

Fig. 9.4 Sequential ABR results of auditory agnosia and later cortical deafness. (**a**) At 5 years old, (**b**) at 29 years old

9.3 Schema of the Auditory Cortex or the Auditory Radiation Lesions in Auditory Agnosia and Cortical Deafness

Figure 9.5 shows an illustration of four patterns of lesions to the bilateral auditory cortex or auditory radiations which result in auditory agnosia due to cerebrovascular lesions in adults. In auditory agnosia caused by herpes simplex encephalitis in children, lesions are commonly localized around the bilateral superior temporal lobes and include the auditory cortices (Fig. 9.5a). However, we have found that in our long-term follow-up of these patients with auditory agnosia, the progression from

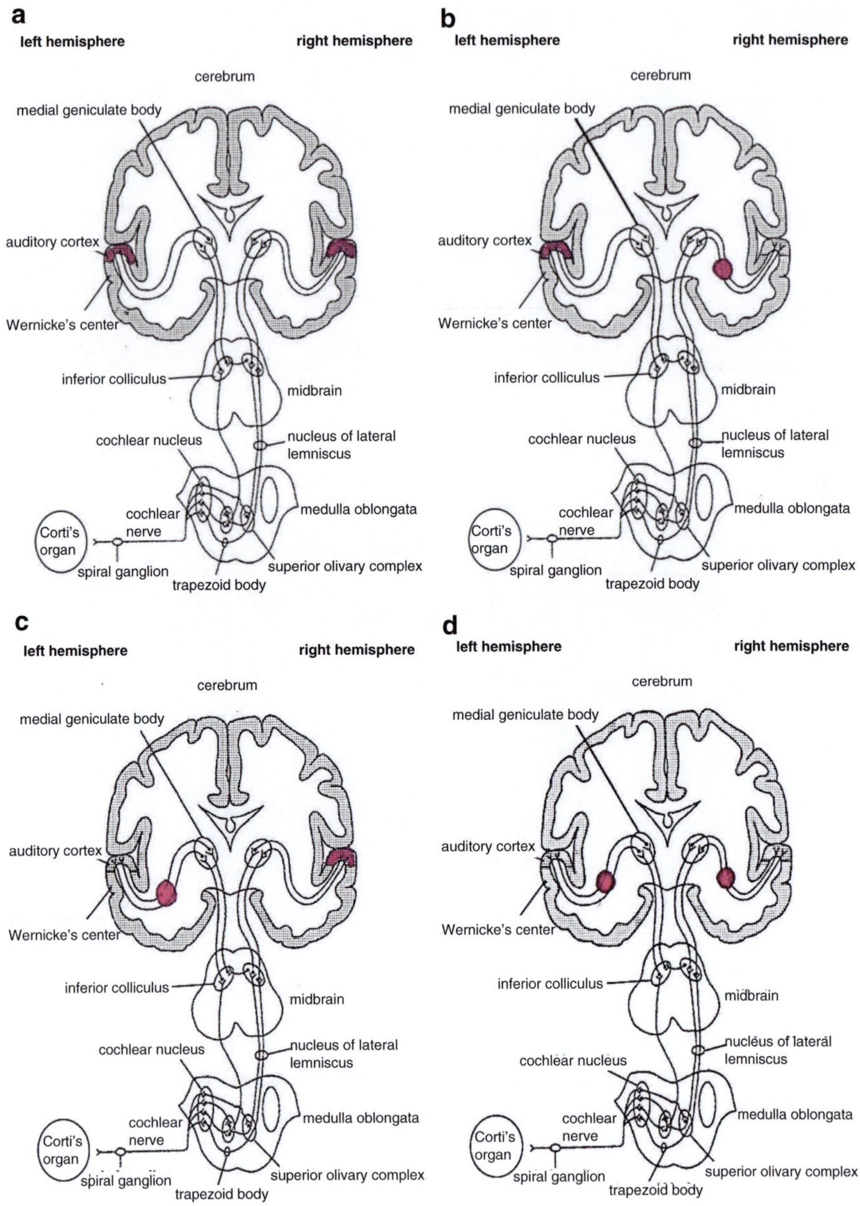

Fig. 9.5 Schema of four lesion patterns in auditory agnosia and cortical deafness. (**a**) Bilateral auditory cortex lesions, (**b**) left auditory cortex lesion and right auditory radiation lesion, (**c**) left auditory radiation lesion and right auditory cortex lesion, (**d**) bilateral auditory radiation lesions

auditory agnosia to cortical deafness may be due to retrograde degeneration of auditory radiation pathways (Fig. 9.5d).

9.4 Cortical Deafness Following Auditory Agnosia

In all of the patients with juvenile auditory agnosia due to bilateral auditory cortex lesions who we have followed, their ABRs consistently displayed normal thresholds and normal waveforms from wave I through wave VII. Although pure tone audiometric findings showed normal or moderately elevated hearing levels, responses to verbal stimuli and environmental sounds were not evaluated. Patients with ongoing auditory agnosia or cortical deafness had difficulty developing auditory perceptual skills and hearing aids or cochlear implants were completely ineffective [1, 2].

This patients' objective audiometric findings (DPOAEs and ABRs) indicated that he maintained normal peripheral end organs of hearing and normal brainstem auditory pathways through his life. It is likely that his total loss of hearing as a teenager was due to retrograde degeneration of auditory radiations or neurons in the medial geniculate body.

Historically, the term "cortical deafness" may have been first used by Henschen in 1918 [3]. This term is often used interchangeably with "central deafness" and may also be synonymous with generalized auditory agnosia [4]. The term "auditory agnosia" has been applied to a group of disorders wherein patients are unable to recognize auditorily presented sounds in the absence of any deficit in processing spoken language, though at times this is difficult to evaluate [5]. The term "cortical deafness" may lead to the misunderstanding that deafness is caused by damage to the auditory cortex only. We propose that subcortical deafness is a subtype of auditory agnosia in that the common loci of lesions suggest significant damage to the bilateral subcortical areas including the medial geniculate bodies (MGBs) in the ascending auditory pathways. The original term of cortical deafness was used because of findings that this type of deafness was associated with damage to the bilateral cortices [6, 7].

As far as communication ability is concerned in juvenile auditory agnosia, all of our patients were not able to develop comprehension of spoken language nor to develop speech. These patients were taught visual communication techniques such as sign language, fingerspelling, or writing and received education via classes for students with multiple learning difficulties at schools for the deaf or at special needs facilities for the physically handicapped. However, all of our patients had poor language skills, including poor vocabulary, difficulty in fostering abstract conceptualizations, and difficulty with syntax acquisition [1, 2]. As such, these long-term residual communication problems cannot be taken lightly and long-term follow-up observations with ongoing specialized support, including educational assistance and counseling appropriate to each individual child's level of development, is indispensable.

References

1. Kaga K, Kaga M, Tamai F, Shindo M. Auditory agnosia in children after herpes encephalitis. Acta Otolaryngol. 2003;123:232–5.
2. Kaga M, Shindo M, Kaga K. Long-term follow-up of auditory agnosia as a sequel of herpes encephalitis in a child. J Child Neurol. 2000;15:626–9.
3. Henschen SE. Über die Hörsphäre. J Psychol Neurol. 1918;22:319–474.
4. Musiek FE, Chermak GE, Cone B. Central deafness: a review of past and current perspectives. Int J Audiol. 2019;58(10):605–17.
5. Poliva O, Bestelmeyer P, Hall M, Bultitude JH, Koller K, Rafal RD. Functional mapping of the human auditory cortex: fMRI investigation of a patient with auditory agnosia from trauma to the inferior colliculus. Cogn Behav Neurol. 2015;28(3):160–80.
6. Akiyoshi R, Kaga K, Shindo M. Subcortical deafness as a subtype of auditory agnosia after injury of bilateral auditory radiations caused by two cerebrovascular accidents-Normal auditory brainstem responses with I-VII waves and abolished consciousness of hearing. Acta Otolaryngol. 2021;141:374–80;
7. Kaga K, Shinjo Y, Enomoto C, Shindo M. A case of cortical deafness and loss of vestibular somatosensory sensations caused by cerebrovascular lesions in bilateral primary auditory cortices, auditory radiations, and postcentral gyruses-complete loss of hearing despite normal DPOAE and ABR. Acta Otolaryngol. 2015;135:389–94.

Part III
Electrically Evoked ABRs (EABRs)

Chapter 10
Electrically Evoked Auditory Brainstem Responses (EABRs), Recording Techniques, Normal (Control) and Abnormal Waveforms of the EABR

Kimitaka Kaga and Chieko Enomoto

Abstract There are two types of EABRs (Electrically evoked Auditory Brainstem Response) which can be recorded following direct stimulation of the cochlear nerve, even from audiometrically deaf patients. One type of EABR consists of recordings taken from the contralateral cochlear promontory of the middle ear by a needle or ball electrode. The other type of EABR, the intracochlear type, is recorded as a result of electrical stimuli applied directly to the CI, during its insertion, again under general anesthesia. This intracochlear type can also be recorded post-CI in the clinic from a patient under deep sleep in a sound conditioned room. The intraoperative recordings of EABRs from an intracochlear electrode show clear and large positive wave potentials which consist of eII, eIII, and eV. Wave eI, from the cochlear nerve, is not evoked because of electrical stimulation itself.

We herein present our recording and stimulus techniques to evoke the EABR which were obtained from multiple subjects over a multi-generational age range: 1-year-old infants to 80-year-old patients.

In addition, we propose that there are four typical types of waveform abnormalities of the EABR which have clinical value in establishing auditory brainstem pathologies. The EABR is also useful to postoperatively determine the effectiveness of a CI.

Keywords EABR · eV · Cochlear implant (CI) · Brainstem

K. Kaga (✉)
National Institute of Sensory Organs, National Hospital Organization, Tokyo Medical Center, Audiology Clinic, Kamio Memorial Hospital, Tokyo, Japan
e-mail: kimitaka.kaga@kankakuki.jp

C. Enomoto
National Institute of Sensory Organs, National Hospital Organization, Tokyo Medical Center, Tokyo, Japan

© Springer Japan KK, part of Springer Nature 2022

K. Kaga (ed.), *ABRs and Electrically Evoked ABRs in Children*, Modern Otology and Neurotology, https://doi.org/10.1007/978-4-431-54189-9_10

10.1 Two Types of EABRs Recordings for Patient

There are two types of EABRs which can be evoked from the clinically deaf patient by electrical pulse stimulation of the cochlear nerve [1]. The purpose of the EABR is to determine if the auditory nerve responds as expected to this electrical stimulation. On this basis, it can be determined, pre-surgically and under anesthesia, if an auditory brainstem or cochlear implant (CI) should be attempted and post-surgically to determine if a CI is working properly. One type of EABR consists of recordings taken from the contralateral cochlear promontory of the middle ear by a needle or ball electrode. The other type of EABR, the intracochlear type, is recorded as a result of electrical stimuli applied directly to the CI, during its insertion, again under general anesthesia. This intracochlear type can also be recorded post-CI in the clinic from a patient under deep sleep in a sound conditioned room.

Historically, the first EABR evoked from stimulating a single-channel CI was reported by Starr et al. in 1979 [2]. The cochlear implanted electrode which was stimulated was inserted into the scala tympani of the cochlea.

CI electrodes available today have at least 12 channels along their lengths, each of which can be independently stimulated. Figure 10.1a is an illustration of the location of a particular five-channel intracochlear electrode in the mid-modiolar section of the cochlea (red circles). Figure 10.1b is a schematic illustrating the intracochlear stimulus channel nodes of the MED-EL's Flex 28 CI electrode.

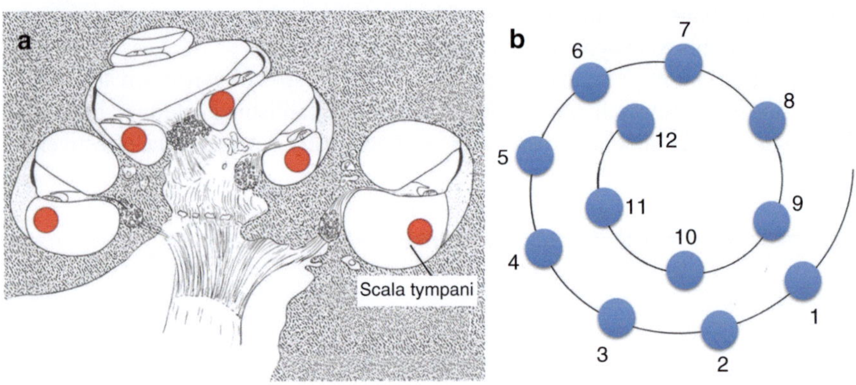

Fig. 10.1 Location of stimulus intracochlear electrodes in the cochlea. A schema of representative location of intracochlear electrodes in the modiolar section of the cochlea is illustrated by red circle (Nomura Y, Atlas of Otology 4th ed., 2017) (**a**) and a schema of cochlear implant intracochlear electrodes of MED-EL's Flex 28 (**b**)

10.2 EABR Recording Protocol

Under general anesthesia, a CI electrode was inserted into the scala tympani of the cochlea. The EABRs were then obtained using the Neuropack Σ (Nihon Kohden Co., Ltd.) system.

10.2.1 Montage of Skin Needle Electrodes for Recording EABRs

We recorded two channels simultaneously of the EABR with skin needle electrodes. The positive electrode was inserted into the skin at the forehead hairline. Two negative electrodes were inserted, one (channel 1) on the mastoid of the non-operated, contralateral, ear and the other (channel 2) on the nape of the neck. Ground was taken at the shoulder on the non-operative side (Fig. 10.2). Channel 2 recordings were often contaminated by myogenic potentials from the neck muscles induced by the electrical stimulation. These simultaneous dual-channel recordings were employed to compare the waveforms and to better differentiate waves eII, eIII, and eV. Electrical artifacts were carefully removed by switching off surrounding devices in the operating room.

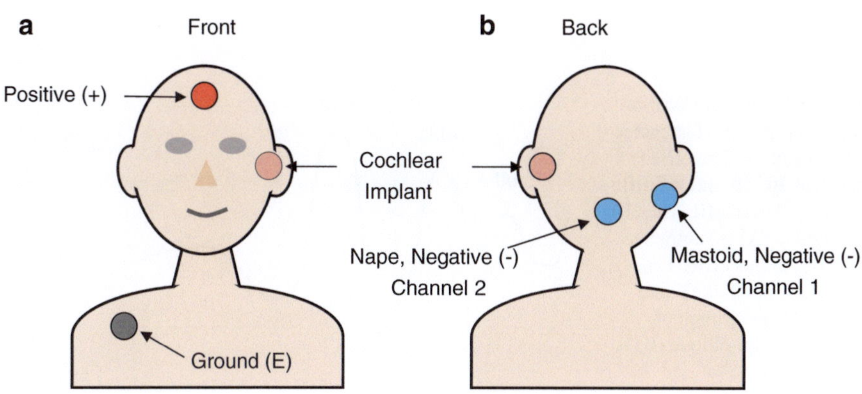

Fig. 10.2 Montage of skin needle electrodes for recording EABRs. Position of skin needle electrodes for simultaneous two-channel recordings in case of a cochlear implant in the left ear. (**a**) front, (**b**) back

10.2.2 Electrical Stimulation from Intracochlear Electrodes

The stimuli used to evoke an EABR were delivered by MED-EL Maestro software to the intracochlear electrodes (CIs) at three stimulus levels: 1000 cu (current units), 800 cu, and 600 cu, with a pulse width of 30 μsecs.

10.2.3 Recording Conditions

For recording EABRs, response frequencies above 1000 Hz and below 100 Hz were high and low pass filtered to remove artifacts and the summed responses to 1000 stimuli were averaged.

10.3 Measurement of the Amplitudes and Latencies of eIII and eV

Figure 10.3 illustrates measurement procedures of each peak latency and amplitude of eIII and eV. The eIIIa is the peak of eIII and the eIIIb is the trough of eIII. Then the eIII amplitude (A) is subtracted by eIIIa minus eIIIb. The peak latency of eIII indicates peak of eIIIa and that of eV indicates the peak of eVa. The eV amplitude (B) is subtracted by eVa minus eVb.

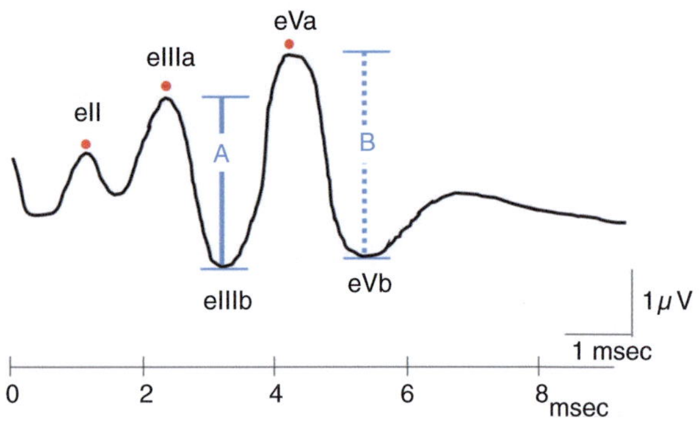

Fig. 10.3 Measurement of the amplitudes and latencies of eIII and eV. The eIIIa is the peak of eIII and the eIIIb is the trough of eIII. The eIII amplitude (A) is subtracted by eIIIa minus eIIIb. The eVa is the peak of eV and the eVb is the trough of eV. The eV amplitude (B) is subtracted by eVa minus eVb

10.4 Typical Waveform of the EABR in Control (Normal) Subjects

Typical EABRs consist of waves eII, eIII, and eV evoked over the analysis time of 10 ms. However, eI was not recorded because the cochlear nerve itself is electrically stimulated.

10.4.1 EABRs Waveforms Recorded from Each of the Twelve Intracochlear Electrodes of an Intracochlear Implant

In Fig. 10.4 EABRs which were recorded from all 12 intracochlear electrodes nodes in a 15-year-old boy are presented. As can be seen, the EABR wave configuration changes from the apical turn (1 ch) to the basal turn (12 ch) of the cochlea as a function of the location of the electrical stimulus at various nodes along the implant. The peak of eII is most clearly defined following from the contralateral mastoid skin electrode (1 ch, a & b) and the peak of eIII is most clearly defined following recordings of the nape skin electrode (2 ch, a & b) which is easily contaminated by muscle artifacts.

10.4.2 Amplitudes and Latencies of EABR Waves eIII and eV Evoked by Independent Stimulation of Each of the Twelve Nodes of the Intracochlear Electrode

Figure 10.5 is a plot of the differences in peak and trough wave amplitudes and latencies evoked from stimulation of each of the 12 implant electrode nodes, i.e., waves eIIIa-eIIIb (■-■) and eVa – eVb (●-●) and peak latency changes of eIIIa (■) and eVa (●). These two graphs illustrate gradient response changes following stimulus of the apical implant node electrode to the basal electrode. The amplitude of eIIIa–eIIIb and eVa – eVb (a) decreases from apical electrode stimulation to basal electrode stimulation and the peak latency of eIIIa and eVa (b) increases from the apical electrode to the basal electrode nodes.

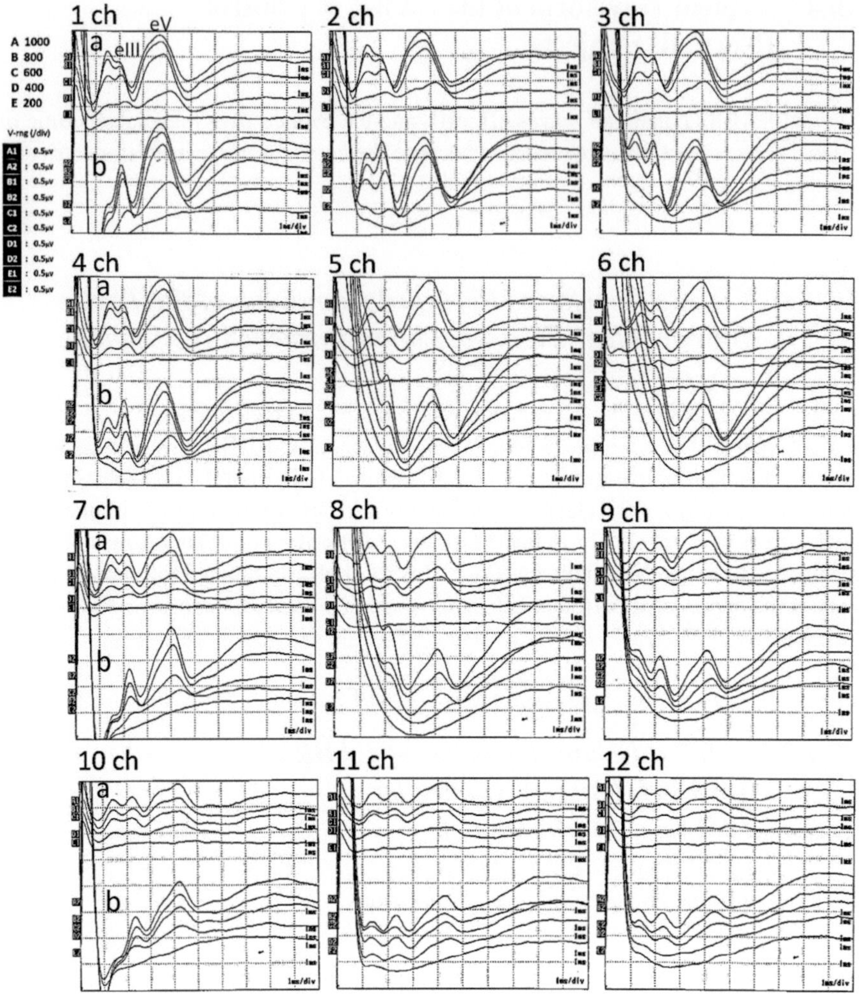

Fig. 10.4 EABRs waveforms recorded from each of the 12 intracochlear electrodes of an intracochlear implant. (**a**) Contralateral mastoid skin electrode and (**b**) the nape skin electrode in each channel

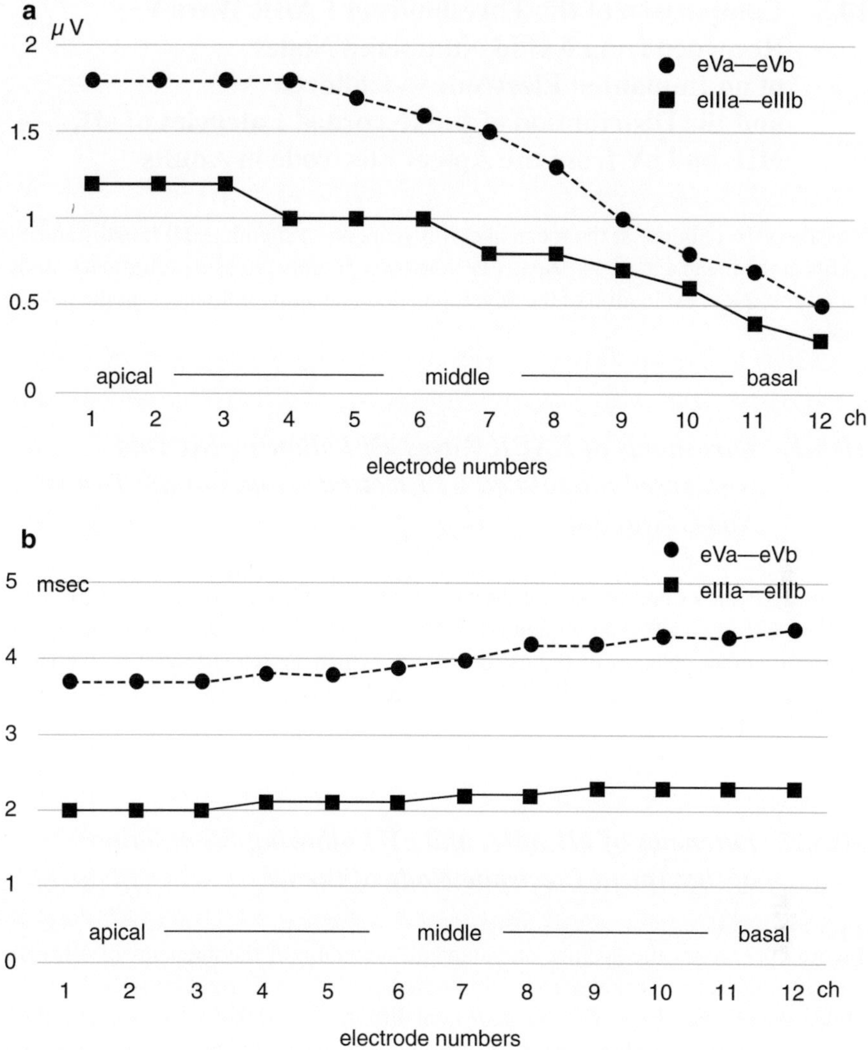

Fig. 10.5 Amplitudes and latencies of EABR waves eIIIa and eV evoked by independent stimulation of each of the 12 nodes of the intracochlear electrode. (**a**) Waves eIIIa-eIIIb (■-■) and eVa-eVb (●-●) from stimulation of each of the 12 implant electrode nodes. (**b**) Peak latency changes of eIIIa (■) and eVa (●) from stimulation of each of the 12 implant electrode nodes

10.5 Comparison of the Thresholds of EABR Wave V Recorded from 6 Odd Numbered Nodes of an Implanted Electrode in Children and the Distribution of the Recorded Latencies of eII, eIII, and eV from the Apical Electrode in Adults

EABRs of 16 children at the mean age of 3 years and 1 month, ±0.9 months and 11 adults at the mean age of 44 years, ±19 years were compared as a preliminary study for a subsequent evaluation of the developmental and aging influences on the EABR waveform.

10.5.1 Thresholds of EABR Waves eV Following Six Odd Numbered Stimulated CI Electrode Nodes of the Twelve Nodes Available

Figure 10.6 shows comparison of the thresholds of EABR waves recorded from six odd numbered nodes of an implanted electrode in children (a) and in adults (b) and reveals gradient changes of the eV thresholds which show the lowest threshold at the apical electrode node and the highest threshold at the basal electrode node in children and adults.

10.5.2 Latencies of eII, eIII, and eV Following Stimulation of the Apical Electrode Node of the CI

Figure 10.7 shows the average and standard deviation of the latencies of eII, eIII, and eV following apical electrode stimulation at 1000 cu (current units) in both the child (a) and adult (b) groups. No statistical difference ($p < 0.05$) was noted in these latencies across the child and adult groups. We then investigated the temporal changes, in detail, of the overall EABR waveform as a result of development and aging.

10.6 Developmental and Aging Influence on EABRs Recorded by Selected Three Stimulus Electrodes as Routine Examination

For this study, three intracochlear CI electrode nodes (1 ch, 6 ch, 12 ch) were stimulated at the apical, middle, and basal turn of the cochlea.

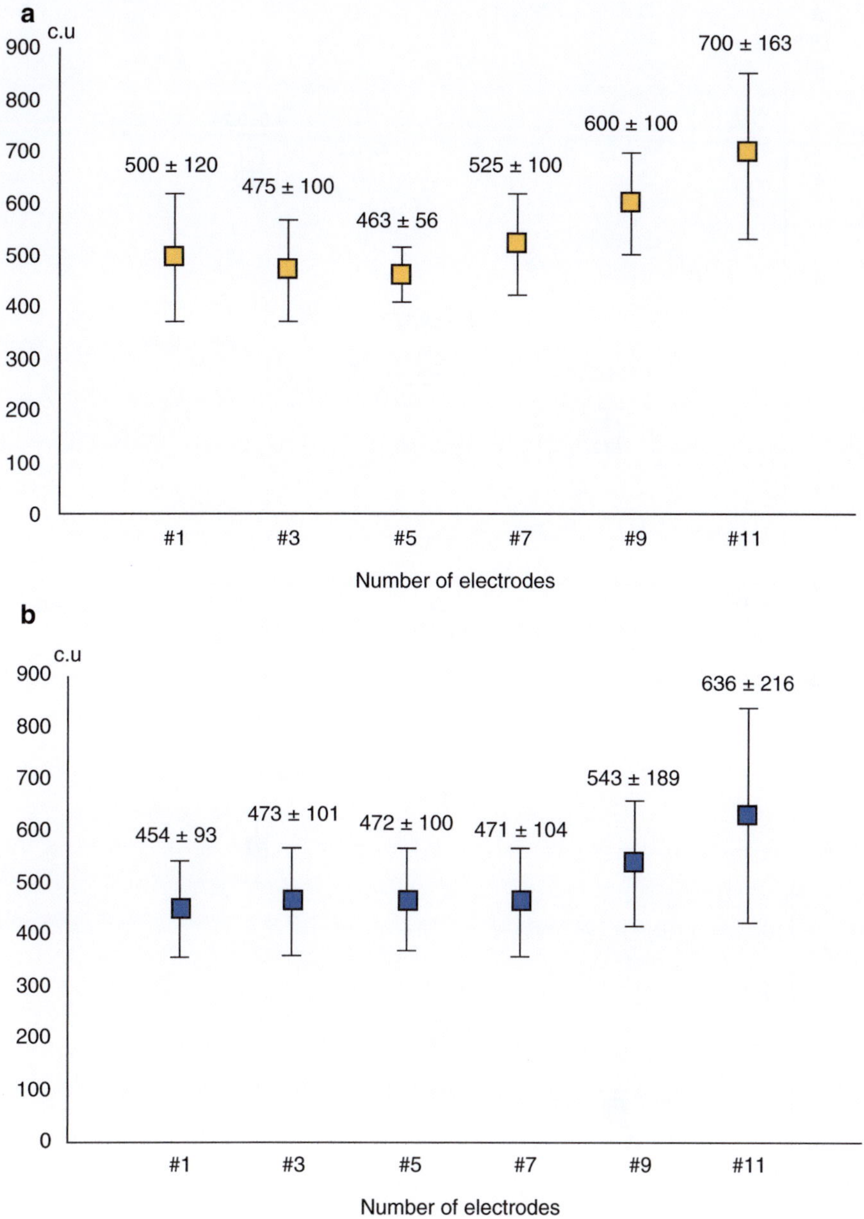

Fig. 10.6 Comparison of the thresholds of EABR wave V recorded from six odd numbered nodes in children (n of 16 at 3 years, 1 month ± 0.9 month) (**a**) and adults (n of 11 at 44 years ± 19 years) (**b**)

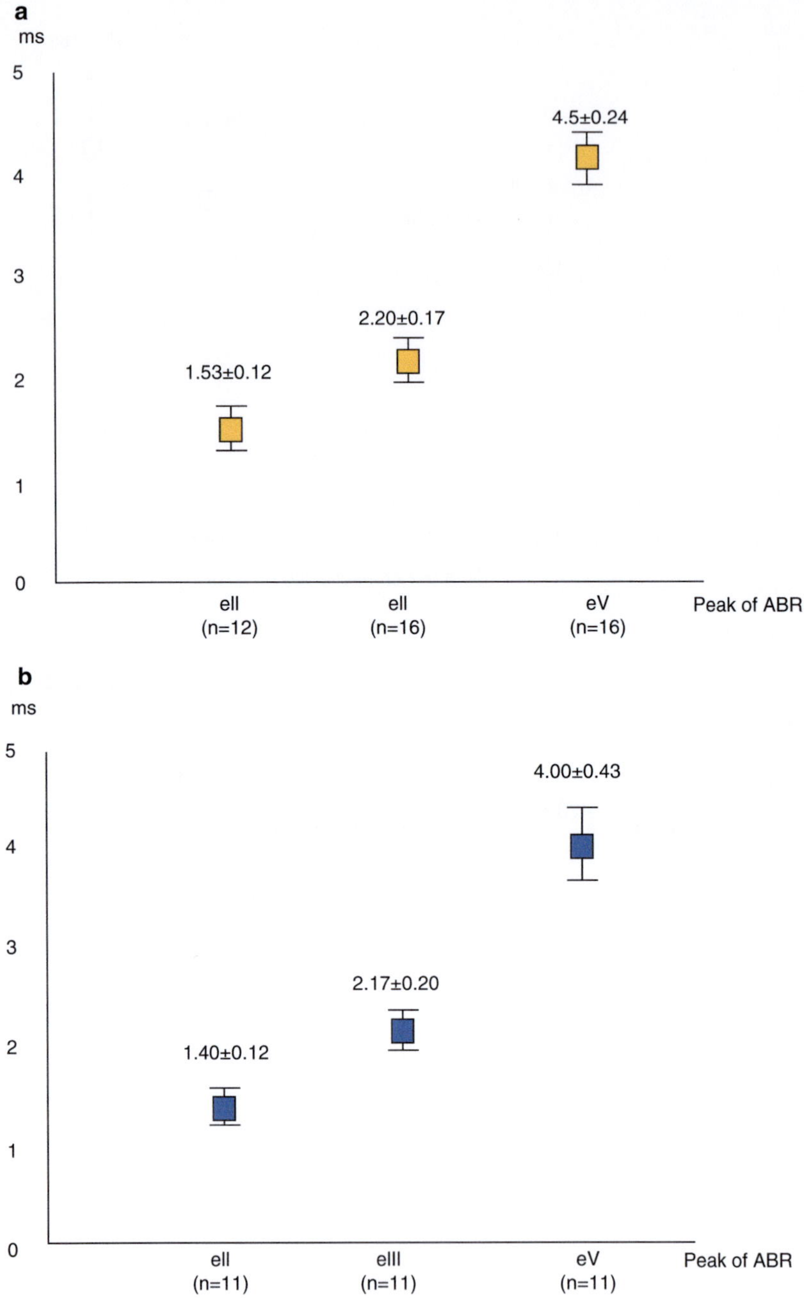

Fig. 10.7 Latencies of eII, eIII, and eV following stimulation at the apical electrode node of the CI (1000 cu). (**a**) Children (n of 16 at 3 years, 1 month ± 0.9 month), (**b**) adults (n of 11 at 44 years ± 19 years)

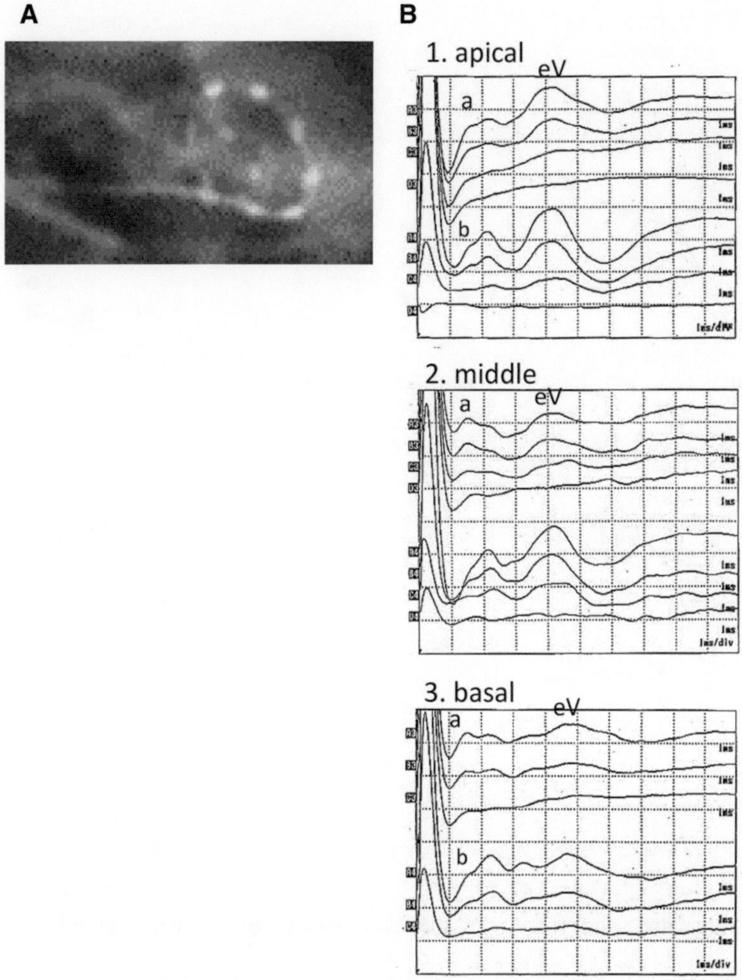

Fig. 10.8 A typical EABR wave configuration of one-year-old female. (**A**) XP of implanted electrodes and (**B**) EABR recorded from three electrode nodes (MED-EL, Co., Ltd., Flex 28). **a**: contralateral mastoid recording (channel 1), **b**: Nape recording (channel 2)

10.6.1 Typical EABR of a One-Year-Old Female

Figure 10.8 shows a typical EABR waveform of one-year-old female recorded from the contralateral skin mastoid electrode and, simultaneously, from the skin nape electrode. Three intracochlear CI electrode nodes (1 ch, 6 ch, 12 ch) were stimulated at the apical, middle, and basal turn of the cochlea. In Fig. 10.9, the amplitudes, in μv, of the evoked eIIIa-eIIIb and eVa-eVb at four different stimulus intensities (cu) are presented (a). Also, the latencies of these responses at different stimulus levels are presented in (b).

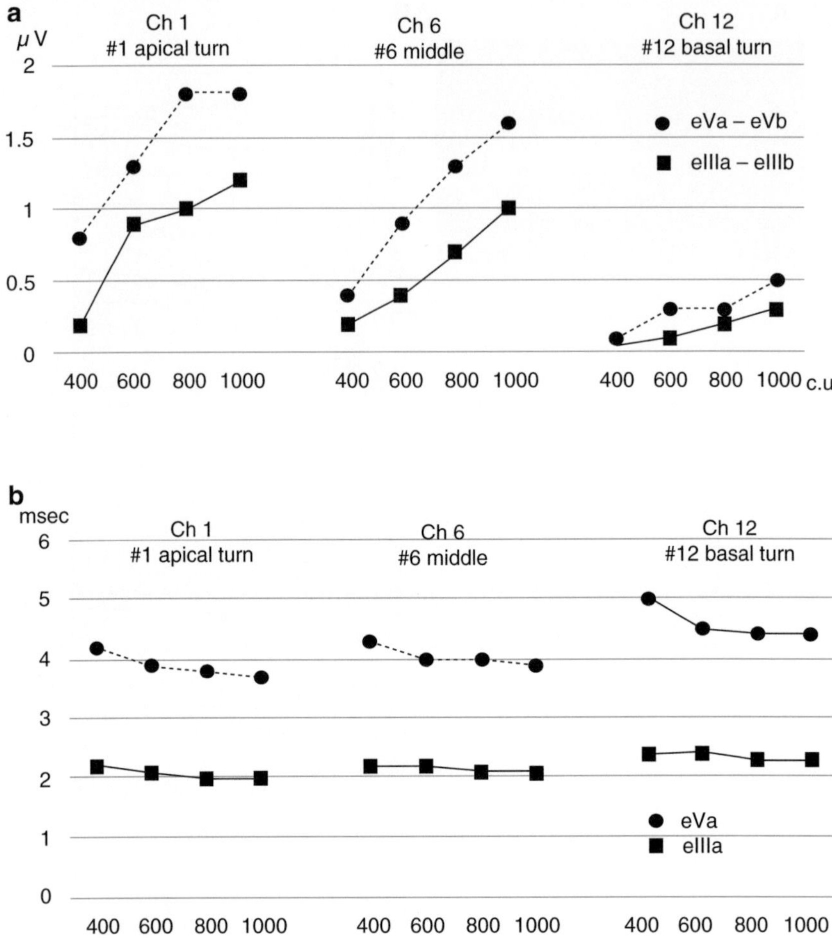

Fig. 10.9 Amplitudes and latencies of Fig. 10.8, the same patient. (**a**) The amplitude of the evoked eIIIa-eIIIb and eVa-eVb at four different stimulus intensities (cu). (**b**) The latencies of the evoked eIIIa-eIIIb and eVa-eVb at four different stimulus intensities (cu)

10.6.2 Comparison of EABR Wave eV Latencies from the Contralateral Mastoid (Channel 1) and Nape Recordings (Channel 2) from Five Different Age Groups: One-Year-Olds, Infants, Children, Adults, Elderly

In our study of the developmental and aging influences on the EABRs of patients over five age groups, we analyzed EABRs recorded retroactively from these five age groups: one-year-olds (n of 7 at 1 year, 6 ± 3 months), infants (n of 23 at

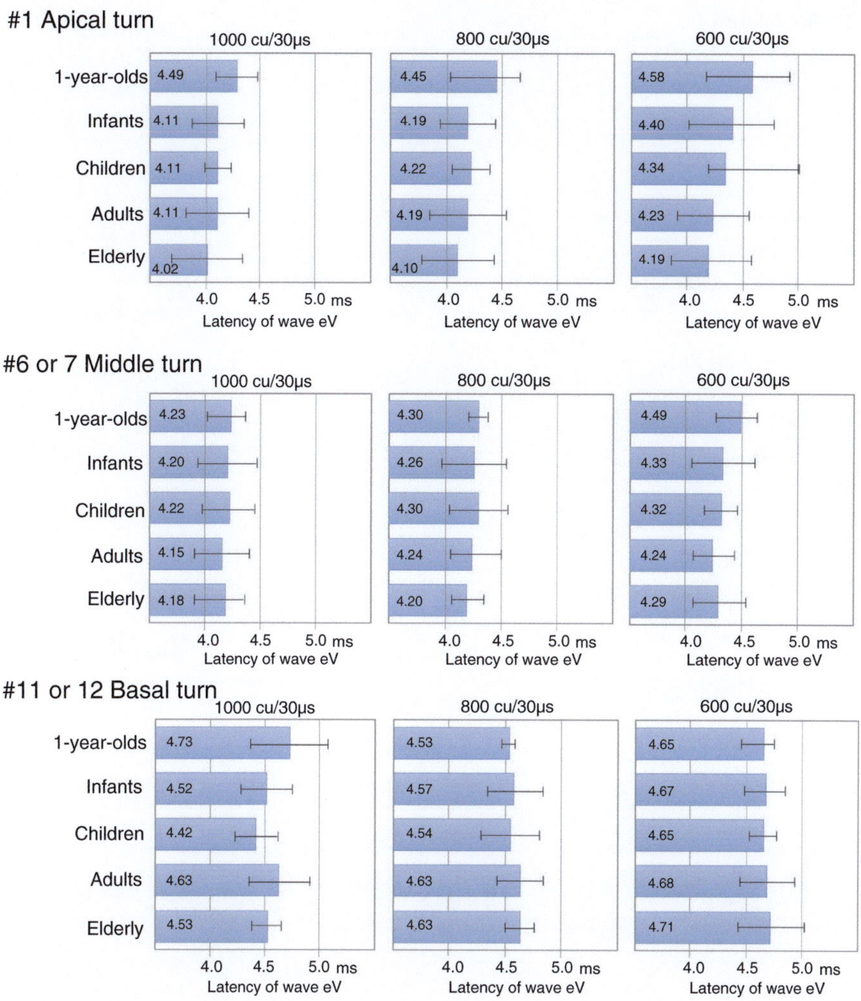

Fig. 10.10 Comparison of eV latencies at three different stimulus intensities in the five different age groups from one-year-olds, infants, children, adults, and elderly. The contralateral mastoid following electrical stimulation of the CI nodes at the apical, middle, and basal turns of the cochlea (channel 1)

3 years, 6 months ±1 year, 1 month), children (n of 9 at 7 years, 6 months ± 1 year, 2 months), adults (11 at 29 years, 0 month ± 15 years, 2 months) and elderly (8 at 80 years, ±6 years, 1 month), 58 patients overall [3]. We were especially interested in documenting age-related changes in the latencies of wave eV of the EABR.

The measured eV (wave V) latencies recorded from the mastoid following electrical stimulation of the CI nodes at the apical, middle, and basal turns of the cochlea (channel 1) are presented for each age group in Fig. 10.10. Simultaneous recordings

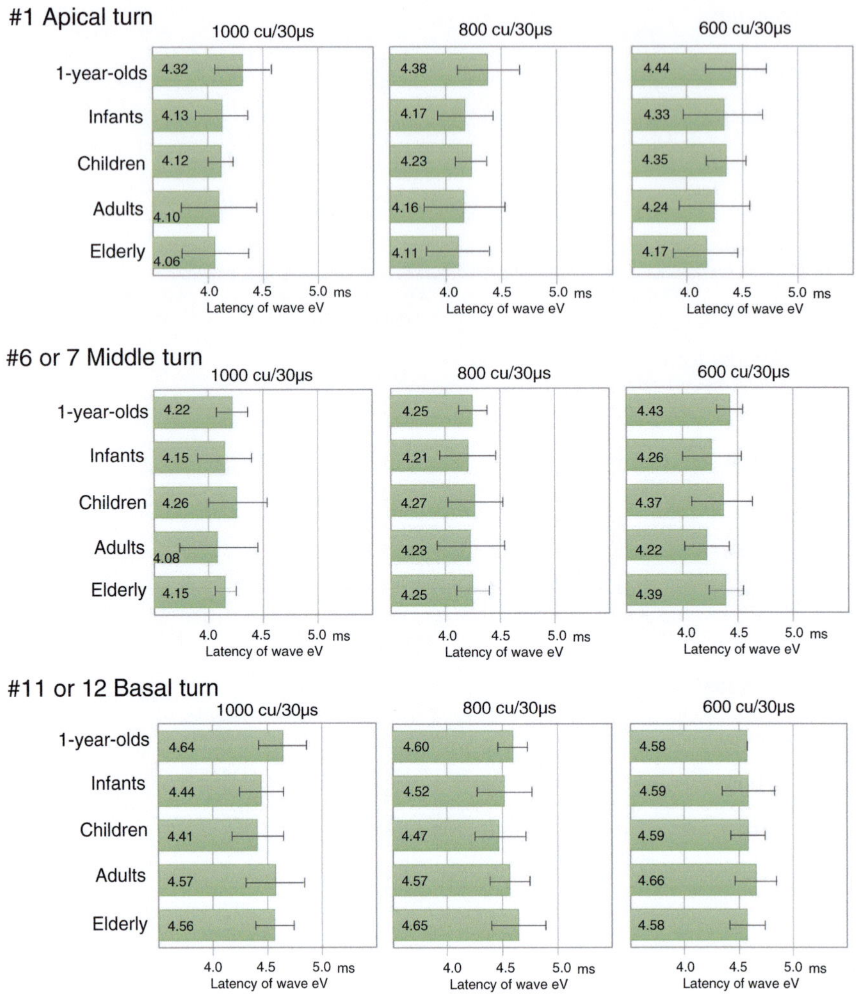

Fig. 10.11 Comparison of eV latencies at three different stimulus intensities in the five different age groups from one-year-olds, infants, children, adults, and elderly. The nape recording (channel 2)

were taken from the nape of the neck of the similarly evoked eV wave latencies for each age group and are shown in Fig. 10.11. Measurements of the various EABR waves recorded from electrodes applied at the mastoid versus recordings taken from the nape of the neck revealed no significant ($p < 0.05$) differences in latencies at three stimulus intensity levels across the age groups [3, 4]. Slight wave eV latency differences were noted following stimulus intensities below 1000 cu and 600 cu except at the basal turn (#11 or #12, nape), ($p < 0.05$). This result suggests that the latency of wave eV increases as the stimulus intensity approaches threshold, a not an unexpected finding.

10.7 Comparison of EABR Waves Recorded from the Bionics and the Cochlear Companies' CI

For reference, EABRs were recorded following stimulation of multi-nodal CIs manufactured by two different companies: Bionics Co., Ltd., Fig. 10.12 and Cochlear Co., Ltd., Fig. 10.13. Recordings were taken from the contralateral

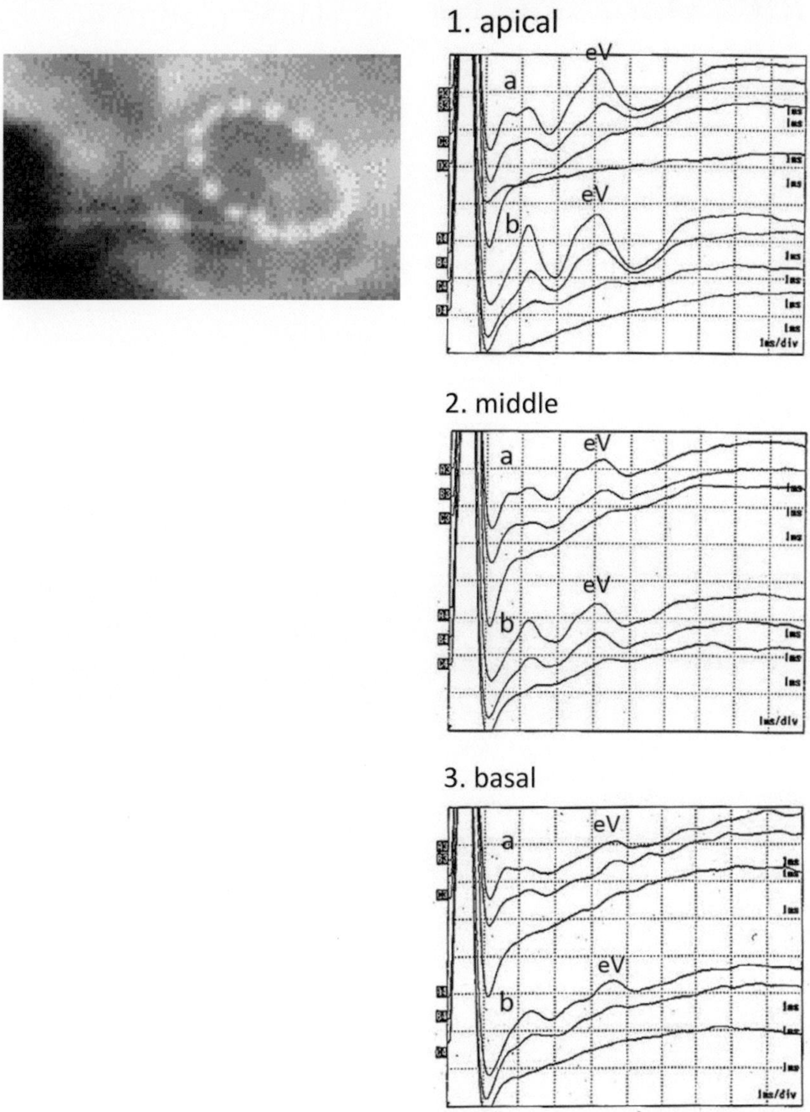

Fig. 10.12 EABRs of Bionics (Co., Ltd.)

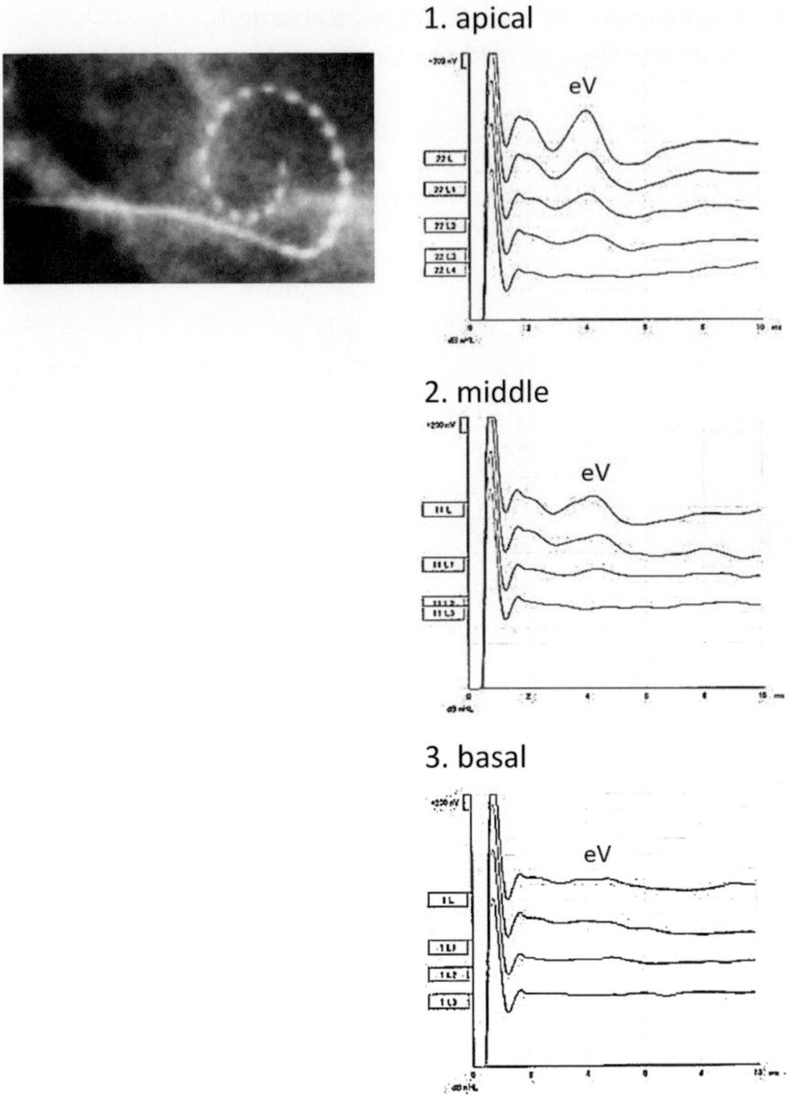

Fig. 10.13 EABRs of Cochlear (Co., Ltd.) recorded from the contralateral skin mastoid electrode

mastoid. Typically, EABRs were evoked by electrical stimuli applied to select nodes of the CI within the scala media, specifically at the apical turn, the middle turn, and the basal turn. These particular CI nodes are chosen to allow for recording efficiency and reduce the time that the patient is under general anesthesia. One caveat of note is that the electrical stimulation was different for each system. The trigger signal by electrical stimulus was sent via the programming interface which was controlled by its own software. Responses were collected from the Bionics (Co., Ltd.) implant by Neuropack software (Nihon Kohden Co., Ltd., Japan) and from the Cochlear (Co., Ltd.) implant by Eclipse software (Intracoustics, Denmark). In general, EABRs of MED-EL (Co., Ltd.), Bionics (Co., Ltd.), and the Cochlear (Co., Ltd.) were very similar. Thus, recordings of EABRs across manufacturers are comparable and reliable for localizing auditory system pathologies, evaluating the post-operation integrity of the CI and assisting in long-term auditory rehabilitation.

10.8 Abnormal Waveform Classification of EABRs During Cochlear Implantation Under General Anesthesia

Valero J. et al. [5] proposed a classification of abnormal waveforms of the EABR in children with auditory nerve hypoplasia in 2012. Their Type I showed a delayed single peak, Type II showed delayed multiple peaks and in Type III all waves were absent. Considering their classification of these three abnormal peak patterns, we propose our own more definitive classification which consists of four types. Type I: prolonged peak latency of eV, Type II: shortened peak latency of eV, Type III: no response, and in Type IV, myogenic potentials are dominant. Our EABRs were recorded during a cochlear implantation under general anesthesia. Figure 10.14 illustrates our schema of these four types and shows the patient's EABR following stimulation of the CI at the node in the apical turn of the cochlea. Generally, abnormal wave configurations of the EABRs are noted in patients with inner ear malformation and/or cochlear nerve deficiencies [6–9].

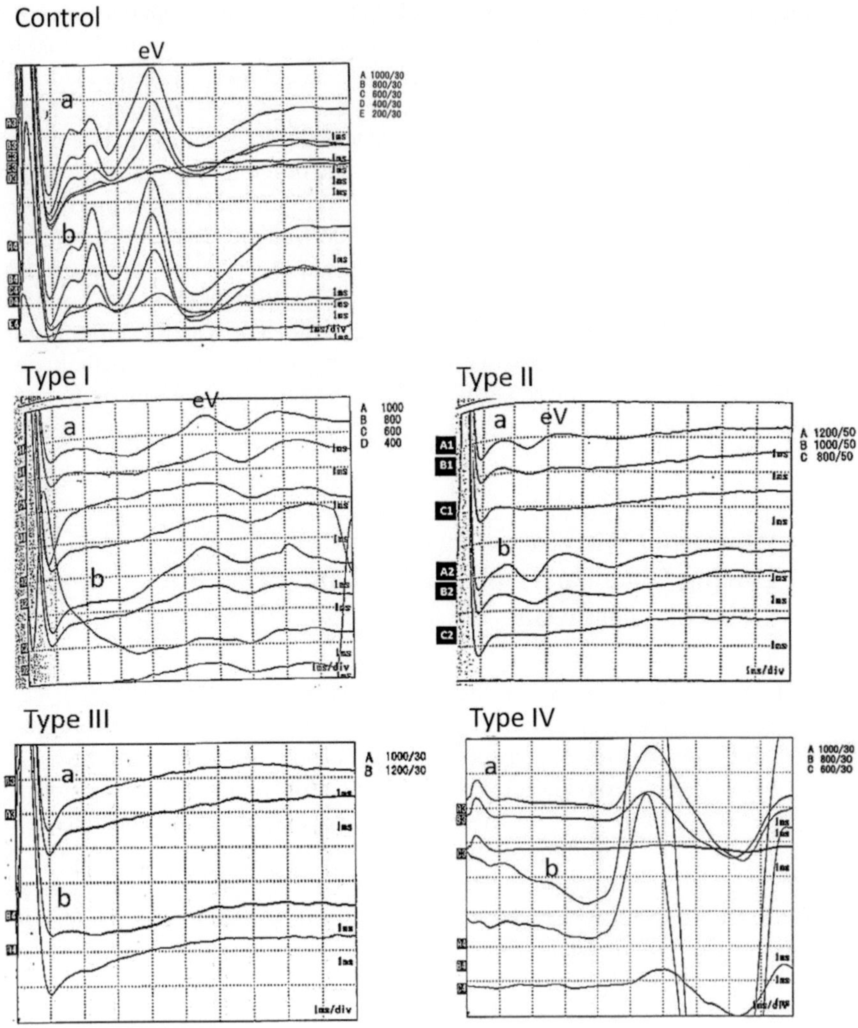

Fig. 10.14 Abnormal wave classification of EABRs during cochlear implantation under general anesthesia. (Apical electrode nodes at 1000 cu). (**a**) channel 1, (**b**) channel 2

References

1. Hall JW 3rd. Electrically evoked auditory responses. In: Handbook of auditory evoked potentials. Boston: Allyn and Bacon; 1992. p. 575–9.
2. Starr A, Brackman DD. Brainstem potentials evoked by electrical stimulations of the cochlea in human subjects. Ann Otol Rhinol Laryngol. 1979;88(4 Pt 1):550–6.
3. Enomoto C, Minami S, Kaga K. EABR measurements during cochlear implantation in one-year-old, infant, child, adult, and elderly patients. Acta Otolaryngol. 2021;141(1):78–82.

4. Hung TV, Sebastian C, Florent B, Francois D, Eric T, Lionel C. The pattern of auditory brainstem response wave V maturation in cochlear-implanted children. Clin Neurophysiol. 2007;118(3):676–89.
5. Valero J, Blaser S, Papsin BC, James AL, Gorden KA. Electrophysiologic and behavioral outcomes of cochlear implantation in children with auditory nerve hypoplasia. Ear Hear. 2012;33(1):3–18.
6. Minami S, Kaga K. EABR of inner ear malformation and cochlear nerve deficiency after cochlear implantation in children. In: Cochlear implantation in children with inner ear malformation and Cochlear nerve deficiency. Singapore: Springer Science; 2017. p. 97–109.
7. Papsin BC. Cochlear implantation in children with anomalous cochleovestibular anatomy. Laryngoscope. 2005;115(S106):1–26.
8. Yamazaki H, Naito Y, Fujiwara K, Moroto S, Yamamoto R, Yamazaki T, Sasaki I. Electrically evoked auditory brainstem response-based evaluation of the special distribution of auditory neuronal tissue in common cavity deformities. Otol Neurotol. 2014;35(8):1394–042.
9. Kaga K, Minami S, Enomoto C. Electrically evoked ABR during cochlear implantation and postoperative development of speech and hearing abilities in infants with common cavity deformity as a type of inner ear malformation. Acta Otolaryngol. 2020;140(1):14–21.

Chapter 11
Inner Ear Malformation and Cochlear Nerve Deficiency

Shujiro B. Minami

Abstract When cochlear implantation is performed in case involving inner ear malformations (IEMs), it is particularly important to perform objective physiological measurements of the cochlear implants. The IEMs can be divided into categories according to the observation of modiolus deficiency and/or cochlear nerve deficiency (CND). Intracochlear electrical auditory brainstem response (EABR) is a reliable and effective way of objectively confirming device function and implant-responsiveness of the cochlear neurons up to the level of the brainstem in cases of inner ear malformation. EABR can often be recorded in cases in which the presence of excessive stimulus artifacts precludes the successful acquisition of ECAP, such as in cases with modiolus deficiency cochlea. This chapter presents a simple grading of IEMs according to the observation of modiolus deficiency and/or CND, intracochlear EABR and outcomes for hearing in terms of the novel grading system.

Keywords EABR · Modiolus deficiency · Cochlear nerve deficiency

11.1 Introduction

It is estimated that 20% of patients with congenital sensorineural hearing loss have varying degrees of inner ear malformation (IEM), identified by using diagnostic imaging. Regarding the classification of inner ear anomalies, Jackler et al. [1] classified cochlear malformations into five groups: complete labyrinthine aplasia (Michel deformity), cochlear aplasia, common cavity, cochlear hypoplasia (CH), and incomplete partition (IP). The classification system of Jackler et al. was based on embryogenesis and developmental arrest. Later, Sennaroglu and Saatci [2] revised the system in 2002; they defined the radiological features of two completely different types of IP anomalies of the cochlea as IP-I and IP-II. Currently, the most

S. B. Minami (✉)
Division of Otolaryngology, National Hospital Organization Tokyo Medical Center, Tokyo, Japan

© Springer Japan KK, part of Springer Nature 2022

K. Kaga (ed.), *ABRs and Electrically Evoked ABRs in Children*, Modern Otology and Neurotology, https://doi.org/10.1007/978-4-431-54189-9_11

widely used classification of IEM is Sennaroglu's classification: cochlear aplasia, common cavity (CC), CH-I, II, III, and IV, IP-I, II, and III, enlarged vestibular aqueduct (EVA), and cochlear aperture abnormality [3]. IEMs are somewhat complicated and difficult to classify in some cases. Adibelli et al. [4] reported that 26.25% of IEMs could not be successfully categorized with existing classification schemes. Cochlear implants (CIs) in various IEMs are still challenging, because it is difficult to predict auditory outcomes. The goal of preoperative imaging is to identify the anatomic variations that affect ear selection, surgical approach, and prognosis. Now, we'd like to propound a novel and simple grading of IEMs. IEMs can be divided into categories according to the observation of modiolus deficiency and/or cochlear nerve deficiency (CND) . Modiolus present-type malformations are CH-III and IV, IP-II, and EVA. Modiolus deficient-type malformations are cochlear aplasia, CC, CH-I and II, and IP-I and III. CND severity can be categorized in one of three ways, according to the MRI findings: (1) A hypoplastic cochlear nerve, (2) absence of cochlear nerve, and (3) absence of vestibulocochlear nerve.

When IEMs are present, it is particularly important to perform objective measurements of the CI, as these measurements will show whether the electrodes are appropriately positioned and whether there is initial failure of the device during surgery. These measurements are also useful for predicting the audiological outcomes after CI implantation, for assisting the speech-processor fitting when behavioral results are difficult to obtain, and for characterizing the pathophysiology of hearing loss. Physiological objective assessment tools measure various aspects of the auditory responses to electrical stimulation through a CI. Electrically evoked compound action potential (ECAP) can be recorded quickly and easily without the need for surface or scalp electrodes and is probably the most widely used measure in clinical settings. In contrast, while electrically evoked auditory brainstem responses (EABR) recordings require the placement of surface electrodes, they can provide information about the auditory pathway up to the level of the brainstem [5]. The purpose of this chapter is to propose a simple grading of IEMs according to the observation of modiolus deficiency and/or CND and investigate intracochlear EABR and outcomes for hearing in terms of the novel grading system.

11.2 A Novel and Simple Grading

11.2.1 Grading According to Observation of Modiolus Deficiency and/or Cochlear Nerve Deficiency

We proposed a simple grading of inner ear malformation (IEM) Grade I: Modiolus present + normal cochlear nerve, Grade II: Modiolus deficiency + normal cochlear nerve, Grade III: Modiolus present + CND, and Grade IV: Modiolus deficiency + CND (Fig. 11.1) [6]. Regarding the classification of cochlear nerves,

		Modiolus			
		Present		Deficiency	
Cochlear nerve in the internal auditory canal	Present	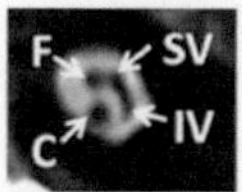 C>F	Grade I	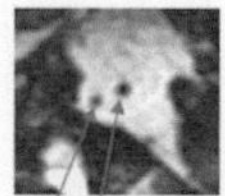 F CV CV>F	Grade II
	Deficiency	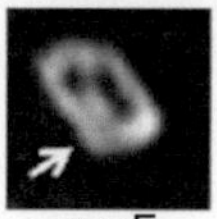 CV<F	Grade III	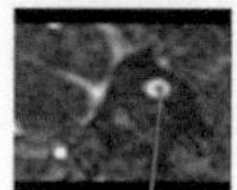 CV<F F	Grade IV

Fig. 11.1 Grading according to observation of modiolus deficiency and/or cochlear nerve deficiency. *C* indicates cochlear nerve, *CV* cochleovestibular nerve, *F* facial nerve, *IV* inferior vestibular nerve, *SV* superior vestibular nerve

cochlear nerves were defined as normal if the cochlear nerves were larger than facial nerves on magnetic resonance imaging (MRI). In the case of modiolus deficient-type malformations, the cochleovestibular nerves (CVN) could enter the cavity without separating into individual nerves. If the CVN size is larger than the facial nerve, it is accepted as normal. The categorization according to this grading system is not difficult, because it is easy to determine via imaging studies whether the modiolus and CND are present or not. In the cases of modiolus deficient-type malformations, it is impossible to determine the cochlear fiber content in the CVN, because the CVN enters the cavity without separating into individual nerves. If the CVN is larger than the facial nerve, it is accepted as normal.

Whether the modiolus and cochlear nerves are present or deficient is an important factor in CI electrode choice. Because the auditory nerve tissues in modiolus deficiency malformations (Grade II or IV) are supposed to be in the inner ear wall, the modiolus hugging type electrodes are not suitable. On the other hand, in the cases with Grade III, it may be better to use modiolus hugging electrodes, because a high intensity may be needed to go through the thin auditory nerve. Thus, this grading system is also useful for the choice of CI electrode, which may result in improved speech discrimination by implant users with IEMs.

11.2.2 Patient Characteristics of Each Different Grade

We divided 60 cases of IEMs with CI surgery into 4 grades according to the observation of modiolus deficiency and/or IAC CND on the side of the first CI and 23 cases (38%) are classified as Grade I, 13 cases (22%) as grade II, 20 cases (33%) as grade III, and 4 cases (7%) as grade IV. Grade I included EVA (65%), IP-II (18%), semicircular canal hypoplasia (13%), and CH-III (4%). Grade II included IP-I (69%), CC (23%), and IP-III (8%). Grade III included cochlear aperture stenosis (35%), inner auditory canal stenosis with normal cochlea (35%), CH-III (20%), CH-IV (5%), and IP-II (5%). Grade IV had IP-I (50%) and CC (50%). The median age of the first cochlear implant surgery is 4 years old (1 year and 8 months old to 68 years old) in Grade I, 2 years old (1 year and 6 months old to 5 years old) in Grade II, 4 years old (1 year and 7 months old to 26 years old) in Grade III, and 2 years old (1 year and 8 months old to 2 years 9 months old) in Grade IV. The second CI on the other side was performed on the 26% of Grade I, 54% of Grade II, 10% of Grade III, and none of Grade IV. The cases who had modiolus present-type malformations (Grade I or III) had the malformations with modiolus on the other side as well. On the other hand, the cases who had modiolus absent-type malformations (Grade II and IV) had the malformations without modiolus or Michel type malformation on the other side. Interestingly, the cases who have modiolus present-type malformations have the modiolus present-type malformations on the other side as well. On the other hand, the cases who have modiolus absent-type malformations have the modiolus absent-type of malformation on the other side. These imply that modiolus deficient-type malformations may be developmental perturbations with similar causes.

11.2.3 EABR Responses and Categories of Auditory Performance (CAP) Scores

Intracochlear EABRs are measured in 15 patients in Grade I, 11 patients in Grade II, 19 patients in Grade III, and four patients in Grade IV. The EABR waves V clearly recognized within 4.5 ms are judged as "typical," and the rest "non-typical." During operation, 93% of Grade I, 36% of Grade II, 23% of Grade III, and 50% of Grade IV patients showed typical EABR waves (Fig. 11.2a). The patients in Grade I show significantly more typical EABRs compared with Grade II, III, and IV ($p < 0.05$). Figure 11.2b shows CAP scores in each grade. 91% of Grade I, 62% of Grade II, 35% of Grade III, and 25% of Grade IV show CAP scores of 4 or more. The percentage of patients with a CAP score of 4 or more is significantly greater for the patients of Grade I compared with those of Grade II, III, and IV ($p < 0.05$). Figure 11.2c–e show CAP scores in the patients who had typical or non-typical EABRs. In Grade II, 75% of patients with typical EABR have CAP scores of 4 or more, compared with 43% of patients with non-typical EABRs. In Grade III, 60% of patients with typical EABR have CAP scores of 4 or more, compared with 29% of patients with non-typical EABRs. In Grade IV, 50% of patients with typical EABR had CAP scores of 4 or more, compared with no patients with non-typical EABR.

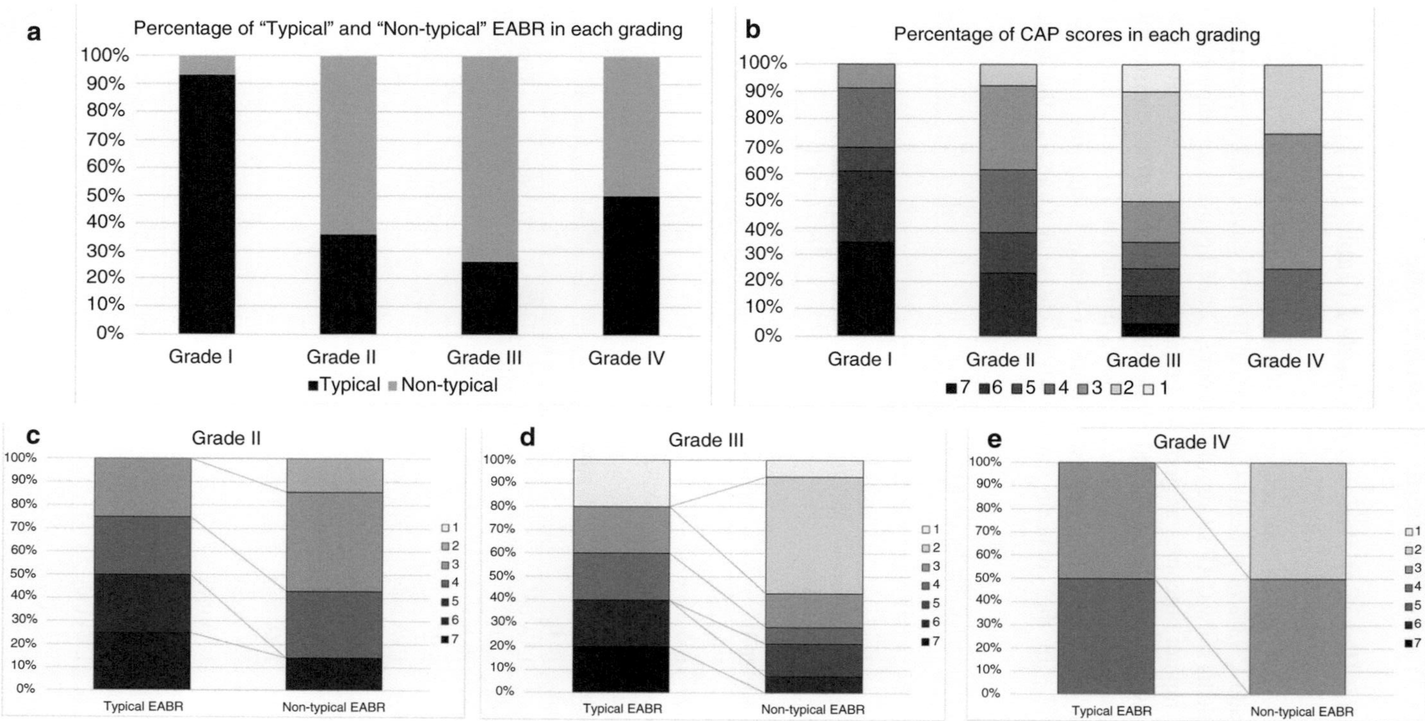

Fig. 11.2 (**a**) Percentage of typical and non-typical electrically evoked auditory brainstem responses (EABR) in each grade. (**b**) Percentage of categories of auditory performance (CAP) scores in each grade. (**c–e**) CAP scores in the patients who had typical or non-typical EABRs in Grade II, III, and IV (Reused with permission from [6])

11.3 EABR Waves of Patients in Each Grade

11.3.1 EABR Waves of Patients in Grade I (Table 11.1)

Grade I includes EVA, IP-II, semicircular canal hypoplasia, and CH-III (Fig. 11.3a). Because in Grade I, 93% of patients show typical EABR waves during operation, and 91% of patients show CAP scores of 4 or more, Grade I patients are expected to have cochlear implant outcomes as good as the patients without malformation. A systematic review reported that at 12 and 24 months post implantation, statistically significant improvement is seen in closed-set word performance for all malformations, with the Mondini/IP-II group, which are in Grade I, showing the most improvement [7]. In the cochlear malformation cases in Grade I, the basal

Table 11.1 Patient characteristics for Grade I

Grade I								
Pt.	Age at first CI (years)	Side of first CI	Type of malformation (first CI)	EABR at first CI	Age at second CI (years)	Side of second CI	Type of malformation (second CI)	EABR at second CI
1	1	Left	IP-II	Typical	–	–	–	–
2	1	Right	IP-II	Typical	–	–	–	–
3	2	Left	EVA only	–	6	Right	EVA only	Typical
4	2	Right	EVA only	–	7	Left	EVA only	–
5	2	Right	CH-III	Typical	–	–	–	–
6	2	Right	SCH	Typical	3	Left	SCH	Typical
7	3	Right	EVA only	Typical	–	–	–	–
8	3	Right	IP-II	–	–	–	–	–
9	3	Right	EVA only	–	7	Left	EVA only	Typical
10	3	Right	SCH	–	–	–	–	–
11	3	Right	IP-II	Typical	–	–	–	–
12	4	Left	EVA only	–	6	Right	EVA only	Typical
13	4	Right	EVA only	Typical	–	–	–	–
14	4	Left	EVA only	Typical	–	–	–	–
15	8	Left	EVA only	–	–	–	–	–
16	11	Left	EVA only	Typical	–	–	–	–
17	14	Left	EVA only	Typical	–	–	–	–
18	14	Left	EVA only	–	–	–	–	–
19	19	Left	EVA only	–	–	–	–	–
20	24	Right	EVA only	Typical	–	–	–	–
21	28	Right	SCH	–	–	–	–	–
22	34	Right	EVA only	–	–	–	–	–
23	68	Right	EVA only	–	71	Left	EVA only	Non-typical

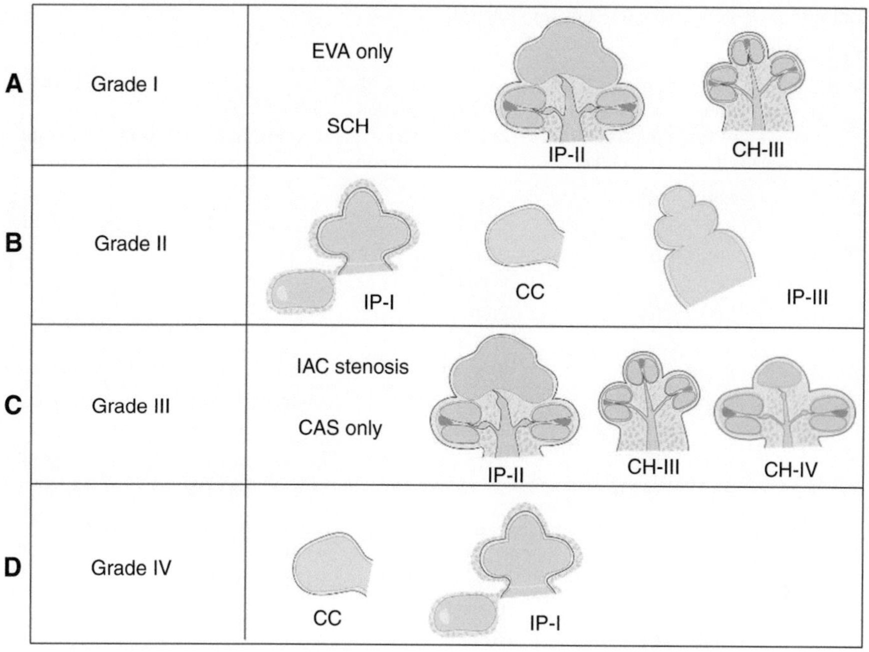

Fig. 11.3 Labeling the cochlear malformations by grading (A: Grade I; B: II, C: III; and D: IV). CAS indicates cochlear aperture stenosis; *CC* common cavity, *CH* cochlear hypoplasia, *EVA* enlarged vestibular aqueduct, *IAC* internal auditory canal, *IP* incomplete partition, *SCH* semicircular canal hypoplasia

electrodes have higher thresholds and longer wave eV latencies than the apical and middle electrodes. These are similar threshold and latency patterns to those observed in the patients without malformations [8].

11.3.2 EABR Waves of Patients in Grade II (Table 11.2)

Grade II includes IP-I, CC, and IP-III (Fig. 11.3b). ECAP recordings depend largely on spinal ganglion cells, which are very often defective in modiolus deficiency-type malformed cochlea. EABR can be obtained in modiolus deficiency-type implant users because the measures are not dependent on the implant having telemetry capabilities and because the wave eV of EABR, which occurs at a later latency than ECAP, is easier to isolate from the stimulus artifacts. The cochlear malformation cases with modiolus deficiency do not exhibit threshold and latency differences between electrodes. The auditory nerve tissues in modiolus deficiency malformations are supposed to be in the inner ear wall, and so the distances from each electrode to the auditory nerve tissue should not be different in modiolus deficiency-type malformations. The modiolus hugging type electrodes are not suitable with the

Table 11.2 Patient characteristics for Grade II

Grade II								
Pt.	Age at first CI (years)	Side of first CI	Type of malformation (first CI)	EABR at first CI	Age at second CI (years)	Side of second CI	Type of malformation (second CI)	EABR at second CI
1	1	Left	IP-I	Non-typical	–	–	–	Non-typical
2	1	Left	IP-I	Non-typical	–	–	–	–
3	1	Left	CC	Non-typical	–	–	–	–
4	1	Right	IP-I	Typical	2	Left	CC	Typical
5	1	Right	CC	Non-typical	4	Right	CC	Typical
6	1	Right	IP-I	Typical	3	Left	CC	Typical
7	2	Right	IP-III	–	13	Left	IP-III	Non-typical
8	2	Left	IP-I	–	5	Right	CC	Typical
9	2	Left	IP-I	Non-typical	4	Right	CH-II	–
10	2	Right	CC	Non-typical	–	–	–	–
11	3	Right	IP-I	–	14	Left	IP-I	–
12	3	Left	IP-I	Non-typical	–	–	–	–
13	5	Right	IP-I	–	–	–	–	–

patients in Grade II. In Grade II, patients with typical EABR showed a tendency to have better CAP scores than patients with non-typical EABRs.

11.3.3 EABR Waves of Patients in Grade III (Table 11.3)

Grade III includes cochlear aperture stenosis, inner auditory canal stenosis with normal cochlea, CH-III, CH-IV, and IP-II (Fig. 11.3c). A good indication for cochlear implantation against cochlear nerve deficiency is obvious auditory response with hearing aids. Because obvious auditory response implies that the cochlear nerve is functionable. Cochlear nerve canal stenosis cases have normal spiral ganglion cells, so ECAP shows good responses with the usual intensity. However, because a high intensity is needed to go through the thin auditory nerve, the EABR threshold is high. In Grade III, patients with typical EABR show a tendency to have better CAP scores than patients with non-typical EABRs. It may be better to use modiolar hugging electrodes, because peri-modiolar electrode placement reduces

Table 11.3 Patient characteristics for Grade III

Grade III								
Pt.	Age at first CI (years)	Side of first CI	Type of malformation (first CI)	EABR at first CI	Age at second CI (years)	Side of second CI	Type of malformation (second CI)	EABR at second CI
1	1	Right	IAC stenosis	Non-typical	–	–	–	–
2	1	Right	IAC stenosis	Non-typical	–	–	–	–
3	2	Left	CH-III	Non-typical	–	–	–	–
4	2	Left	CAS only	Non-typical	–	–	–	–
5	2	Right	IAC stenosis	Non-typical	3	Left	IAC stenosis	Non-typical
6	2	Right	CH-IV	Typical	–	–	–	–
7	2	Right	IAC stenosis	Non-typical	–	–	–	–
8	2	Left	CAS only	Non-typical	–	–	–	–
9	4	Left	CAS only	Non-typical	–	–	–	–
10	4	Right	IAC stenosis	Non-typical	–	–	–	–
11	4	Right	CAS only	Non-typical	–	–	–	–
12	5	Right	CH-III	Typical	–	–	–	–
13	5	Left	CAS only	Non-typical	–	–	–	–
14	6	Left	IP-II	Typical	–	–	–	–
15	8	Right	CAS only	–	–	–	–	–
16	10	Left	CAS only	Non-typical	–	–	–	–
17	11	Right	IAC stenosis	Non-typical	–	–	–	–
18	15	Left	IAC stenosis	Typical	–	–	–	–
19	17	Left	CH-III	Non-typical	–	–	–	–
20	26	Left	CH-III	Non-typical	27	Right	CH-III	Typical

the spread of excitation of CI stimulation. These reduce nerve stimulation thresholds may result in improved speech discrimination by implant users with modiolus presence and cochlear nerve deficiency. Because about half of the children in Grades III go to classes for the multiply handicapped, we have to exercise caution due to the possible comorbidity of developmental disabilities.

Table 11.4 Patient characteristics for Grade IV

Grade IV								
Pt.	Age at first CI (years)	Side of first CI	Type of malformation (first CI)	EABR at first CI	Age at second CI (years)	Side of second CI	Type of malformation (second CI)	EABR at second CI
1	1	Left	CC	Typical	3	Right	CC	Typical
2	2	Left	IP-I	Non-typical	–	–	–	–
3	2	Right	IP-I	Non-typical	5	Left	IP-I	Typical
4	2	Right	CC	Non-typical	–	–	–	–

11.3.4 EABR Waves of Patients in Grade IV (Table 11.4)

Grade IV includes IP-I and CC (Fig. 11.3d). This type of malformation is challenging. We think good vestibular functions in the cases of Grade IV can be an indication for CI. In the case of internal auditory canal stenosis, vestibular evaluation helps us to determine the neural connection between inner ear and brain. It is possible that vestibular nerves can obtain the function of auditory nerve via auditory stimulation plasticity. In Grade IV, patients with typical EABR show a tendency to have better CAP scores than patients with non-typical EABRs. Because more than half of the children in Grades IV go to classes for the multiply handicapped, we have to exercise caution due to the possible comorbidity of developmental disabilities.

References

1. Jackler RK, Luxford WM, House WF. Congenital malformations of the inner ear: a classification based on embryogenesis. Laryngoscope. 1987;97(3 Pt 2 Suppl 40):2–14.
2. Sennaroglu L, Saatci I. A new classification for cochleovestibular malformations. Laryngoscope. 2002;112(12):2230–41. https://doi.org/10.1097/00005537-200212000-00019.
3. Sennaroglu L, Bajin MD. Classification and current Management of Inner ear Malformations. Balkan Med J. 2017;34(5):397–411. https://doi.org/10.4274/balkanmedj.2017.0367.
4. Adibelli ZH, Isayeva L, Koc AM, Catli T, Adibelli H, Olgun L. The new classification system for inner ear malformations: the INCAV system. Acta Otolaryngol. 2017;137(3):246–52. https://doi.org/10.1080/00016489.2016.1247498.
5. Minami SB, Takegoshi H, Shinjo Y, Enomoto C, Kaga K. Usefulness of measuring electrically evoked auditory brainstem responses in children with inner ear malformations during cochlear implantation. Acta Otolaryngol. 2015;135(10):1007–15. https://doi.org/10.3109/00016489.2015.1048377.
6. Minami SB, Yamamoto N, Hosoya M, Enomoto C, Kato H, Kaga K. Cochlear Implantation in Cases of Inner Ear Malformation: A Novel and Simple Grading, Intracochlear EABR, and

Outcomes of Hearing. Otology & Neurotology. 2020;42(2):e117–23. https://doi.org/10.1097/mao.0000000000002879.

7. Farhood Z, Nguyen SA, Miller SC, Holcomb MA, Meyer TA, Rizk HG. Cochlear implantation in inner ear malformations: systematic review of speech perception outcomes and intraoperative findings. Otolaryngol Head Neck Surg. 2017;156(5):783–93. https://doi.org/10.1177/0194599817696502.
8. Enomoto C, Minami S, Kaga K. EABR measurements during cochlear implantation in one-year-old, infant, child, adult, and elderly patients. Acta Otolaryngol. 2020:1–5. https://doi.org/10.1080/00016489.2020.1826576.

Chapter 12
Auditory Neuropathy

Makoto Hosoya, Shujiro B. Minami, and Kimitaka Kaga

Abstract Recording electrical auditory brainstem responses (EABRs) is useful for investigating the pathophysiology of hearing loss as well as for predicting the outcomes of cochlear implantation. In this chapter, we review the applications of EABR in hearing loss and auditory neuropathy.

Auditory neuropathy (or auditory neuropathy spectrum disease) is a heterogeneous disease characterized by absent or abnormal auditory nerve function but normal hair cell function. Clinically, patients with auditory neuropathy lack the auditory brainstem response (ABR) induced by auditory stimulation. Some patients with auditory neuropathy have severe-to-profound hearing loss and undergo cochlear implantation surgery. While they lack ordinal sound-evoked ABR, cochlear implant-mediated EABR may be present in several patients.

Herein, we present examples of EABR in patients with auditory neuropathy and discuss the importance of EABR in this field. Moreover, we review previous reports of EABR waveforms and propose a new system for classification of EABR patterns in patients with auditory neuropathy by combining the different pathophysiological mechanisms of this heterogeneous disease.

Keywords Auditory neuropathy · Cochlear implant · EABR · DIAPH3
OTOF · OPA1

M. Hosoya (✉)
Department of Otolaryngology, Keio University, School of Medicine, Tokyo, Japan

S. B. Minami
Department of Otolaryngology, National Hospital Organization, Tokyo Medical Center, Tokyo, Japan

K. Kaga
National Institute of Sensory Organs, National Hospital Organization, Tokyo Medical Center, Audiology Clinic, Kamio Memorial Hospital, Tokyo, Japan
e-mail: kimitaka.kaga@kankakuki.jp

© Springer Japan KK, part of Springer Nature 2022

K. Kaga (ed.), *ABRs and Electrically Evoked ABRs in Children*, Modern Otology and Neurotology, https://doi.org/10.1007/978-4-431-54189-9_12

12.1 Introduction

Auditory neuropathy (AN) is characterized by absent or abnormal auditory nerve function with normal sensory hair cell function. Clinically, AN presents as sensorineural hearing loss accompanied by impaired speech discrimination as predicted from patients' hearing level, which is characterized by preserved otoacoustic emissions (OAE) and disturbed auditory brainstem response (ABR) [1, 2]. This disease entity has been expanded to be called auditory neuropathy spectrum disorder (ANSD).

Hearing levels in patients with AN/ANSD are variable, ranging from normal hearing to profound hearing loss. Patients with AN who have severe or profound hearing loss may be candidates for cochlear implantation. While ABR waveforms are absent in patients with AN, cochlear implant (CI)-mediated electrical ABR (EABR) may be evoked. In this chapter, we elaborate the pathophysiology of AN, especially from a genetic viewpoint, and discuss several examples of CI-evoked EABR waveforms. Moreover, we propose a new classification of the EABR waveform typical of AN, which would help to understand the pathophysiology of this heterogeneous disease.

12.2 Auditory Neuropathy

12.2.1 Pathophysiology of Auditory Neuropathy

Auditory perception is the process by which mechanical sound waves are detected by the cochlea and converted into neuronal electrical impulses that are consequently perceived by the brain. In the cochlea, sensory hair cells convert mechanosensory sound waves into neural electrical pulses, which eventually reach the auditory cortex of the brain. This afferent transmission of the neural electrical pulses is achieved by the sophisticated interaction between the inner hair cells and spiral ganglion neurons. In patients with AN, synaptic transmission or neuronal transmission through the spiral ganglion neurons is disturbed. This disturbance can have congenital or acquired causes. Genetic mutations are the most well-understood cause of congenital AN. Chronic inflammatory demyelinating polyneuropathy (CIDP) is an example of acquired AN caused by demyelinating diseases. In the following sections, we present the pathophysiology and the genes associated with AN.

12.2.2 Genetics of Auditory Neuropathy

Genetic causes of AN include mutations in *OTOF* [3], *DIPH3* [4], *CACNA1D* [5], *OPA1* [6], *PJVK* [7], *MPZ* [8], and *ATP1A3* [9] genes. Such cases of AN can be stratified into two types based on the roles of their encoding proteins (Fig. 12.1):

pre-synaptic neuropathy and post-synaptic neuropathy [10] (type II, distal neuropathy or type I, proximal neuropathy [11]).

The most frequently occurring type of pre-synaptic neuropathy is AN, which is caused by an *OTOF* mutation. The transmembrane protein OTOFERLIN, which is encoded by the *OTOF* gene, is critical for pre-synaptic vesicle fusion at the ribbon synapses between inner hair cells and spiral ganglion neurons. Thus, *OTOF* mutation-induced AN is thought to be caused by pre-synaptic disruption. Another example of pre-synaptic neuropathy is AN caused by *CACNA1D* mutation. *CACNA1D* encodes the voltage-gated calcium channel subunit, alpha1 D, also known as Cav1.3. *CACNA1D* mutations associated with loss of function lead to impaired synaptic transmission between the inner hair cells and spiral ganglion

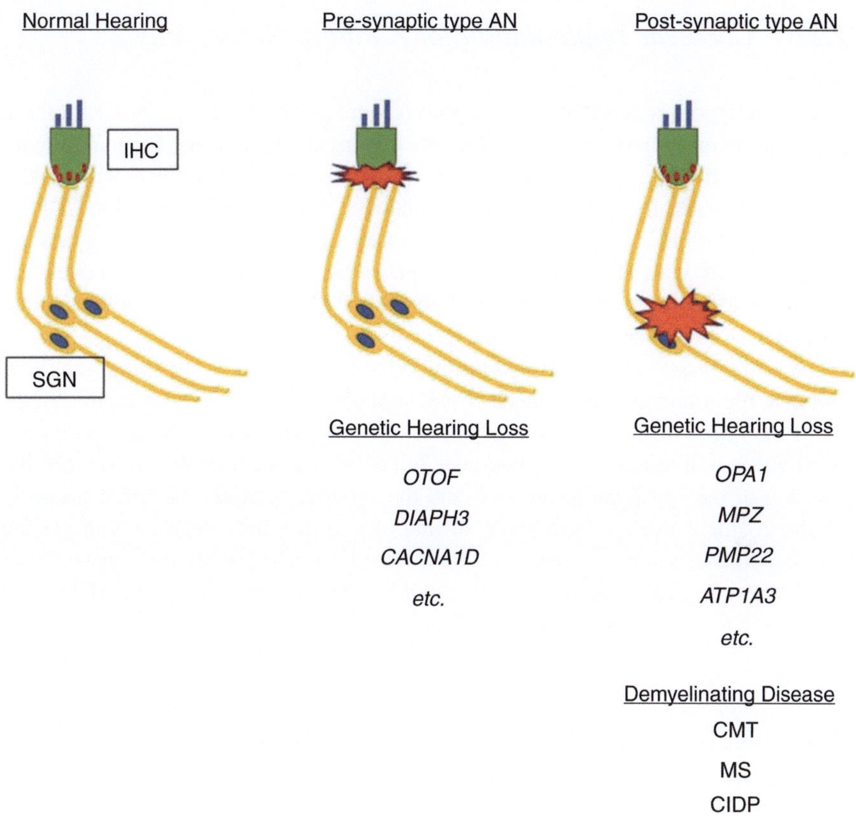

Fig. 12.1 Pre- and post-synaptic auditory neuropathy (AN). In pre-synaptic AN, the inner hair cells or synapses between the inner hair cells and spiral ganglions are disturbed. *OTOF* and *DIAPH3* are the causative genes of this type of AN. In post-synaptic AN, the proximal synapse between the inner hair cells and spiral ganglions (mainly spiral ganglion neuron itself or myelin) is disturbed. *OPA1*, *MPZ*, and *PMP22* are the causative genes of this type of AN, which may also be caused by demyelinating diseases. *IHC* inner hair cell, *SGN* spiral ganglion neuron, *CMT* Charcot–Marie–Tooth disease, *MS* multiple sclerosis, *CIDP* Chronic inflammatory demyelination polyneuropathy

neurons. *DIAPH3* mutation also causes pre-synaptic AN due to disturbance of inner hair cell function, while sparing outer hair cell function.

A well-known example of post-synaptic neuropathy is AN caused by an *OPA1* mutation. The *OPA1* gene encodes the OPA1 protein, which is crucial for mitochondrial functioning. It is hypothesized that this mutation results in the degeneration of terminal axons of spiral ganglion neurons, ultimately leading to post-synaptic neuropathy. AN caused by *MPZ* mutation is another example of post-synaptic neuropathy. *MPZ* genes encode myelin protein zero. *MPZ* mutation causes the dysfunction of the myelin of spiral ganglion neurons and leads to disturbance in the neuronal transmission of spiral ganglion neurons.

12.2.3 Cochlear Implantation for Auditory Neuropathy

It has been hypothesized that patients with AN are poor candidates for CI. In these patients, transmission of the signal from the electrical stimulation of the spiral ganglion provided by the CI may be affected. However, studies of subjects with ANSD have shown generally positive, though somewhat variable, outcomes for CI [12–21]. Recent studies have suggested that the exact site of the lesion causing hearing loss in patients with AN is important in predicting CI outcomes. Moreover, the recent understanding of the genetic background of AN has allowed a more accurate prediction of CI outcomes in some cases.

The CI bypasses synaptic transition by directly stimulating the spiral ganglion, leading to the transmission of the electrical signal to the brain. Therefore, the condition of the organ of Corti or of the synapses between the hair cells and spiral ganglion neuron will not affect the outcomes of cochlear implantation. Conversely, the condition of the spiral ganglion itself and the synapse between the spiral ganglion and the cochlear nucleus, midbrain, or auditory cortex may negatively affect the electrical transmission of sound provided by a CI since it does not bypass these sites. Therefore, patients with a genetic mutation that can be bypassed by a CI would be expected to have good outcomes [10].

12.3 Electrical Auditory Brainstem Responses and Auditory Neuropathy

12.3.1 The Usefulness of Electrical Auditory Brainstem Responses in Auditory Neuropathy

EABR can be used for measuring neuronal activity in the cochlear nerve after CI placement, and the clinical usefulness of recording EABR has been reported [22–24]. Despite the lack of ABR, EABR can be detected in patients with AN. However, the expected waveforms depend on the pathophysiology of the disease. In this section, we present an overview of the CI-evoked EABR observed in patients with AN.

EABR can be recorded in these patients; to date, several reports have shown the usefulness of recording EABR patients with AN who use a CI.

Thus far, electrophysiological investigations have been performed using EABR analysis in patients with AN [14, 25–29]. Runge et al. showed reduced suprathreshold amplitude of wave V in patients with AN and residual dyssynchronous neuronal activity in the central auditory pathway [26]. Walton et al. reported the relationship between speech perception after CI placement and EABR waveforms in children with AN. They concluded that patients with abnormal EABR waveforms had significantly worse speech outcomes [28]. Jeong et al. reported that among patients with ANSD, the group eliciting EABR response showed relatively good results after CI placement, while the nonresponsive group demonstrated variable results [29]. These reports suggest that EABR waveforms are a predictor of postoperative outcomes in patients with AN or ANSD who undergo CI placement, as shown in other hearing loss patients.

However, given the heterogeneity of the potential causes of AN, reports about the EABR in AN with definitive cause are limited, and there is no classification of patients according to the waveforms of EABR. In the following section, we will review previous studies of EABR waveforms in patients of AN with known pathophysiology, including genetic investigations. Moreover, we will attempt to classify these patients by combining the pathophysiological mechanism and EABR waveforms.

12.3.2 Electrical Auditory Brainstem Responses in Genetic Auditory Neuropathy

As shown below, several reports about EABR recorded in AN or ANSD show the variety of EABR waveforms observed in this disease. Studying EABR evoked in patients with AN with a confirmed genetic mutation is a reasonable approach because genetic testing provides the pathophysiological mechanism and the origin of the disturbance in neuronal transmission. Theoretically, as genetic AN can be divided into two types, CI-evoked EABR waveforms can be categorized depending on pre- and post-synaptic types, with normal and elongated EABR corresponding to the pre- and post-synaptic types, respectively. In cases of pre-synaptic AN, the EABR waveform is expected to be normal because the pre-synaptic function can be bypassed by the direct electrical stimulation of spiral ganglion neurons provided by the CI, and the post-synaptic neuronal transmission of spiral ganglion neurons is not disturbed in this type. Conversely, in post-synaptic AN, electrical stimulation of spiral ganglion neurons cannot be bypassed by the pathogenic neurons. Therefore, the EABR waveform would be elongated or absent. However, several reports have suggested that there are exceptions to this theory.

To date, studies of EABR in patients with genetically caused AN have focused on *DIAPH3* [11], *OTOF* [30], *OPA1* [31], and *ATP1A3* [9] mutations. Among these cases, only a trans-tympanic EABR was recorded in patients with *ATP1A3* mutations. Han et al. reported that not perfect but replicable trans-tympanic EABR was recorded in the two AN patients with *ATP1A3* mutation [9]. In the following section, we discuss the gene mutations in which a CI-evoked EABR has been reported: *DIAPH3*, *OTOF*, and *OPA1*.

12.3.3 Electrical Auditory Brainstem Responses in Patients with DIAPH3 Mutation

Starr et al. reported a dominantly inherited AN kindred [11], and the gene responsible for this autosomal dominant AN (*AUNA1*) kindred was mapped to 13q14–21 in 2004 [32]. In 2010, *DIAPH3* mutations were identified in this kindred [4]. *DIAPH3* is one of the three human orthologs of Drosophila diaphanous. A mutation in *DIAPH1* causes an autosomal dominant nonsyndromic sensorineural hearing loss (DFNA1) [33]. It has been reported that mouse lines overexpressing *Diaph3* in hair cells provide some interesting clues about its function. In these mutants, the hair bundle morphology of inner, but not of outer hair cells, was disrupted [34]. Therefore, it was hypothesized that this disturbance of inner hair cell hair bundle morphology leads to pre-synaptic AN in patients with *DIAPH3* mutations.

In 2004, Starr et al. reported EABR waveforms in three patients with CI. The EABR of the three patients showed a normal wave V but no ABR response [11]. They concluded that the locus of the auditory abnormality involved only the auditory periphery, sparing the ganglion cells and their axons to a great extent, based on their observation of ABR and EABR. This conclusion was supported by findings from a mutant mouse model [34]. This would be an example in which the hypothesized pathophysiological mechanism of AN obtained through clinical observation of EABR waveforms could be proven genetically and biochemically, thus indicating the clinical usefulness of measuring EABR.

12.3.4 Electrical Auditory Brainstem Responses in Patients with OTOF Mutations

OTOF mutations were first reported as a genetic cause of DFNB9 nonsyndromic hearing loss [35]. *OTOF* mutations account for 1.4–5% of autosomal recessive nonsyndromic hearing impairment cases [36–43]. Patients carrying two mutant alleles of *OTOF* show a severe-to-profound congenital hearing loss. In the first 1 or 2 years after birth, they show preserved OAE without an ABR response, leading to the diagnosis of AN. The *OTOF* gene encodes the trans-membranous protein OTOFERLIN, whose expression has been reported in the inner and outer hair cells of the rodent cochlea [35, 44]. OTOFERLIN plays an important role in synaptic transmission at the afferent ribbon synapses between the inner hair cells and spiral ganglion neurons. In pre-synaptic lesions, OTOFERLIN acts as one of the key molecules for vesicle fusion with the pre-synaptic membrane of the inner hair cells [45]. Thus, it is thought that AN caused by an *OTOF* mutation is caused by a disturbance of synaptic function (pre-synaptic AN) between the inner hair cells and the spiral ganglion neuron [46].

CI placement is a valuable treatment option for profound-to-severe hearing loss in patients with AN. AN caused by *OTOF* mutations is thought to be a better indication for cochlear implantation [47–49] since the electrode can directly stimulate the auditory nerves, bypassing the impaired synapses.

Hosoya et al. reported the CI-evoked EABR waveforms obtained from patients with *OTOF* mutations [30]. While AN caused by *OTOF* mutation is thought to be caused by the disturbance of ribbon synapses between the inner hair cells and spiral ganglion cells, leading to pre-synaptic AN that can be bypassed by the CI, the waveform obtained from patients with *OTOF* mutations showed a distinct elongated form (Fig. 12.2). This observation indicated that *OTOF* mutations cause delayed (or slowed) post-synaptic neurotransmission, while the presumed pathophysiological mechanism involves reduced pre-synaptic transmission between the hair cells and spiral ganglion neurons.

This observation may suggest that pre-synaptic AN can affect the post-synaptic neurotransmission due to secondary reasons such as developmental delay or degeneration of spiral ganglion neurons caused by loss or decrease in neuronal stimulation of the spiral ganglion, at least in some conditions. We hypothesized that these possible secondary changes could be detected by recording long-term changes in EABR in the patients with *OTOF* mutations, since CI stimulation would improve the post-synaptic function by electrically stimulating the spiral ganglion neurons.

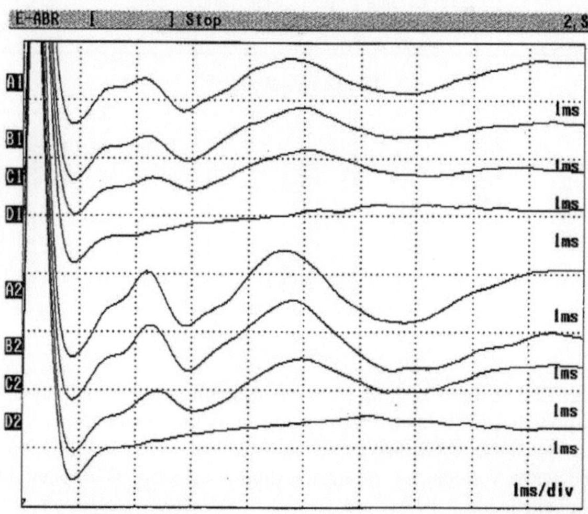

Fig. 12.2 Example of an electrical auditory brainstem response (EABR) waveform in a patient with *OTOF* mutation. In patients with *OTOF* mutations, elongated EABR waveforms are observed

Moreover, we hypothesized that long-term CI stimulation would improve this elongated waveform.

In this context, we examined the long-term changes in EABR evoked in patients with *OTOF* mutations. To evaluate the changes brought by long-term auditory stimulation after CI placement, we analyzed EABRs in case #1 (82 months after the first CI surgery) and case #4 (8 months after the first CI surgery) of a previous paper when these patients underwent a second CI placement (Fig. 12.3). We found a tendency for the latencies of waves III and V to shorten in response to long-term CI stimulation. We also found that the EABR latency of the side where the second CI was placed was longer than that of the first CI side, which received stimulation during the preceding several months until the second CI surgery.

Nerve development is promoted by increasing electrical pre- and post-synaptic stimulation, improving firing synchrony. The disturbed synchrony observed in *OTOF* mutations could be caused by insufficient pre-synaptic stimulation and/or delayed pre- and post-synaptic neural network maturation. Our observations, limited by the small number of cases, revealed a tendency toward shorter post-CI wave III and V latencies. While it is possible that neuronal maturation mediated by CI caused this change, a larger-scale study with follow-up analysis will need to be carried out in the future.

It is also possible that *OTOF* mutation disturbs neurotransmission in not only hair cell-spiral ganglion synapses but also in the cochlear nucleus or other more

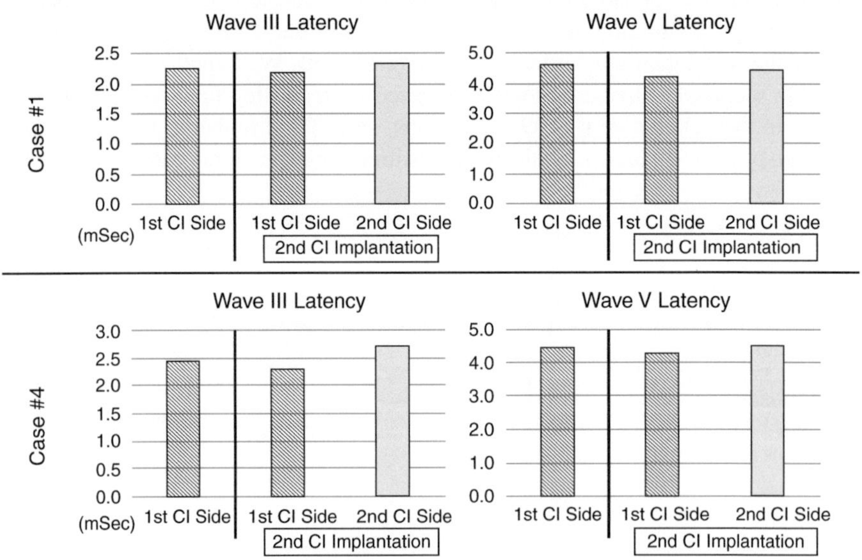

Fig. 12.3 Effects of long-term cochlear implant (CI) stimulation on evoked auditory brainstem response (EABR) latencies in patients with *OTOF* mutations. Two cases with a previous CI on one side and a recent CI surgery on the other side were identified; note the tendencies of both wave III and wave V latencies to shorten after long-term CI implantation as compared to the recently implanted side

central components of the auditory pathway. A more detailed study of the auditory pathway in primates will also need to be carried out in the near future.

12.3.5 *Electrical Auditory Brainstem Responses in Patients with* OPA1 *Mutations*

OPA1 is another AN causative gene [50–52] and is also associated with optic neuropathy [6]. Hearing loss caused by *OPA1* mutations starts in childhood or adolescence, usually following the onset of visual symptoms [53]. The *OPA1* gene encodes the OPA1 protein, a mitochondrial protein that belongs to the dynamin family [54]. OPA1 plays an important role in the formation and maintenance of mitochondrial network and morphology, including promoting fusion of the inner mitochondrial membrane, maintaining the integrity and structure of the mitochondrial cristae, and maintaining membrane potential and oxidative phosphorylation [55–57].

In previous study on a mouse model reported that *Opa1* is essential for normal mitochondrial fusion balance, which is important for the normal neuron dendritic morphology [58]. Therefore, haploinsufficiency of the OPA1 protein leads to a disturbance in the dendritic morphology of retinal ganglion cells and causes optic neuropathy. It has been hypothesized that AN in patients carrying *OPA1* missense mutations is also caused by disordered synchrony in auditory nerve fiber activity resulting from neural degeneration affecting the terminal dendrites of the spiral ganglion, similar to what occurs in the retinal ganglion [31].

Santarelli et al. reported the EABR waveforms of patients with *OPA1* mutations [31]. Findings from six patients with CI indicated that the most common pattern of EABR in patients with *OPA1* is elongated wave V latency from apical to basal electrodes, while an electrically evoked compound action potential was not detected in most patients. The authors concluded that this discrepancy would reflect the hypothesized pathological mechanisms of *OPA1*, in which degeneration of the distal portion of the auditory nerve fibers occurs. In this condition, the CI's electrical stimulation can evoke an EABR as it bypasses the site of the degenerated terminus of the spiral ganglion neuron. They also mentioned that their findings are also consistent with a mouse model showing dendritic pruning of the optic nerve fibers at the very early stage of the disorder [58].

12.3.6 *Electrical Auditory Brainstem Responses in Patients with Demyelinating Disease*

Finally, we have included other examples of EABR recordings in cases of AN. Several demyelinating diseases can cause AN disease [59], including Charcot–Marie–Tooth disease [1], multiple sclerosis, and CIDP [60].

Charcot–Marie–Tooth disease is a well-known cause of AN. In this disease, AN is caused by the demyelination of the spiral ganglion neuron. CIDP is another myelinating disease that causes AN [60, 61]. It is a chronic or relapsing motor and sensory neuropathy, with inflammation and demyelination of the peripheral nerve [62]. CIDP is closely related to Guillain–Barré syndrome, and is considered the chronic counterpart of that acute disease. In these demyelinating diseases, the neurotransmission of the spiral ganglion could be disturbed over the entire length. Thus, the effect of CI placement is hypothesized to be limited.

Mowry et al. reported a case of a patient with CIDP in which an EABR was recorded [61]. The patient did not demonstrate a consistent EABR response, which led to the conclusion that the CIDP axonopathy caused the absence of the EABR waveform.

12.3.7 New Classification for Electrical Auditory Brainstem Responses in Auditory Neuropathy

We reviewed the various EABR waveforms seen in AN and their causes. While variable EABR waveforms have been reported in AN, they can be divided into four patterns based on the combination of the affected point (pre- or post-synaptic) and waveforms. Here, we propose a new classification of EABR observed in AN (Fig. 12.4). Pre-synaptic AN is expected to show a normal EABR waveform. However, we report that an elongated waveform is observed in cases of *OTOF* mutation. Therefore, in this new classification, we propose that this pre-synaptic AN should be divided into two groups: Group A and Group B. Pre-synaptic AN with normal EABR would be classified into Group A. AN with *DIAPH3* mutation would be a good example of Group A. This group would be composed of "pure" pre-synaptic AN. Pre-synaptic AN with abnormal EABR would therefore be classified into Group B, such as AN due to *OTOF* mutation. Group B AN is mainly caused by a pre-synaptic neurotransmission disturbance, which may lead to the secondary neuronal transmission disturbance detected in EABR measurement. In this new classification, we propose that post-synaptic AN can be divided into two groups: Group C and Group D. Post-synaptic AN in which an EABR is detected would be classified into Group C. CI-mediated electrical stimulation could bypass the site of lesions in this group. Post-synaptic AN with absent EABR would thus be classified into Group D. Most demyelinating diseases would be included in this group.

We believe that this simple classification would be useful for understanding the EABR variability observed in patients with AN. As mentioned above, theoretically, pre-synaptic AN will show a normal EABR (Group A), and post-synaptic AN will have an absence of EABR (Group D). However, this theory is not always true; therefore, AN classified into Group B or Group C requires a careful pathophysiological evaluation. While there is a small number of studies of EABR recorded in patients with AN, we hope that this new classification will help in understanding the relationship between EABR waveforms and the pathophysiology of the different AN types.

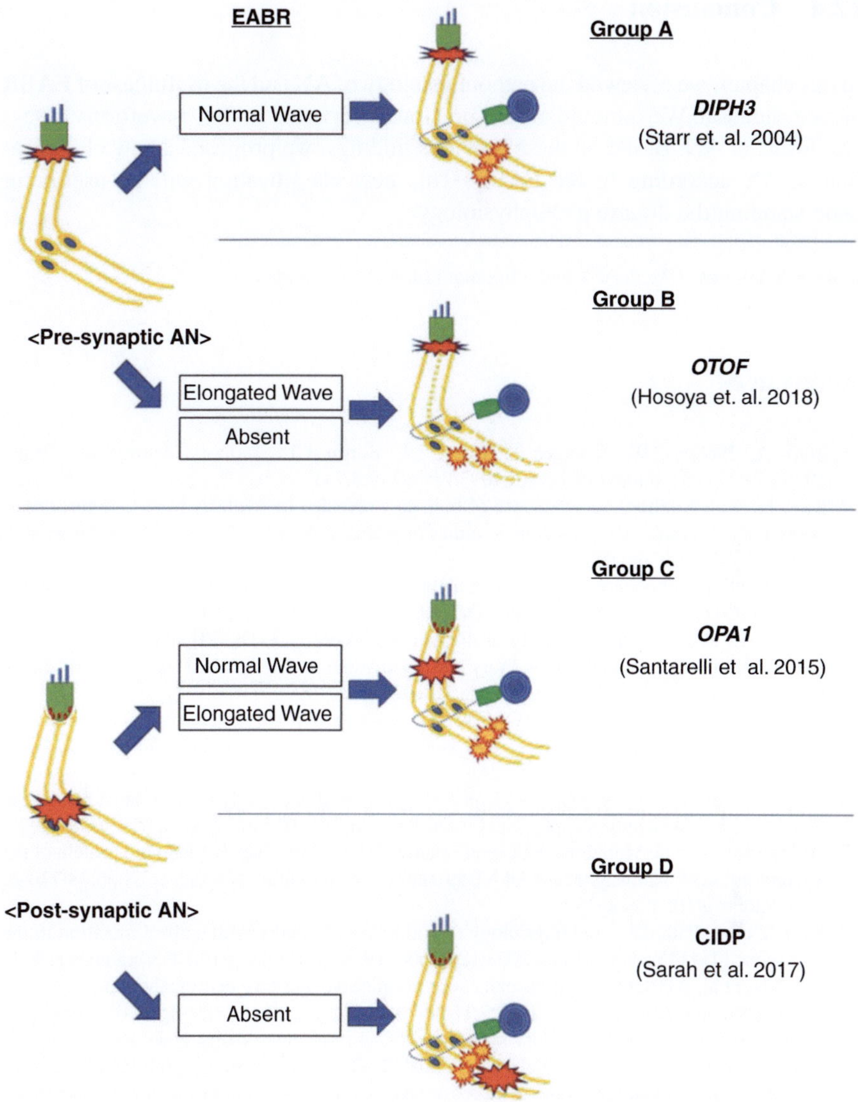

Fig. 12.4 The proposed new electrical auditory brainstem response (EABR) waveform classification. We propose a new EABR waveform classification for patients with auditory neuropathy (AN) based on the pathophysiological mechanisms underlying each AN and EABR waveform. *CIDP* Chronic inflammatory demyelination polyneuropathy

12.4 Conclusion

In this chapter, we reviewed the pathophysiology of AN and the usefulness of EABR in its evaluation. We summarized the previously reported EABR waveforms in several forms of AN. Based on these previous findings, we proposed a new classification of AN according to the EABR. This new classification will be useful for understanding the disease pathophysiology.

Acknowledgments We thank Chieko Enomoto for technical support.

References

1. Starr A, Picton TW, Sininger Y, Hood LJ, Berlin CI. Auditory neuropathy. Brain. 1996;119:741–53. https://doi.org/10.1093/brain/119.3.741.
2. Kaga K, et al. Auditory nerve disease of both ears revealed by auditory brainstem responses, electrocochleography and otoacoustic emissions. Scand Audiol. 1996;25:233–8. https://doi.org/10.3109/01050399609074960.
3. Varga R, et al. Non-syndromic recessive auditory neuropathy is the result of mutations in the otoferlin (OTOF) gene. J Med Genet. 2003;40:45–50. https://doi.org/10.1136/jmg.40.1.45.
4. Schoen CJ, et al. Increased activity of diaphanous homolog 3 (DIAPH3)/diaphanous causes hearing defects in humans with auditory neuropathy and in drosophila. Proc Natl Acad Sci U S A. 2010;107:13396–401. https://doi.org/10.1073/pnas.1003027107.
5. Baig SM, et al. Loss of ca(v)1.3 (CACNA1D) function in a human channelopathy with bradycardia and congenital deafness. Nat Neurosci. 2011;14:77–84. https://doi.org/10.1038/nn.2694.
6. Delettre C, et al. Nuclear gene OPA1, encoding a mitochondrial dynamin-related protein, is mutated in dominant optic atrophy. Nat Genet. 2000;26:207–10. https://doi.org/10.1038/79936.
7. Delmaghani S, et al. Mutations in the gene encoding pejvakin, a newly identified protein of the afferent auditory pathway, cause DFNB59 auditory neuropathy. Nat Genet. 2006;38:770–8. https://doi.org/10.1038/ng1829.
8. Starr A, et al. Pathology and physiology of auditory neuropathy with a novel mutation in the MPZ gene (Tyr145->Ser). Brain. 2003;126:1604–19. https://doi.org/10.1093/brain/awg156.
9. Han KH, et al. ATP1A3 mutations can cause progressive auditory neuropathy: a new gene of auditory synaptopathy. Sci Rep. 2017;7:16504. https://doi.org/10.1038/s41598-017-16676-9.
10. Shearer AE, Hansen MR. Auditory synaptopathy, auditory neuropathy, and cochlear implantation. Laryngoscope Investig Otolaryngol. 2019;4:429–40. https://doi.org/10.1002/lio2.288.
11. Starr A, et al. A dominantly inherited progressive deafness affecting distal auditory nerve and hair cells. J Assoc Res Otolaryngol. 2004;5:411–26. https://doi.org/10.1007/s10162-004-5014-5.
12. Rance G, Barker EJ. Speech and language outcomes in children with auditory neuropathy/dys-synchrony managed with either cochlear implants or hearing aids. Int J Audiol. 2009;48:313–20. https://doi.org/10.1080/14992020802665959.
13. Trautwein PG, Sininger YS, Nelson R. Cochlear implantation of auditory neuropathy. J Am Acad Audiol. 2000;11:309–15.
14. Shallop JK, Peterson A, Facer GW, Fabry LB, Driscoll CL. Cochlear implants in five cases of auditory neuropathy: postoperative findings and progress. Laryngoscope. 2001;111:555–62. https://doi.org/10.1097/00005537-200104000-00001.
15. Rance G, Barker EJ. Speech perception in children with auditory neuropathy/dyssynchrony managed with either hearing AIDS or cochlear implants. Otol Neurotol. 2008;29:179–82. https://doi.org/10.1097/mao.0b013e31815e92fd.

16. Mason JC, De Michele A, Stevens C, Ruth RA, Hashisaki GT. Cochlear implantation in patients with auditory neuropathy of varied etiologies. Laryngoscope. 2003;113:45–9. https://doi.org/10.1097/00005537-200301000-00009.
17. Teagle HF, et al. Cochlear implantation in children with auditory neuropathy spectrum disorder. Ear Hear. 2010;31:325–35. https://doi.org/10.1097/AUD.0b013e3181ce693b.
18. Kontorinis G, et al. Cochlear implantation in children with auditory neuropathy spectrum disorders. Cochlear Implants Int. 2014;15(Suppl 1):S51–4. https://doi.org/10.1179/1467010014Z.000000000157.
19. Humphriss R, et al. Does cochlear implantation improve speech recognition in children with auditory neuropathy spectrum disorder? A systematic review. Int J Audiol. 2013;52:442–54. https://doi.org/10.3109/14992027.2013.786190.
20. Ji F, et al. Determination of benefits of cochlear implantation in children with auditory neuropathy. PLoS One. 2015;10:e0127566. https://doi.org/10.1371/journal.pone.0127566.
21. Harrison RV, Gordon KA, Papsin BC, Negandhi J, James AL. Auditory neuropathy spectrum disorder (ANSD) and cochlear implantation. Int J Pediatr Otorhinolaryngol. 2015;79:1980–7. https://doi.org/10.1016/j.ijporl.2015.10.006.
22. Minami SB, Takegoshi H, Shinjo Y, Enomoto C, Kaga K. Usefulness of measuring electrically evoked auditory brainstem responses in children with inner ear malformations during cochlear implantation. Acta Otolaryngol. 2015;135:1007–15. https://doi.org/10.3109/00016489.2015.1048377.
23. Bierer JA, Faulkner KF, Tremblay KL. Identifying cochlear implant channels with poor electrode-neuron interfaces: electrically evoked auditory brain stem responses measured with the partial tripolar configuration. Ear Hear. 2011;32:436–44. https://doi.org/10.1097/AUD.0b013e3181ff33ab.
24. Enomoto C, Minami S, Kaga K. EABR measurements during cochlear implantation in one-year-old, infant, child, adult, and elderly patients. Acta Otolaryngol. 2020;1-5 https://doi.org/10.1080/00016489.2020.1826576.
25. Buss E, et al. Outcome of cochlear implantation in pediatric auditory neuropathy. Otol Neurotol. 2002;23:328–32.
26. Runge-Samuelson CL, Drake S, Wackym PA. Quantitative analysis of electrically evoked auditory brainstem responses in implanted children with auditory neuropathy/dyssynchrony. Otol Neurotol. 2008;29:174–8. https://doi.org/10.1097/mao.0b013e31815aee4b.
27. Jeong SW, Kim LS, Kim BY, Bae WY, Kim JR. Cochlear implantation in children with auditory neuropathy: outcomes and rationale. Acta Otolaryngol Suppl. 2007;36-43 https://doi.org/10.1080/03655230701624848.
28. Walton J, Gibson WP, Sanli H, Prelog K. Predicting cochlear implant outcomes in children with auditory neuropathy. Otol Neurotol. 2008;29:302–9. https://doi.org/10.1097/MAO.0b013e318164d0f6.
29. Jeon JH, et al. Relationship between electrically evoked auditory brainstem response and auditory performance after cochlear implant in patients with auditory neuropathy spectrum disorder. Otol Neurotol. 2013;34:1261–6. https://doi.org/10.1097/MAO.0b013e318291c632.
30. Hosoya M, Minami SB, Enomoto C, Matsunaga T, Kaga K. Elongated EABR wave latencies observed in patients with auditory neuropathy caused by OTOF mutation. Laryngoscope Investig Otolaryngol. 2018;3:388–93. https://doi.org/10.1002/lio2.210.
31. Santarelli R, et al. OPA1-related auditory neuropathy: site of lesion and outcome of cochlear implantation. Brain. 2015;138:563–76. https://doi.org/10.1093/brain/awu378.
32. Kim TB, et al. A gene responsible for autosomal dominant auditory neuropathy (AUNA1) maps to 13q14-21. J Med Genet. 2004;41:872–6. https://doi.org/10.1136/jmg.2004.020628.
33. Lynch ED, et al. Nonsyndromic deafness DFNA1 associated with mutation of a human homolog of the drosophila gene diaphanous. Science. 1997;278:1315–8.
34. Schoen CJ, Burmeister M, Lesperance MM. Diaphanous homolog 3 (Diap3) overexpression causes progressive hearing loss and inner hair cell defects in a transgenic mouse model of human deafness. PLoS One. 2013;8:e56520. https://doi.org/10.1371/journal.pone.0056520.

35. Yasunaga S, et al. A mutation in OTOF, encoding otoferlin, a FER-1-like protein, causes DFNB9, a nonsyndromic form of deafness. Nat Genet. 1999;21:363–9. https://doi.org/10.1038/7693.
36. Choi BY, et al. Identities and frequencies of mutations of the otoferlin gene (OTOF) causing DFNB9 deafness in Pakistan. Clin Genet. 2009;75:237–43. https://doi.org/10.1111/j.1399-0004.2008.01128.x.
37. Duman D, Sirmaci A, Cengiz FB, Ozdag H, Tekin M. Screening of 38 genes identifies mutations in 62% of families with nonsyndromic deafness in Turkey. Genet Test Mol Biomarkers. 2011;15:29–33. https://doi.org/10.1089/gtmb.2010.0120.
38. Hutchin T, et al. Assessment of the genetic causes of recessive childhood non-syndromic deafness in the UK - implications for genetic testing. Clin Genet. 2005;68:506–12. https://doi.org/10.1111/j.1399-0004.2005.00539.x.
39. Iwasa Y, et al. OTOF mutation screening in Japanese severe to profound recessive hearing loss patients. BMC Med Genet. 2013;14:95. https://doi.org/10.1186/1471-2350-14-95.
40. Jin YJ, Park J, Kim AR, Rah YC, Choi BY. Identification of a novel splice site variant of OTOF in the Korean nonsyndromic hearing loss population with low prevalence of the OTOF mutations. Int J Pediatr Otorhinolaryngol. 2014;78:1030–5. https://doi.org/10.1016/j.ijporl.2014.03.033.
41. Mahdieh N, et al. Screening of OTOF mutations in Iran: a novel mutation and review. Int J Pediatr Otorhinolaryngol. 2012;76:1610–5. https://doi.org/10.1016/j.ijporl.2012.07.030.
42. Rodriguez-Ballesteros M, et al. A multicenter study on the prevalence and spectrum of mutations in the otoferlin gene (OTOF) in subjects with nonsyndromic hearing impairment and auditory neuropathy. Hum Mutat. 2008;29:823–31. https://doi.org/10.1002/humu.20708.
43. Romanos J, et al. Novel OTOF mutations in Brazilian patients with auditory neuropathy. J Hum Genet. 2009;54:382–5. https://doi.org/10.1038/jhg.2009.45.
44. Schug N, et al. Differential expression of otoferlin in brain, vestibular system, immature and mature cochlea of the rat. Eur J Neurosci. 2006;24:3372–80. https://doi.org/10.1111/j.1460-9568.2006.05225.x.
45. Roux I, et al. Otoferlin, defective in a human deafness form, is essential for exocytosis at the auditory ribbon synapse. Cell. 2006;127:277–89. https://doi.org/10.1016/j.cell.2006.08.040.
46. Moser T, Starr A. Auditory neuropathy--neural and synaptic mechanisms. Nat Rev Neurol. 2016;12:135–49. https://doi.org/10.1038/nrneurol.2016.10.
47. Rouillon I, et al. Results of cochlear implantation in two children with mutations in the OTOF gene. Int J Pediatr Otorhinolaryngol. 2006;70:689–96. https://doi.org/10.1016/j.ijporl.2005.09.006.
48. Wu CC, et al. Timing of cochlear implantation in auditory neuropathy patients with OTOF mutations: our experience with 10 patients. Clin Otolaryngol. 2017; https://doi.org/10.1111/coa.12949.
49. Rodriguez-Ballesteros M, et al. Auditory neuropathy in patients carrying mutations in the otoferlin gene (OTOF). Hum Mutat. 2003;22:451–6. https://doi.org/10.1002/humu.10274.
50. Amati-Bonneau P, et al. OPA1 R445H mutation in optic atrophy associated with sensorineural deafness. Ann Neurol. 2005;58:958–63. https://doi.org/10.1002/ana.20681.
51. Huang T, Santarelli R, Starr A. Mutation of OPA1 gene causes deafness by affecting function of auditory nerve terminals. Brain Res. 2009;1300:97–104. https://doi.org/10.1016/j.brainres.2009.08.083.
52. Santarelli R. Information from cochlear potentials and genetic mutations helps localize the lesion site in auditory neuropathy. Genome Med. 2010;2:91. https://doi.org/10.1186/gm212.
53. Yu-Wai-Man P, et al. Multi-system neurological disease is common in patients with OPA1 mutations. Brain. 2010;133:771–86. https://doi.org/10.1093/brain/awq007.
54. Alexander C, et al. OPA1, encoding a dynamin-related GTPase, is mutated in autosomal dominant optic atrophy linked to chromosome 3q28. Nat Genet. 2000;26:211–5. https://doi.org/10.1038/79944.
55. Olichon A, et al. Mitochondrial dynamics and disease, OPA1. Biochim Biophys Acta. 2006;1763:500–9. https://doi.org/10.1016/j.bbamcr.2006.04.003.

56. Frezza C, et al. OPA1 controls apoptotic cristae remodeling independently from mitochondrial fusion. Cell. 2006;126:177–89. https://doi.org/10.1016/j.cell.2006.06.025.
57. Lodi R, et al. Deficit of in vivo mitochondrial ATP production in OPA1-related dominant optic atrophy. Ann Neurol. 2004;56:719–23. https://doi.org/10.1002/ana.20278.
58. Williams PA, Morgan JE, Votruba M. Opa1 deficiency in a mouse model of dominant optic atrophy leads to retinal ganglion cell dendropathy. Brain. 2010;133:2942–51. https://doi.org/10.1093/brain/awq218.
59. Rance G, Starr A. Pathophysiological mechanisms and functional hearing consequences of auditory neuropathy. Brain. 2015;138:3141–58. https://doi.org/10.1093/brain/awv270.
60. Norrix LW, Velenovsky DS. Auditory neuropathy spectrum disorder: a review. J Speech Lang Hear Res. 2014;57:1564–76. https://doi.org/10.1044/2014_JSLHR-H-13-0213.
61. Mowry SE, King S. Cochlear implantation in chronic demyelinating inflammatory polyneuropathy. Cochlear Implants Int. 2017;18:116–20. https://doi.org/10.1080/14670100.2016.1264115.
62. McCombe PA, Pollard JD, McLeod JG. Chronic inflammatory demyelinating polyradiculoneuropathy. A clinical and electrophysiological study of 92 cases. Brain. 1987;110(Pt 6):1617–30. https://doi.org/10.1093/brain/110.6.1617.

Part IV
Particular Topics

Chapter 13
Common Cavity Deformity

Kimitaka Kaga

Abstract Common cavity (CC) deformity is a severe inner ear malformation accompanied by profound hearing loss. However, the cochlear nerve distribution in the CC is unknown in this deformity. We studied the electrically evoked auditory brainstem response (EABR) during cochlear implant surgery and the postoperative development of speech and hearing ability in children with CC deformity to determine the presence or absence of physiological auditory function in this type of severe inner ear malformation. Nine children who were congenitally deaf with profound hearing loss were found to have CC deformities by temporal bone computed tomography (CT) and magnetic resonance imaging (MRI). All of these children underwent cochlear implant surgery. Their EABRs were recorded during cochlear implant surgery and their postoperative development of speech and hearing ability was evaluated periodically as they aged. Their modes of communication and their educational levels were assessed on multiple followed ups. All of the nine children with CC deformities showed that their eV mean peak latencies of their EABRs were 3.9 ± 0.2 ms which were the same as the controls and the eV mean peak thresholds were twice as high compared with controls and they showed marked improvement of their postoperative hearing thresholds of between 30 and 40 dBSNL.

Keywords Common cavity deformity · Cochlear implant · EABR · Cochleovestibular nerve

13.1 Definition and Embryological View

Common cavity (CC) deformities are characterized by a bag-shaped cavity within the temporal bone due to the absence of the cochlea, semicircular canals, and otolith organs and they are a severe type of inner ear malformation resulting in

K. Kaga (✉)
National Institute of Sensory Organs, National Hospital Organization, Tokyo Medical Center, Audiology Clinic, Kamio Memorial Hospital, Tokyo, Japan
e-mail: kimitaka.kaga@kankakuki.jp

© Springer Japan KK, part of Springer Nature 2022

K. Kaga (ed.), *ABRs and Electrically Evoked ABRs in Children*, Modern Otology and Neurotology, https://doi.org/10.1007/978-4-431-54189-9_13

profound hearing loss [1, 2]. Morphologically, the number of sensory cells and cochlear and vestibular nerves that are still extant in the CC is unknown. Functionally, auditory function can be evaluated objectively in infants with CC deformities by recording their EABRs during cochlear implantation and vestibular function can be evaluated by recording the vestibular ocular reflex. Infants with CC deformities have a round or ovoid appearance with an internal auditory canal (IAC) opening into the brainstem. This indicates an interruption in the development of the vestibule. If there is a well-developed cochleovestibular nerve (CVN), patients with CC deformity may benefit from cochlear implantation [3]. Sennaroglu et al. reported that patients with CC deformity but with a well-developed CVN, without branching into the cochlear and vestibular nerve, benefited from cochlear implantation [4].

13.2 CT and MRI of Common Cavity Deformities

Nine infants were studied, by temporal bone CT and MRI, who were congenitally profoundly deaf (Table 13.1) and were shown to have CCs with suspected cochlear nerve deformities (CND) (Figs. 13.1 and 13.2) [5].

13.3 EABRs of Common Cavity Deformities

We studied the eV peak latencies and thresholds of EABRs during cochlear implantation to determine the distribution of cochlear neurons, the brainstem transmission time and followed up on the postoperative development of speech and hearing abilities in children with CC deformities. We also investigated the relationship between the auditory capabilities and the educational settings of these children with this type of severe inner malformation as a follow-up of our previous vestibular study on the vestibular ocular reflex and gross motor development [6].

All of these deformed CC children underwent cochlear implantation using implants from MED-EL, except for case 3 for which an implant from Cochlear (Nucleus CI522) was used. In the case of implants from MED-EL, electrodes of different lengths were chosen to match the size of the CC and were inserted by labyrinthotomy (80%) or by a round window approach (20%) with fluoroscopic visualization to determine optimal positioning within the cochlea (Table 13.1).

Table 13.1 Profiles of nine infants with CC deformities and cochlear nerve deficiencies at cochlear implantation including facial nerve stimulation during the adjustment of postoperative programming parameters

Case	Present age	Gender	Implanted ear	Age of cochlear implantation	Cochlear nerve deficiency by CT	Surgical approach	Electrode length (mm)	Gusher	CAP	EABR	Postoperative facial nerve stimulation at programming
1	14 years 5 months	F	R	2 years 8 months	+	Labyrinthotomy	31.5	(−)	(+)	(+)	(+)
2	11 years 5 months	M	R	1 year 10 months		Labyrinthotomy	31.5	(−)	(−)	(+)	(−)
			L	4 years 6 months		Labyrinthotomy	24	(−)	(−)	(+)	(−)
3	8 years 11 months	F	R	5 years 3 months		Labyrinthotomy	25	(−)	(+)	(+)	(+)
			L	2 years 1 months		Round window	25	(+)	(+)		(−)
4	7 years 5 months	F	R	1 year 8 months	+	Labyrinthotomy	24	(−)	(−)	(+)	(−)
			L	3 years 2 months	+	Labyrinthotomy	31.5	(−)	(−)	(+)	(+)
5	9 years 11 months	F	L	2 years 1 months	+	Labyrinthotomy	31.5	(−)	(+)	(+)	(−)
6	7 years 2 months	F	R	1 year 8 months	+	Round window	24	(−)	(−)	(+)	(+)
			L	2 years 11 monts	+	Labyrinthotomy	24	(−)	(−)	(+)	(+)
7	6 years 3 months	F	R	1 year 8 months		Round window	24	(−)	(−)	(+)	(+)
			L	3 years 3 months		Labyrinthotomy	24	(−)	(−)	(+)	(+)
8	5 years 2 months	M	L	1 year 8 months	+	Labyrinthotomy	31.5	(−)	(−)	(+)	(+)
9	3 years 6 months	F	R	1 year 6 months		Labyrinthotomy	24	(−)	(+)	(+)	(−)
			L	2 years 7 months		Labyrinthotomy	24	(−)	(−)	(+)	(−)
Appearance rate								7%	33%	100%	53%

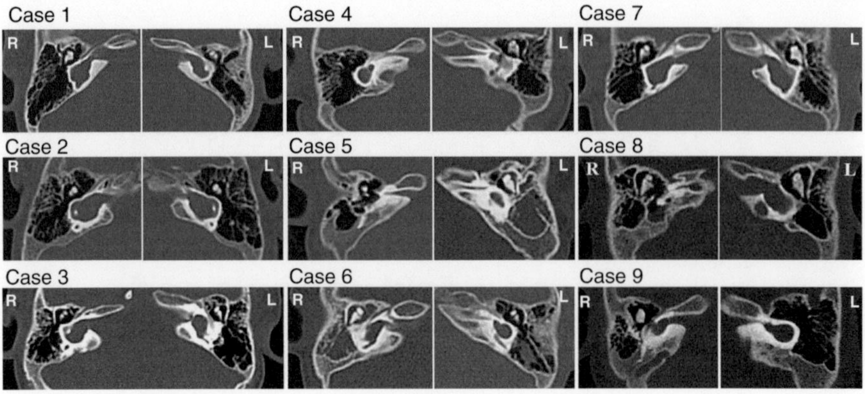

Fig. 13.1 CT imaging of the temporal bones of nine infants with CC deformities with or without cochlear nerve deficiencies. The magnitudes of the cavities and the diameters of the internal auditory canals are different in each case

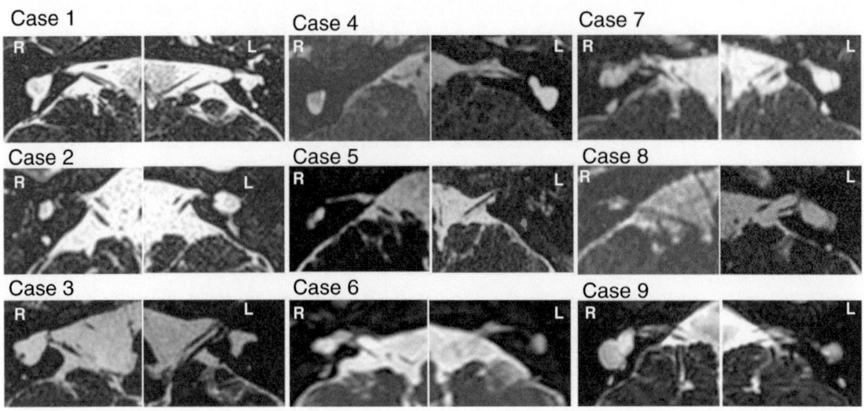

Fig. 13.2 MR imaging of the temporal bones of nine infants with CC deformities and their eighth nerve

Figure 13.3a illustrates comparison of wave configuration between ABR and EABR. Figure 13.3b shows typical EABR wave configuration changes, in a control patient, at the tip of the electrode (distal, #1, apical side), the middle electrode (#6, middle turn), and the end (proximal) electrode (#12, round window side in the basal turn) at different stimulation levels of the different electrode locations using MED-EL's Flex 28 electrodes. Figure 13.4 shows all of the EABR wave configurations at the tip electrode of the unilateral ear in nine infants with CC deformities for comparison. The eV peak latencies of the nine infants are not significantly different across all electrode positions; however, the EABR wave configurations varied among these infants.

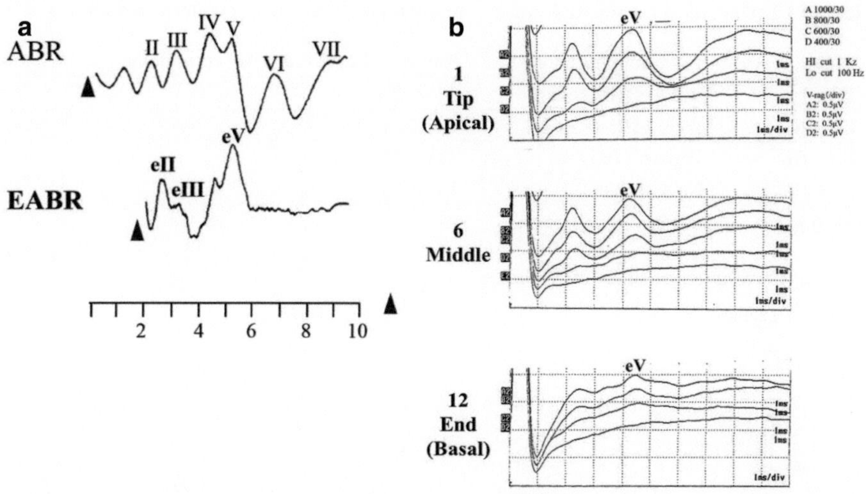

Fig. 13.3 EABR recordings. (**a**) Comparison of wave configurations between the EABR and the ABR. (**b**) Typical recordings of EABR in a control subject with normal cochlear anatomy using MED-EL's Flex 28 electrodes

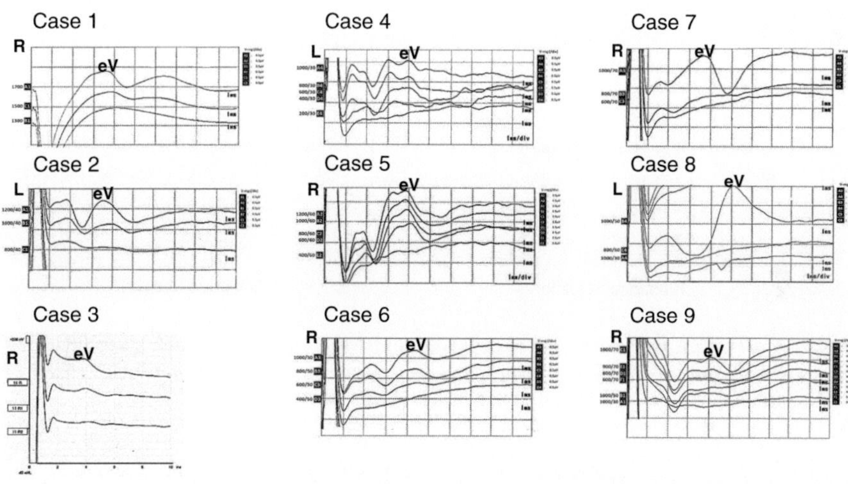

Fig. 13.4 Typical EABR wave configuration changes at the tip of the cochlear implant electrode using MED-EL's Flex 28 electrode in nine infants with CC deformities except Cochlear's CI522 in Case 3. The peak latency of eV is around 4.0 ms except in Case 8 which is 5.0 ms

In Table 13.2, the wave configuration patterns of nine infants with CC deformities and the difference in wave configuration are classified into four types depending on the presence of waves eII, eIII, and eV. Type III of wave eV could only be evoked in 50.0% of the recorded EABRs.

Table 13.2 Classification of EABR wave configurations in nine infants with CC deformities

Type	Wave configuration	Number of EABR at 1000 current unit
Type I	Wave eII, eIII, eV	5 (35.7%)
Type II	Wave eIII, eV only	1 (7.1%)
Type III	Wave eV only	7 (50.0%)
Type IV	No response	1 (7.1%)

($n = 9$ for 14 electrodes)

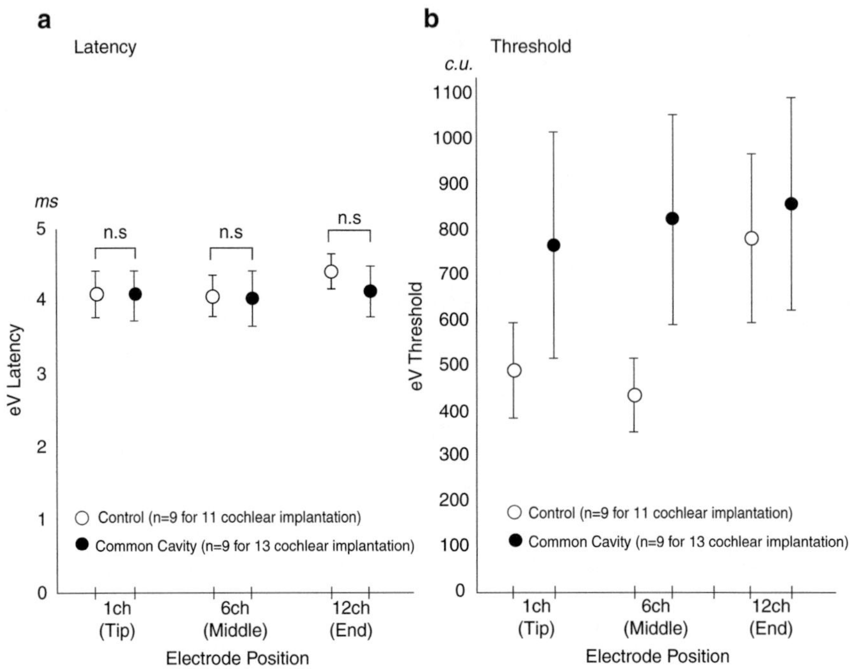

Fig. 13.5 Comparison of latencies and thresholds of EABRs between the common cavity deformities and control groups. Comparison of eV wave peak latency (**a**) and thresholds (**b**) of 13 EABRs in infants with CC deformities and of 11 EABRs in nine controls

13.4 Latencies and Thresholds of EABRs

Figure 13.5 shows a comparison of eV peak latencies and thresholds in CC deformity cases versus controls. The eV peak latencies at the tip, middle, and end electrodes of the cochlear implants in 13 of the cochlear implants from nine infants with CC deformities are not significantly different from those in 11 cochlear implants of nine controls, except at the end, most distal, electrode (Tip = 4.1 ± 03 ms, Middle = 4.1 ± 0.3 s, End = 4.4 ± 0.2 ms) (Fig. 13.5a). However, the eV peak thresholds at the tip and middle electrodes in 13 cochlear implants of nine infants with CC deformities are twice as high as those from 11 cochlear implants of nine controls

(Fig. 13.5b). A comparison of the eV peak latencies does not show a significant difference but those of the eV peak thresholds do ($p < 0.05$).

13.5 Postoperative Hearing and Speech Development

Visual reinforcement audiometry (VRA) in nine infants prior to cochlear implantation with CC deformities was conducted to evaluate hearing thresholds. All of these infants showed markedly elevated thresholds. However, after cochlear implantation, all these infants demonstrated only mild threshold elevations bilaterally or from the ear with implantation (◢ indicates right ear and ◣ indicates left ear) (Fig. 13.6).

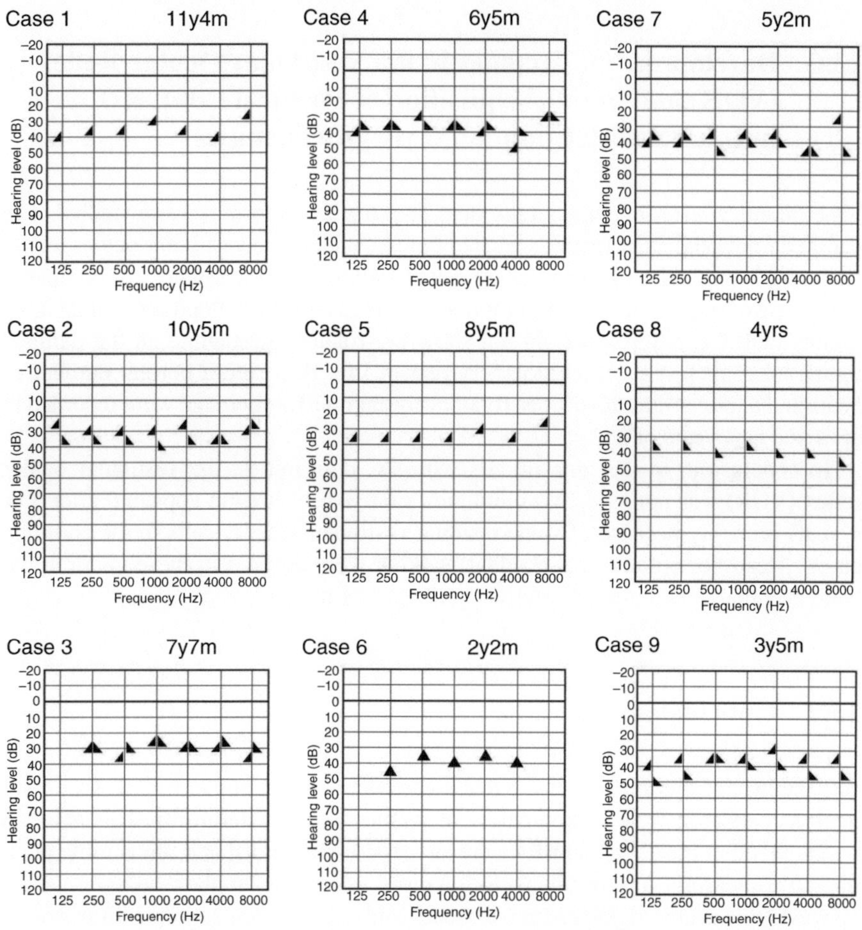

Fig. 13.6 VRA's thresholds after cochlear implantation in nine infants with CC deformities

Postoperative speech ability and the educational settings of these children were monitored periodically by observing their articulation, vocabulary, and sentence construction during conversation. It was possible to examine only case 3 using the Wechsler preschool and primary scale of intelligence (WPPSI). At the age of six, she showed a verbal intelligence quotient (IQ) of 95, a performance IQ of 93, and a total IQ of 95. Her parents choose to enroll her in an ordinary mainstream primary school. Her articulation was good, and her speech and hearing abilities were close to those of children of the same age. However, at the age of nine, her speech discrimination fell to 45% and her short sentence recognition rate fell to 30%. However, the same measurements from the other eight children did not fare so well [5].

Presently, the educational setting for seven of these children is a school for the deaf. Another child is enrolled in a kindergarten which provides auditory verbal therapy, and the other is mainstreaming in primary school.

13.6 Developmental Changes in the Vestibular Ocular Reflex (VOR) and in the Acquisition of Postural Control in Infants with Common Cavity Deformities

Nine infants who were congenitally deaf due to a CC deformity were studied. The damped rotational chair test was carried out to evaluate the vestibular ocular reflex. Acquisition of head control and independent walking in these infants was compared with those of normal infant's development of gross motor development. All the nine infants with CC deformities did not show per-rotatory nystagmus in the damped rotational chair test at around the first year of life. However, a normal number of beats and a longer duration of per-rotatory nystagmus for their age were recorded at around 3 or 4 years of age.

In conclusion, in the nine infants with CC deformities, the vestibular ocular reflex (VOR) was not evident around their first year of life but appeared after 3 or 4 years probably because of some residual vestibular sensory cells in the common cavity. Head control and independent walking were delayed in these children but were eventually acquired via central vestibular compensation [6, 7].

13.7 Conclusion

The findings of this study indicate that some cochlear neurons as well as vestibular neurons persist in the common cavity of infants with this deformity. This is based on the fact that the eV of EABRs were successfully recorded and remarkable postoperative hearing improvement following a cochlear implant was achieved. However, the acquired postoperative speech and auditory perception abilities varied among these patients, probably because of the free insertion of the electrode array within the cavity and the twofold higher thresholds of the EABRs and the obscure relationship between the tonotopic distribution of residual auditory neural tissue within the inner surface of the cavity.

References

1. Jackler RK, Luxford WM, House WF. Congenital malformations of the inner ear: a classification based on embryogenesis. Laryngoscope. 1987;97(S40):2–14.
2. Sennaroglu L, Saatci I. A new classification for chochleovestibular malformations. Laryngoscope. 2002;112(12):2230–41.
3. Sennaroglu L. Histopathology of inner ear malformations: do we have enough evidence to explain pathophysiology? Cochlear Implants Int. 2016;17(1):3–20.
4. Sennaroglu L, Gursel B, Sennaroglu G, Yucei E, Saatch I. Vestibular stimulation after cochlear implantation in common cavity deformity. Otolaryngol Head Neck Surg. 2001;125(4):408–10.
5. Kaga K, Minami S, Enomoto C. Electrically evoked ABR during cochlear implantation and postoperative development of speech and hearing abilities in infants with common cavity deformity as a type of inner ear malformation. Acta Otolaryngol. 2020;140(1):14–21.
6. Kaga K, Kimura Y, Minami S. Development of vestibular ocular reflex and gross motor function in infants with common cavity deformity as a type of inner ear malformation. Acta Otolaryngol. 2019;139(4):361–6.
7. Kaga K, Yulian J. Chapter 11. Vestibular-evoked myogenic potential after cochlear implantation. In: Kaga K, editor. Cochlear implantation in children with inner ear malformation and cochlear nerve deficiency. Singapore: Springer; 2017. p. 139–46.

Chapter 14
Galvanic VEMP

Kimitaka Kaga

Abstract Vestibular-evoked myogenic potentials (VEMPs), induced by loud and brief auditory stimuli, are far-field potentials recorded by surface electrodes and which can be used clinically to assess vestibular function. There are two types of sound-evoked VEMPs: cervical (cVEMPs) recorded by EMG (electromyographically) from the sternocleidomastoid muscle (SCM); ocular (oVEMPs) recorded from the activity of the extraocular muscles, again by EMG, taken from just below the eye. Both types of VEMPs are evoked by loud auditory stimuli such as clicks, short tone bursts (air conduction stimulation (ACS) or auditory conducted sounds) or by physically tapping the subject. Each of these recorded potentials have been used to specifically evaluate the integrity of the vestibular systems' saccule and utricle afferents and also the inferior and superior vestibular nerves. cVEMPs, provoked by ACS, reflect the integrity of saccular afferents, whereas oVEMPs provoked by ACS reflect the integrity of utricular afferents.

Galvanic vestibular stimulation (GVS) has also been found to elicit biphasic EMG responses from SCM via the vestibular nerve but not from the otolith organs. Galvanic stimulation can elicit VEMPs and may enable the differentiation of retrolabyrinthine lesions from labyrinthine lesions in the vestibular neuronal system.

Keywords Galvanic vestibular stimulation · Vestibular nerve · Vestibular-evoked myogenic potentials (VEMPs) · Sternocleidomastoid muscle (SCM) · Interaural asymmetry ratio (IAR)

K. Kaga (✉)
National Institute of Sensory Organs, National Hospital Organization, Tokyo Medical Center, Audiology Clinic, Kamio Memorial Hospital, Tokyo, Japan
e-mail: kimitaka.kaga@kankakuki.jp

© Springer Japan KK, part of Springer Nature 2022

K. Kaga (ed.), *ABRs and Electrically Evoked ABRs in Children*, Modern Otology and Neurotology, https://doi.org/10.1007/978-4-431-54189-9_14

14.1 Auditory VEMPs and Galvanic (Electrically Stimulated) VEMP

Three types of stimuli have been used to elicit VEMPs: ACS (clicks and tone bursts), bone conducted vibration (BCV) (tapping), and GVS. GVS has been used as a non-mechanical means to activate the vestibular apparatus [1, 2].

Murofusi et al. reported that patients who had no myogenic responses from the sternocleidomastoid muscle (SCM), evoked by clicks or galvanic stimulation, are likely to have retrolabyrinthine lesions while patients who had no response to clicks but normal responses to galvanic stimulation did not. These results did not correlate with the caloric response. Therefore, they speculated that galvanic vestibular stimulation might have stimulated only the neurons of the otolith organs [2, 3].

The neural pathway of the sound-evoked vestibulocollic reflex (cVEMP) is illustrated in Fig. 14.1.

Of the vestibular end-organs in mammals, the macula of the saccule seems to respond especially well to air-conducted sound. The hair cells on the saccular macula, the type I hair cells around the striola, seem to be the most sensitive. What then is the neural pathway of the sound-evoked vestibulocollic reflex?

The primary afferents from the saccule are mainly found in the inferior vestibular nerve. Therefore, inputs to the vestibular system from sound stimulation are mostly transmitted via the inferior vestibular nerve. According to Kushiro et al. [4], the saccular afferents in cats have inhibitory projections to the ipsilateral motoneurons of the SCM but no contralateral projections. These authors also showed that this projection was mediated via the medial vestibulospinal tract. Based on these findings, the neural pathway of the air-conducted sound-evoked cVEMP reflex recorded from the SCM is thought to be as shown as in Fig.14.1. The cVEMPs are clearly

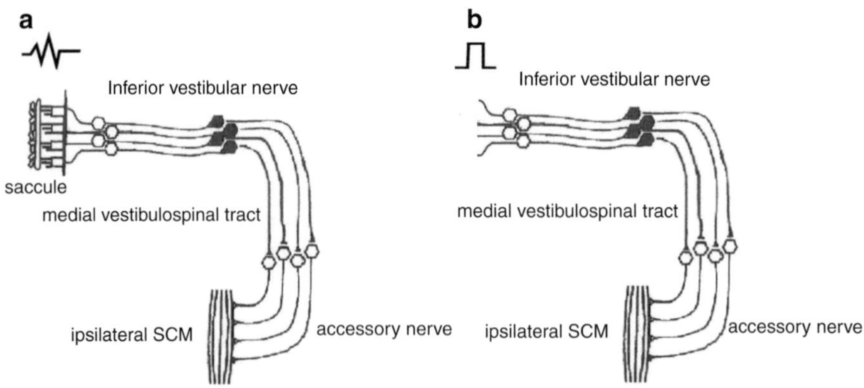

Fig. 14.1 Pathways of air-conducted sound-evoked vestibulocollic (otolith-sternocleidomastoid) reflexes. SCM, sternocleidomastoid muscle. (**a**) cVEMP response pathway; (**b**) Galvanic VEMP (GVS) response pathway [2]

ipsilateral-dominant. Therefore, the supposed neural pathway corresponds well with the results of cVEMP studies in humans.

Assuming that bone-conducted sound stimulates the utricular macula as well as the saccular macula, cVEMPS to bone-conducted sound might have some features different from those of cVEMPS to air-conducted sound. Utricular afferents have not only inhibitory projections to the ipsilateral motoneurons of the SCM but also excitatory projections to the contralateral motoneurons of the SCM [4]. When one uses bone-conducted sound as the stimulus, one should bear in mind that the neural pathways of cVEMPs to air-conducted sound are different.

When sound is presented to the ear, there is a real possibility of the coexistence of a so-called "sound-evoked cochleocollic reflex." However, any direct projection from the cochlear nucleus to the motoneurons of the SCM is unknown. Therefore, the sound-evoked cochleocollic reflex, if any, would be transmitted via the reticular formation which would result in a significantly longer response latency than that of the sound-evoked vestibulocollic reflex. Furthermore, the cochleocollic reflex would be evoked bilaterally [5–7].

14.2 Stimulation and Recording of Galvanic VEMPs

14.2.1 Recording

The active, recording, electrode is placed on the mid-body of the SCM. The indifferent electrode is placed on the lateral end of the ipsilateral upper sternum. The ground electrode is placed onto the middle of the forehead.

14.2.2 Galvanic Stimulation

The stimulus electrodes for galvanic vestibular stimulus (GVS) are placed on the ipsilateral mastoid. These make up the cathode while the other electrodes (the anode) are placed on the forehead (Fig.14.2). In our practice, we apply a 3 mA, 1 msec galvanic pulse stimulation to the vestibular nerve. The thresholds of responses evoked by this stimulation are determined by the EMG activity of the sternocleidomastoid muscle which is amplified and bandpass-filtered (20–2000 Hz). Response analysis time is 50 ms and the stimulation presentation rate is 5 Hz. Responses to 50 stimuli are twice averaged, with and without contraction of the SCM by the rotation of the neck. Contraction of the SCM, i.e., by turning the head fully to one side, potentiates the response. When these galvanic stimuli are applied, subjects feel a slight tapping sensation but no pain [2, 8, 9].

In order to remove the artifacts caused by the electrical stimulation, the average responses obtained without contraction of the SCM are subtracted from the average

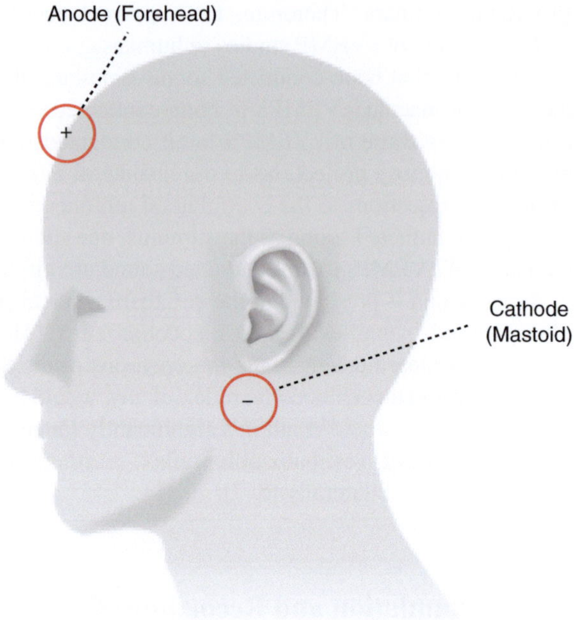

Fig. 14.2 Location of galvanic stimulus electrodes

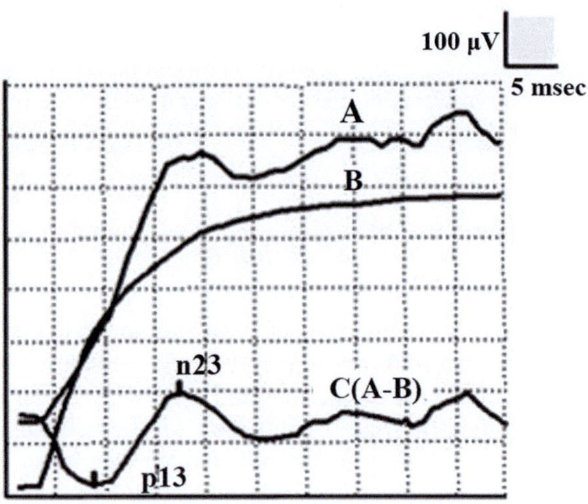

Fig. 14.3 GVS responses from a subject. A. shofws the reflex response with SCM contraction. B. shows the reflex response without SCM contraction. C. is the result of subtracting B. from A. which removes artifacts revealing the actual GVS potentials

responses obtained with contraction of the SCM (Fig.14.3) [8, 9]. Electromyogram waveforms are monitored during the recording session. Then the muscular tonus of the bilateral SCMs is stabilized at the same level, no contraction, and recordings are again taken and averaged as above. Subtraction of the averaged response obtained *without* contraction of the SCM from the average obtained *with* contraction of the SCM further removes the electrical stimulus artifact. Our methodology is the same as that reported by Watson and Colebatch (1998), and Watson et al. (1998) [8, 9].

The interaural asymmetry ratio (IAR) is another important parameter for evaluating the vestibular function of both labyrinths. The calculation method for obtaining the IAR (i.e., the latency of p13) is as follows: $|Lr-Ll| / (Lr + Ll) \times 100\%$. Lr is the p13 latency from the right ear, Ll is the p13 latency from the left ear, and $|Lr-Ll|$ is the absolute value of (Lr–Ll) [10, 11]. Then the distribution of the latencies of p13 (mean latency 11.7 ± 3.0 SD) is calculated. The latency of n23 (mean latency 17.8 ± 3.4 SD) and the amplitude of p13-n23 are determined using the same method. In electrophysiological measurements such as that of the VEMP, the symmetry of results between across the ears is important; a lack of the symmetry across the ears may be a sign of a unilateral deficit in the vestibular function or system. The value of the IAR lies between 0 and 1. The closer the IAR approaches 0, the better the symmetry between the right and left ears. Conversely, if the IAR is close to 1, the worse the symmetry between the right and left ears [12].

14.3 Typical Response of Galvanic VEMP

All of our normal-hearing subjects showed biphasic responses. In this study we named the first positive peak recorded following galvanic stimulation as "p13," and the first negative peak following galvanic stimulation as "n23." Amongst our subjects, we found that the average latency of p13 was 11.7 ms ± 3.0 ms. The latency of n23 was 17.8 ms ± 3.4 ms. The amplitude of p13-n23 was 147.0 μV ± 69.0 μV. The statistical data are shown in Table 14.1. Our recordings of the responses of the SCM with and without contraction and the waves after subtraction are shown in Fig. 14.3. The IARs of p13 and n23 latencies, and their amplitudes, are respectively 0.12 ms ± 0.09 ms, 0.08 ms ± 0.08 ms, and 0.16 μV ± 0.10 μV. The statistical data are shown in Table 14.2 [12].

Table 14.1 Means and standard deviations (SD) of the latencies of p13 and n23 and their amplitudes from all ears

N = 31 (ears)	p13 latency (ms)	n23 latency (ms)	Amplitude (μV)
Mean	11.7	17.8	147.0
SD	3.0	3.4	69.0

Table 14.2 Interaural asymmetry ratios IARs of p13 and n23 latencies and amplitudes in 15 subjects

IAR (*N* = 15 subjects)	Mean	SD
Latency p13	0.12	0.09
Latency n23	0.08	0.08
Amplitude (–)	0.16	0.10

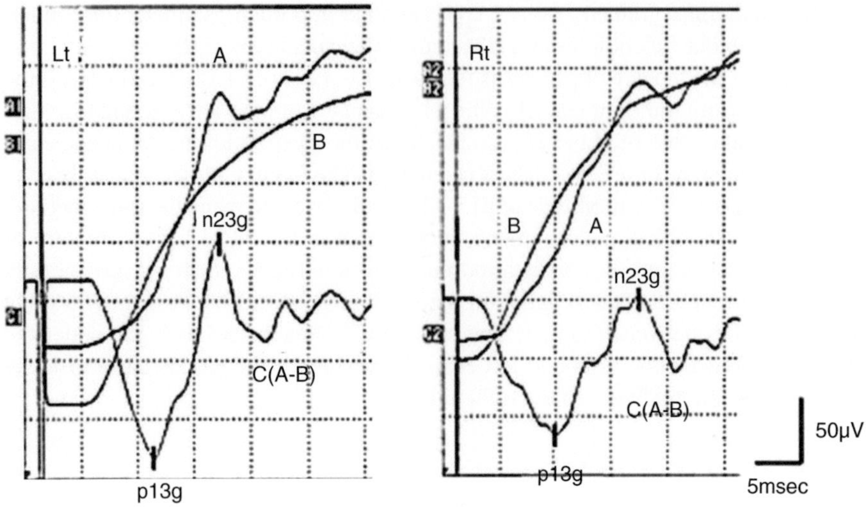

Fig. 14.4 GVEMPs from a patient with auditory neuropathy

14.4 Galvanic VEMP in Auditory Neuropathy

The use of galvanic stimulation together with ACS or BCV stimulation may enable the differentiation of labyrinthine lesions from retrolabyrinthine lesions. The accurate determination of the location of lesions is useful for studying the pathophysiology of vestibular diseases. From the data of our normal subjects, we can differentiate GVS elicited VEMPs in the clinical determination of vestibular neuropathy complicated by auditory neuropathy.

Murofushi et al. found that the combined use of click and galvanic stimuli was useful for the differential diagnosis of labyrinthine lesions versus retrolabyrinthine lesions of the vestibular system in patients with vestibular deficits [2, 13, 14].

Kimura and Kaga found half of their patients with auditory neuropathy who had normal DPOAEs but absent ABRs, had no evoked galvanic VEMPs but the other half had normal galvanic VEMPs (Fig.14.4) [15]. They supported the finding that vestibular neuropathy is complicated by auditory neuropathy. Thus, the galvanic VEMP is a reliable way to demonstrate that vestibular neuropathy is a synaptic pathophysiology between the vestibular hair cells and its afferents [15].

14.5 Galvanic VEMPs from Cochlear Implants

With cochlear implants, external sound stimuli are converted to electrical currents in a speech processor and these currents are conducted by electrodes along the cochlear implant by magnetic conduction. Thus, VEMPs recorded by stimulation of the cochlear implant can be regarded as a particular type of GVEMP.

Jin et al. compared VEMPs before and after surgery [16]. Before implant surgery, 6 of the 12 children showed normal VEMPs, 1 showed a decrease in the amplitude of VEMPs, and 5 showed no VEMPs. After surgery, with the cochlear implant switched off, 11 showed no VEMPs and 1 showed decreased VEMPs. These results reveal that even normal VEMPs disappear owing to trauma following electrode insertion. With the cochlear implant switched on, 4 children showed normal VEMPs, but 8 did not (Fig. 14.5). This can be explained by the fact that these 4 children's inferior vestibular nerves were stimulated by the spread of electrical current from the cochlear implant. We questioned why one-third of these children with cochlear implants showed VEMPs but others did not. Later, Jin et al. demonstrated that VEMPs evoked by cochlear implants may be related to an electrical current intensity at a comfortable level (C level), particularly in channels that are closer to the apical turn of the cochlea [17].

The patients who showed no VEMPs with the cochlear implant switched on may require higher current intensities to elicit clear VEMPs (if they need to be recorded). However, it is difficult to increase current intensity in such children because they feel pain or facial nerve stimulation when the current intensity is higher than the C level.

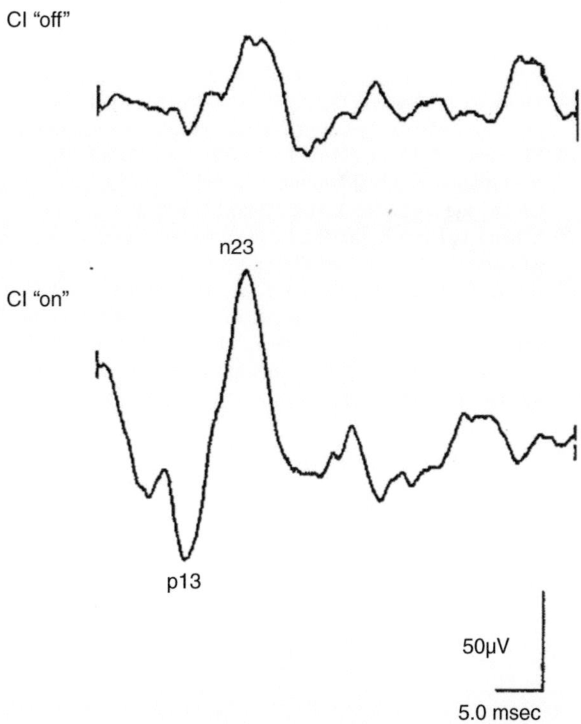

Fig. 14.5 Changes in VEMPs before and after cochlear implantation. Switched-off cochlear implant (CI "off") after surgery and switched-on (CI "on") after surgery

References

1. Camis M. The physiology of vestibular apparatus. London: Oxford University Press; 1903. p. 209–12.
2. Murofusi T, Kaga K. editors. Vestibular evoked myogenic potential. Its basis and clinical applications. Tokyo: Springer; 2009.
3. Murofushi T, Monobe H, Ochiai A, Ozeki H. The site of the lesion in "vestibular neuritis": study by galvanic VEMP. Neurology. 2003;61:417–8.
4. Kushiro K, Zakir M, Ogawa Y, et al. Saccular and utricular inputs to sternocleidomastoid motoneurons of decerebrate cat. Exp Brain Res. 1999;126:410–6.
5. Colebathc JG, Halmagyi GM. Vestibular evoked potentials in human neck muscles before and after unilateral vestibular deafferentation. Neurology. 1992;42:1635–6.
6. Welgampola MS, Colebatch JG. Characteristics and clinical application of vestibular-evoked myogenic potentials. Neurology. 2005;64:1682–8.
7. McCue MP, Guinan JJ Jr. Acoustically responsive fibers in the vestibular nerve of the cat. J Neurosci. 1994;14:6058–70.
8. Watson SRD, Colebatch JG. Vestibulocollic reflexes evoked by short-duration galvanic stimulation in man. J Physiol. 1998;513:587–97.
9. Watson SRD, Fagan P, Colebatch JG. Galvanic stimulation evokes short latency EMG responses in sternocleidomastoid which are abolished by selective vestibular nerve section. Electroenceph Clin Neurophyisol. 1998;109:471–4.
10. Murofushi T, Shimizu K, Takegoshi H, Cheng PW. Diagnostic value of prolonged latencies in the vestibular evoked myogenic potential. Arch Otolaryngol Head Neck Surg. 2001;127(9):1069–72.
11. Oh SY, Kim JS, Yang TH, Shin BS, Jeong SK. Cervical and ocular vestibular-evoked myogenic potentials in vestibular neuritis: comparison between air- and bone-conducted stimulation. J Neurol. 2013;260(8):2102–9.
12. Cheng Y, Kimura Y, Kaga K. A study on vestibular-evoked myogenic potentials via galvanic vestibular stimulation in normal people. J. Otol. 2018;13:16–9.
13. Murofusi T, Curthoys IS, Topple AN, Colebatch JG, Halmagyi GM. Responses of Guinea pig primary vestibular neurons to clicks. Exp Brain Res. 1995;103:174–8.
14. Murofushi T, Halmagyi GM, Yavor RA, Colebatch JG. Absent vestibular evoked potentials in vestibular neurolabyrinthitis: an indicator of inferior vestibular nerve involvement? Acta Otolaryngol Head Neck Surg. 1996;122:845–8.
15. Kimura Y, Kaga K. Vestibular neuropathy in patients with auditory neuropathy revealed by galvanic VEMP. Otol Jpn. 2021;31:161–7
16. Jin Y, Nakamura M, Shinjo Y, et al. Vestimular-evoked myogenic potentials in cochlear implant children. Acta Otolaryngol (Stockh). 2006;126:164–9.
17. Jin Y, Shinjo Y, Akamatsu Y, et al. Vestibular evoked myogenic potentials evoked by multichannel cochlear implant-influence of C levels. Acta Otolaryngol (Stockh). 2008;128:284–90.

Index

© Springer Japan KK, part of Springer Nature 2022

K. Kaga (ed.), *ABRs and Electrically Evoked ABRs in Children*, Modern Otology and Neurotology, https://doi.org/10.1007/978-4-431-54189-9

MIX
Papier aus verantwortungsvollen Quellen
Paper from responsible sources
FSC® C105338

If you have any concerns about our products,
you can contact us on
ProductSafety@springernature.com

In case Publisher is established outside the EU,
the EU authorized representative is:
Springer Nature Customer Service Center GmbH
Europaplatz 3, 69115 Heidelberg, Germany

Printed by Libri Plureos GmbH
in Hamburg, Germany